Genetic Disorders Sourcebook,
    1st Edition
Genetic Disorders Sourcebook,
    2nd Edition
Head Trauma Sourcebook
Headache Sourcebook
Health Insurance Sourcebook
Health Reference Series Cumulative
    Index 1999
Healthy Aging Sourcebook
Healthy Children Sourcebook
Healthy Heart Sourcebook for Women
Heart Diseases & Disorders
    Sourcebook, 2nd Edition
Household Safety Sourcebook
Immune System Disorders Sourcebook
Infant & Toddler Health Sourcebook
Injury & Trauma Sourcebook
Kidney & Urinary Tract Diseases &
    Disorders Sourcebook
Learning Disabilities Sourcebook,
    1st Edition
Learning Disabilities Sourcebook,
    2nd Edition
Liver Disorders Sourcebook
Leukemia Sourcebook
Lung Disorders Sourcebook
Medical Tests Sourcebook
Men's Health Concerns Sourcebook
Mental Health Disorders Sourcebook,
    1st Edition
Mental Health Disorders Sourcebook,
    2nd Edition
Mental Retardation Sourcebook
Movement Disorders Sourcebook
Obesity Sourcebook
Ophthalmic Disorders Sourcebook,
    1st Edition
Oral Health Sourcebook
Osteoporosis Sourcebook
Pain Sourcebook, 1st Edition
Pain Sourcebook, 2nd Edition
Pediatric Cancer Sourcebook
Physical & Mental Issues in Aging
    Sourcebook

Podiatry Sourcebook
Pregnancy & Birth Sourcebook
Prostate Cancer
Public Health Sourcebook
Reconstructive & Cosmetic Surgery
    Sourcebook
Rehabilitation Sourcebook
Respiratory Diseases & Disorders
    Sourcebook
Sexually Transmitted Diseases
    Sourcebook, 1st Edition
Sexually Transmitted Diseases
    Sourcebook, 2nd Edition
Skin Disorders Sourcebook
Sleep Disorders Sourcebook
Sports Injuries Sourcebook, 1st Edition
Sports Injuries Sourcebook, 2nd Edition
Stress-Related Disorders Sourcebook
Stroke Sourcebook
Substance Abuse Sourcebook
Surgery Sourcebook
Transplantation Sourcebook
Traveler's Health Sourcebook
Vegetarian Sourcebook
Women's Health Concerns Sourcebook
Workplace Health & Safety Sourcebook
Worldwide Health Sourcebook

## Teen Health Series

Diet Information for Teens
Drug Information for Teens
Mental Health Information
    for Teens
Sexual Health Information
    for Teens
Skin Health Information
    for Teens
Sports Injuries Information
    for Teens

# Stroke
## SOURCEBOOK

# Health Reference Series

*First Edition*

# Stroke
## SOURCEBOOK

*Basic Consumer Health Information about
Stroke, Including Ischemic, Hemorrhagic,
Transient Ischemic Attack (TIA), and
Pediatric Stroke, Stroke Triggers and Risks,
Diagnostic Tests, Treatments, and
Rehabilitation Information*

*Along with Stroke Prevention Guidelines,
Legal and Financial Information, a Glossary,
and a Directory of Additional Resources*

*Edited by*
**Joyce Brennfleck Shannon**

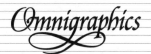

615 Griswold Street • Detroit, MI 48226

Bibliographic Note

Because this page cannot legibly accommodate all the copyright notices, the Bibliographic Note portion of the Preface constitutes an extension of the copyright notice.

Edited by Joyce Brennfleck Shannon

Health Reference Series

Karen Bellenir, *Managing Editor*
David A. Cooke, MD, *Medical Consultant*
Elizabeth Barbour, *Permissions Associate*
Dawn Matthews, *Verification Assistant*
Laura Pleva Nielsen, *Index Editor*
EdIndex, Services for Publishers, *Indexers*

\* \* \*

Omnigraphics, Inc.

Matthew P. Barbour, *Senior Vice President*
Kay Gill, *Vice President—Directories*
Kevin Hayes, *Operations Manager*
Leif Gruenberg, *Development Manager*
David P. Bianco, *Marketing Consultant*

\* \* \*

Peter E. Ruffner, *Publisher*

Frederick G. Ruffner, Jr., *Chairman*

Copyright © 2003 Omnigraphics, Inc.

ISBN0-7808-0630-1

Library of Congress Cataloging-in-Publication Data

Stroke sourcebook : basic consumer health information about stroke, including
    ischemic, hemorrhagic, transient ischemic attack (TIA), and pediatric stroke, stroke
    triggers and risks, diagnostic tests, treatments, and rehabilitation information; along
    with stroke prevention guidelines, legal and financial information, a glossary, and a
    directory of additional resources / edited by Joyce Brennfleck Shannon.-- 1st ed.
        p. cm. -- (Health reference series)
    Includes index.
    ISBN 0-7808-0630-1
        1. Cerebrovascular disease--Popular works. I. Shannon, Joyce Brennfleck. II. Health
    reference series (Unnumbered)

    RC388.5.S8566 2003
    616.8'1--dc21

                                                                    2003043309

Electronic or mechanical reproduction, including photography, recording, or any other information storage and retrieval system for the purpose of resale is strictly prohibited without permission in writing from the publisher.

The information in this publication was compiled from the sources cited and from other sources considered reliable. While every possible effort has been made to ensure reliability, the publisher will not assume liability for damages caused by inaccuracies in the data, and makes no warranty, express or implied, on the accuracy of the information contained herein.

(∞)

This book is printed on acid-free paper meeting the ANSI Z39.48 Standard. The infinity symbol that appears above indicates that the paper in this book meets that standard.

Printed in the United States

# Table of Contents

## Part III: Diagnosis and Treatments for Stroke

## Part IV: Stroke Recovery and Rehabilitation

## Part V: Stroke Prevention

## Part VI: Legal and Financial Information for Stroke Survivors

## Part VII: Additional Help and Information

# *Preface*

## About This Book

A stroke, or brain attack, is an emergency. From the onset of stroke symptoms, time is precious. Getting emergency help within three hours can mean the difference between severe brain damage and a full or partial recovery. Stroke is the third leading cause of death and the number one cause of adult disability in this country.

This *Sourcebook* provides health information about stroke, its causes, health risk factors, diagnosis, and treatments. Readers will learn about transient ischemic attack, ischemic, hemorrhagic, and pediatric stroke, the importance of fast response to stroke symptoms, and rehabilitation for patients with tips for caregivers. Prevention guidelines are included, along with legal and financial information, a glossary, and a listing of additional resources.

## How to Use This Book

This book is divided into parts and chapters. Parts focus on broad areas of interest. Chapters are devoted to single topics within a part.

*Part I: The Basics of Stroke* presents the distinctive signs of stroke; statistics and information about the cost of stroke in the U.S.; types of stroke including ischemic, hemorrhagic, and transient ischemic attack (TIA); stroke in children; and how to seek care following a stroke.

*Part II: Stroke Triggers and Risks* describes the many possible causes of stroke including atherosclerosis, cardiovascular disease, diabetes, hypertension, obesity, and sleep disorders. Recurrent stroke risks and tests that help predict stroke risk are also reviewed.

*Part III: Diagnosis and Treatments for Stroke* explains the medical tests used in the diagnosis of stroke, acute management of stroke, stroke scales that evaluate effects of stroke, surgical treatment of stroke, and access to treatment for stroke—always emphasizing the necessity of fast treatment.

*Part IV: Stroke Recovery and Rehabilitation* gives practical advice about discharge planning and rehabilitation, including physical, occupational, and speech therapy. It also provides information about life at home, nutrition, activities of daily living (ADLs), and tips for caregivers.

*Part V: Stroke Prevention* reviews prevention treatment, programs, and guidelines including carotid endarterectomy, cholesterol control, *Take Your Pulse America*™, the DASH diet, drug therapy, community-based interventions, and current legislation and research aimed at stroke prevention.

*Part VI: Legal and Financial Information for Stroke Survivors* offers information about disability benefits, seeking work when disabled, and how to prepare advance directives and living wills.

*Part VII: Additional Help and Information* includes a glossary of important terms and a directory of on-line resources and organizations able to provide additional information.

## Bibliographic Note

This volume contains documents and excerpts from publications issued by the following U.S. government agencies: Agency for Healthcare Research and Quality (AHRQ); Brain Attack Coalition; Centers for Disease Control and Prevention (CDC); Health and Human Services—Office on Women's Health (HHS-OWH); National Center for Research Resources (NCRR); National Heart, Lung, and Blood Institute (NHLBI); National Institute of Neurological Disorders and Stroke (NINDS); National Institute on Aging (NIA); National Institute on Deafness and Other Communication Disorders (NIDCD);

National Institutes of Health (NIH); National Recreation and Park Association; Social Security Administration (SSA); U.S. Department of Justice (DOJ); U.S. Department of Veterans Affairs; and U.S. Food and Drug Administration (FDA).

In addition, this volume contains copyrighted documents from the following organizations and individuals: A.D.A.M., Inc.; AgeNet, Inc.; American Academy of Physical Medicine and Rehabilitation (AAPM&R); American Heart Association (AHA); American Occupational Therapy Association, Inc. (AOTA); American Parkinson Disease Association, Inc. (APDA); American Physical Therapy Association (APTA); Associated Press (AP); Doctor's Guide Publishing Limited; Internet Stroke Center; Joyce Dreslin; Lippincott, Williams, and Wilkins; Maryland State Medical Society; Massachusetts Medical Society; National Aphasia Association (NAA); National Stroke Association (NSA); Research Center for Stroke and Heart Disease; United Press International (UPI); University of Maryland Medical System; and University of Pittsburgh Medical Center News Bureau.

Full citation information is provided on the first page of each chapter. Every effort has been made to secure all necessary rights to reprint the copyrighted material. If any omissions have been made, please contact Omnigraphics to make corrections for future editions.

## *Acknowledgements*

Special thanks go to the many organizations, agencies, and individuals who have contributed materials for this *Sourcebook* and to the managing editor Karen Bellenir, medical consultant Dr. David Cooke, permissions specialist Liz Barbour, verification assistant Dawn Matthews, indexer Edward J. Prucha, and document engineer Bruce Bellenir.

## *Note from the Editor*

This book is part of Omnigraphics' *Health Reference Series*. The *Series* provides basic information about a broad range of medical concerns. It is not intended to serve as a tool for diagnosing illness, in prescribing treatments, or as a substitute for the physician/patient relationship. All persons concerned about medical symptoms or the possibility of disease are encouraged to seek professional care from an appropriate health care provider.

## Our Advisory Board

The *Health Reference Series* is reviewed by an Advisory Board comprised of librarians from public, academic, and medical libraries. We would like to thank the following board members for providing guidance to the development of this series:

Dr. Lynda Baker, Associate Professor of Library and Information Science, Wayne State University, Detroit, MI

Nancy Bulgarelli, William Beaumont Hospital Library, Royal Oak, MI

Karen Imarisio, Bloomfield Township Public Library, Bloomfield Township, MI

Karen Morgan, Mardigian Library, University of Michigan-Dearborn, Dearborn, MI

Rosemary Orlando, St. Clair Shores Public Library, St. Clair Shores, MI

## Medical Consultant

Medical consultation services are provided to the *Health Reference Series* editors by David A. Cooke, MD. Dr. Cooke is a graduate of Brandeis University, and he received his M.D. degree from the University of Michigan. He completed residency training at the University of Wisconsin Hospital and Clinics. He is board-certified in Internal Medicine. Dr. Cooke currently works as part of the University of Michigan Health System and practices in Brighton, MI. In his free time, he enjoys writing, science fiction, and spending time with his family.

## Health Reference Series *Update Policy*

The inaugural book in the *Health Reference Series* was the first edition of *Cancer Sourcebook* published in 1989. Since then, the *Series* has been enthusiastically received by librarians and in the medical community. In order to maintain the standard of providing high-quality health information for the layperson the editorial staff at Omnigraphics felt it was necessary to implement a policy of updating volumes when warranted.

Medical researchers have been making tremendous strides, and it is the purpose of the *Health Reference Series* to stay current with the most recent advances. Each decision to update a volume will be made on an individual basis. Some of the considerations will include how much new information is available and the feedback we receive from people who use the books. If there is a topic you would like to see added to the update list, or an area of medical concern you feel has not been adequately addressed, please write to:

Editor
*Health Reference Series*
Omnigraphics, Inc.
615 Griswold Street
Detroit, MI 48226
E-mail: editorial@omnigraphics.com

# Part One

# The Basics of Stroke

# Chapter 1

# *Know Stroke:*
# *Know the Signs, Act in Time*

## Know Stroke

Stroke is the third leading cause of death in the United States and a leading cause of serious, long-term disability in adults. About 600,000 new strokes are reported in the U.S. each year. The good news is that treatments are available that can greatly reduce the damage caused by a stroke. However, you need to recognize the symptoms of a stroke and get to a hospital quickly. Getting treatment within 60 minutes can prevent disability.

### *What Is a Stroke?*

A stroke, sometimes called a "brain attack," occurs when blood flow to the brain is interrupted. When a stroke occurs, brain cells in the immediate area begin to die because they stop getting the oxygen and nutrients they need to function.

### *What Causes a Stroke?*

There are two major kinds of stroke. The first, called an ischemic stroke, is caused by a blood clot which blocks or plugs a blood vessel or artery in the brain. About 80 percent of all strokes are ischemic. The second, known as a hemorrhagic stroke, is caused by a blood vessel

"Know Stroke. Know the Signs. Act in Time," National Institute of Neurological Disorders and Stroke (NINDS), reviewed July 1, 2001.

in the brain that breaks and bleeds into the brain. About 20 percent of strokes are hemorrhagic.

### *What Disabilities Can Result from a Stroke?*

Although stroke is a disease of the brain, it can affect the entire body. The effects of a stroke range from mild to severe and can include paralysis, problems with thinking, problems with speaking, and emotional problems. Patients may also experience pain or numbness after a stroke.

## Know the Signs

Because stroke injures the brain, you may not realize that you are having a stroke. To a bystander, someone having a stroke may just look unaware or confused. Stroke victims have the best chance if someone around them recognizes the symptoms and acts quickly.

### *What Are the Symptoms of a Stroke?*

The symptoms of stroke are distinct because they happen quickly:

- Sudden numbness or weakness of the face, arm, or leg (especially on one side of the body)
- Sudden confusion, trouble speaking or understanding speech
- Sudden trouble seeing in one or both eyes
- Sudden trouble walking, dizziness, loss of balance or coordination
- Sudden severe headache with no known cause

### *What Should a Bystander Do?*

If you believe someone is having a stroke—if he or she suddenly loses the ability to speak, or move an arm or leg on one side, or experiences facial paralysis on one side—call 911 immediately.

## Act in Time

Stroke is a medical emergency. Every minute counts when someone is having a stroke. The longer blood flow is cut off to the brain, the greater the damage. Immediate treatment can save people's lives and enhance their chances for successful recovery.

### Why Is There a Need to Act Fast?

Ischemic strokes, the most common type of strokes, can be treated with a drug called tissue plasminogen activator (tPA), that dissolves blood clots obstructing blood flow to the brain. The window of opportunity to start treating stroke patients is three hours, but to be evaluated and receive treatment, patients need to get to the hospital within 60 minutes.

### What Is the Benefit of Treatment?

A five-year study by the National Institute of Neurological Disorders and Stroke (NINDS) found that some stroke patients who received tPA within three hours of the start of stroke symptoms were at least 30 percent more likely to recover with little or no disability after three months.

### What Can I Do to Prevent a Stroke?

The best treatment for stroke is prevention. There are several risk factors that increase your chances of having a stroke:

- High blood pressure
- Heart disease
- Smoking
- Diabetes
- High cholesterol

If you smoke—quit. If you have high blood pressure, heart disease, diabetes, or high cholesterol, getting them under control—and keeping them under control—will greatly reduce your chances of having a stroke.

# Chapter 2

# *Stroke Statistics in the U.S.*

## *Stroke Is the Third Leading Cause of Death in the U.S.*

**Table 2.1.** Leading Causes of Death, U.S., 2000

| Cause of Death | Number |
|---|---|
| Total | 2,404,624 |
| 1. Heart disease* | 709,894 |
| 2. Cancer | 551,833 |
| 3. Stroke (Cerebrovascular disease) | 166,028 |
| 4. COPD (chronic obstructive pulmonary disease) and allied conditions** | 123,550 |
| 5. Accidents | 93,592 |
| 6. Diabetes | 68,662 |
| 7. Influenza and pneumonia | 67,024 |
| 8. Alzheimer's disease | 49,044 |
| 9. Nephritis | 37,672 |
| 10. Septicemia | 31,613 |
| All other causes of death | 505,712 |

*Includes 529,659 deaths from coronary heart disease.

**Chronic lower respiratory diseases.

---

This chapter includes excerpts from "Morbidity and Mortality: 2002 Chart Book on Cardiovascular, Lung, and Blood Diseases," National Heart, Lung, and Blood Institute, May 2002; excerpts from "Fact Book Fiscal Year 2001," National Heart, Lung, and Blood Institute, February 2002; and "State-Specific Mortality from Stroke and Distribution of Place of Death—United States, 1999," *Morbidity and Mortality Weekly Report*, May 24, 2002/51(20); 429-433, Centers for Disease Control and Prevention (CDC).

**Table 2.2.** Leading Causes of Death by Age and Rank, U.S., 2000

| | Rank | | | | |
|---|---|---|---|---|---|
| Cause of Death | 1-24 | 25-44 | 45-64 | 65-84 | 85+ |
| Heart disease | 5 | 3 | 2 | 1 | 1 |
| Cancer | 4 | 2 | 1 | 2 | 2 |
| Cerebrovascular disease (Stroke) | 9 | 8 | 4 | 3 | 3 |
| Accidents | 1 | 1 | 3 | 9 | 9 |
| COPD and allied conditions* | 8 | -- | 5 | 4 | 6 |
| Influenza and pneumonia | 7 | 10 | -- | 6 | 4 |
| Diabetes mellitus | -- | 9 | 6 | 5 | 7 |

*Chronic lower respiratory diseases

## Age-Adjusted Death Rates for Stroke by Race/Ethnicity and Sex, U.S., 1985-1999

Between 1985 and 1999, stroke mortality declined for all groups. The decrease was modest among Asian males and American Indian females.

### Death Rates for Stroke 2000

In 2000, stroke mortality was higher in blacks than in whites at all ages. Within race groups, it was higher in males than in females.

### Disease Statistics from Fact Book Fiscal Year 2001

Cardiovascular, lung, and blood diseases constitute a large morbidity, mortality, and economic burden on individuals, families, and the Nation. Common forms are atherosclerosis, hypertension, COPD, and blood-clotting disorders—embolisms and thromboses. The most serious atherosclerotic diseases are CHD (coronary heart disease), as manifested by heart attack and angina pectoris, and cerebrovascular disease as manifested by stroke.

In 1999, cardiovascular, lung, and blood diseases accounted for 1,187,000 deaths and 50 percent of all deaths in the United States. The projected economic cost in 2002 for these diseases is expected to be $456 billion, 23 percent of the total economic costs of illness, injuries, and death. Of all diseases, heart disease is the leading cause of death, cerebrovascular disease is third (behind cancer, and COPD (including

**Table 2.3.** Male: Deaths/100,000 Population

| Year | Black | White* | American Indian | Hispanic | Asian |
|------|-------|--------|-----------------|----------|-------|
| 1985 | 114.3 | 74.6 | 49.4 | 55.3 | 65.6 |
| 1986 | 111.9 | 73.2 | 48.4 | 54.2 | 65.2 |
| 1987 | 109.6 | 72.0 | 47.5 | 53.2 | 65.7 |
| 1988 | 107.3 | 70.7 | 46.6 | 52.2 | 64.2 |
| 1989 | 105.1 | 69.5 | 45.7 | 51.2 | 63.8 |
| 1990 | 102.9 | 68.3 | 44.9 | 50.2 | 63.3 |
| 1991 | 100.8 | 67.1 | 44.0 | 49.3 | 62.9 |
| 1992 | 98.7 | 65.9 | 43.2 | 48.3 | 62.4 |
| 1993 | 96.6 | 64.7 | 42.4 | 47.4 | 62.0 |
| 1994 | 94.6 | 63.6 | 41.6 | 46.5 | 61.5 |
| 1995 | 92.7 | 62.5 | 40.8 | 45.6 | 61.1 |
| 1996 | 90.7 | 61.4 | 40.0 | 44.7 | 60.6 |
| 1997 | 88.9 | 60.3 | 39.3 | 43.9 | 60.2 |
| 1998 | 87.0 | 59.3 | 38.5 | 43.1 | 59.8 |
| 1999 | 85.2 | 58.2 | 37.8 | 42.2 | 59.3 |

*Non-Hispanic

Note: Each line is a log linear regression derived from the actual rates.

**Table 2.4.** Female: Deaths/100,000 Population

| Year | Black | White* | American Indian | Hispanic | Asian |
|------|-------|--------|-----------------|----------|-------|
| 1985 | 97.1 | 68.3 | 43.5 | 48.5 | 57.1 |
| 1986 | 95.2 | 67.4 | 43.1 | 47.4 | 56.3 |
| 1987 | 93.3 | 66.5 | 42.7 | 46.4 | 55.6 |
| 1988 | 91.5 | 65.6 | 42.3 | 45.3 | 54.9 |
| 1989 | 89.7 | 64.7 | 41.9 | 44.3 | 54.2 |
| 1990 | 88.0 | 63.8 | 41.5 | 43.3 | 53.4 |
| 1991 | 86.3 | 63.0 | 41.2 | 42.3 | 52.7 |
| 1992 | 84.6 | 62.1 | 40.8 | 41.4 | 52.0 |
| 1993 | 82.9 | 61.3 | 40.4 | 40.5 | 51.4 |
| 1994 | 81.3 | 60.4 | 40.1 | 39.5 | 50.7 |
| 1995 | 79.7 | 59.6 | 39.7 | 38.7 | 50.0 |
| 1996 | 78.2 | 58.8 | 39.3 | 37.8 | 49.4 |
| 1997 | 76.6 | 58.0 | 39.0 | 36.9 | 48.7 |
| 1998 | 75.2 | 57.2 | 38.6 | 36.1 | 48.1 |
| 1999 | 73.7 | 56.5 | 38.3 | 35.3 | 47.4 |

*Non-Hispanic

Note: Each line is a log linear regression derived from the actual rates.

**Table 2.5.** Death Rates for Stroke by Age, Race, and Sex, U.S., 2000

Deaths/100,000

| Ages | White Male | White Female | Black Male | Black Female |
|------|------------|--------------|------------|--------------|
| 35-44 | 4.4 | 4.5 | 14.3 | 13.7 |
| 45-54 | 13.4 | 11.2 | 49.9 | 38.4 |
| 55-64 | 39.7 | 29.9 | 118.6 | 74.6 |
| 65-74 | 134.3 | 108.5 | 256.3 | 187.9 |
| 75-84 | 465.4 | 440.1 | 632.4 | 563.1 |

asthma) ranks fourth. Cardiovascular and lung diseases account for three of the five leading causes of death and four of the five leading causes of infant death. Hypertension, heart disease, asthma, and chronic bronchitis are especially prevalent and account for substantial morbidity in Americans. Increases in prevalence have been greatest for asthma and congestive heart failure (CHF).

The purpose of the biomedical research conducted by the NHLBI is to contribute to the prevention and treatment of cardiovascular, lung, and blood diseases. Nation disease statistics show that by mid-century, morbidity and mortality from these diseases had reached record high levels. Since then, however, substantial improvements have been achieved, especially over the past 30 years, as shown by the significant decline in mortality rates. Because many of these diseases begin early in life, their early detection and control can reduce the risk of disability and delay death. Although important advances have been made in the treatment and control of cardiovascular, lung, and blood diseases, these diseases continue to be a major burden on the Nation.

## *Cardiovascular Diseases*

- In 1999, CVD caused 959,000 deaths—40 percent of all deaths.

- The annual number of deaths from CVD increased substantially between 1900 and 1970. This trend ended even though the population continues to increase and age.

- Total CVD mortality from all ages combined, measured by the crude death rate, changed from an increasing to a decreasing trend with a peak in 1968. By 1995, the rate achieved was similar to the rate in 1936.

- Cerebrovascular disease, the third leading cause of death, accounted for 167,000 deaths in 1999.

- Among minority groups, heart disease ranks first, and stroke ranks fifth or higher as the leading causes of death.

- The steep decline in age-adjusted death rate for CVD means a substantial reduction in annual risk of death for an individual of any age. The smaller reduction in crude death rate reflects the impact of an aging population that is growing over time, so that the overall national mortality burden of CVD remains at a high level compared with other causes of death.

- Between 1985 and 1999, death rates for heart disease and stroke declined for men and women in all racial/ethnic groups.

- Substantial improvements have been made in the treatment of CVD. Since 1975, case-fatality rates from hospitalized AMI, stroke, cardiac dysrhythmia, and CHF patients declined appreciably.

- In 1999, an estimated 61.8 million persons in the United States had some form of CVD; 50 million had hypertension, and almost 13 million had CHD.

- Since the 1960s, there has been a substantial reduction in the prevalence of CVD risk factors: hypertension, smoking, and high cholesterol, but not overweight.

- A 1988–94 national survey showed that many more people with hypertension (systolic BP [blood pressure] > 160 mmHg or diastolic BP > 95 mmHg or on antihypertensive medication) were aware of their condition and had it treated and controlled compared with individuals with hypertension in previous years.

- A 1991–94 national survey showed only 27 percent of hypertensive patients (systolic BP > 140 mmHg or diastolic BP > 90 mmHg or on antihypertensive medication) had their condition under control.

- The estimate of economic cost of CVD is expected to be $329 billion in 2002:

  - $199 billion in direct health expenditures
  - $31 billion in indirect cost of morbidity
  - $99 billion in indirect cost of mortality

11

**Figure 2.1.** *Deaths from Cardiovascular Diseases, U.S., 1999*

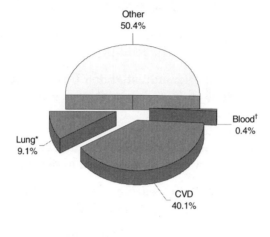

Other
50.4%

Blood[†]
0.4%

Lung*
9.1%

CVD
40.1%

Total Cardiovascular, Lung, and
Blood Diseases 49.6%

* Excludes deaths from pulmonary heart disease.
† Excludes deaths from blood-clotting disorders and
pulmonary embolism (10.4%).

**Figure 2.2.** *Deaths from Blood Diseases, U.S., 1999*

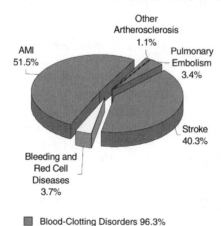

Other
Artherosclerosis
1.1%

Pulmonary
Embolism
3.4%

AMI
51.5%

Stroke
40.3%

Bleeding and
Red Cell
Diseases
3.7%

Blood-Clotting Disorders 96.3%

Note: Numbers may not add to total due to rounding.
Source: Estimated by the NHLBI from Vital Statistics of
the United States, NCHS.

12

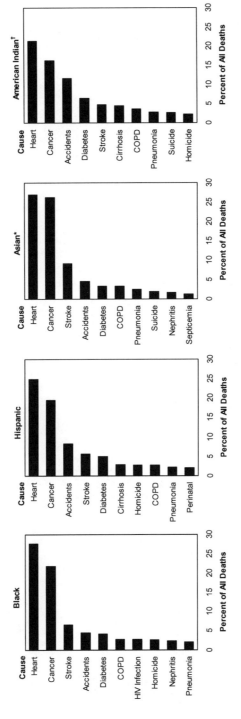

**Figure2.3.** *Ten Leading Causes of Death among Minority Groups, U.S., 1999*

\* Includes deaths among individuals of Asian extraction and Asian-Pacific Islanders.

† Includes deaths among Aleuts and Eskimos.

Source: Vital Statistics of the United States, NCHS.

**Table 2.6.** Number, Rate*, and Place of Stroke-Related Deaths,[1] by Selected Characteristics—United States, 1999

| Characteristic | No. | Rate | Place of death | | | | |
|---|---|---|---|---|---|---|---|
| | | | Pretransport | DOA[2] | ED[3] | In hospital | Data missing |
| **Age group (yrs)** | | | | | | | |
| 0-34 | 976 | (0.7) | 11.6% | 1.1% | 10.7% | 75.5% | 1.1% |
| 35-44 | 2,574 | (5.7) | 14.7% | 1.9% | 9.4% | 73.5% | 0.5% |
| 45-54 | 5,563 | (15.5) | 15.7% | 1.0% | 6.9% | 75.7% | 0.7% |
| 55-64 | 9,652 | (41.3) | 19.5% | 0.7% | 5.5% | 73.6% | 0.6% |
| 65-74 | 24,092 | (132.2) | 30.2% | 0.5% | 4.3% | 64.2% | 0.7% |
| 75-84 | 57,427 | (472.8) | 45.8% | 0.5% | 3.2% | 50.0% | 0.5% |
| ≥85 | 67,080 | (1,606.7) | 63.9% | 0.5% | 2.1% | 33.2% | 0.4% |
| **Race/ethnicity** | | | | | | | |
| White | 144,827 | (166.7) | 50.1% | 0.5% | 2.9% | 46.0% | 0.5% |
| Black | 18,884 | (225.2) | 32.2% | 1.1% | 5.8% | 59.9% | 0.9% |
| American Indian/Alaska Native | 546 | (99.6) | 35.7% | 0.7% | 3.5% | 59.9% | 0.2% |
| Asian/Pacific Islander | 3,109 | (123.9) | 28.6% | 0.4% | 4.1% | 66.2% | 0.8% |
| Hispanic | 5,907 | (100.6) | 30.8% | 0.3% | 4.8% | 63.6% | 0.4% |
| Non-Hispanic[4] | 161,459 | (179.4) | 48.2% | 0.6% | 3.2% | 47.4% | 0.5% |

14

**Sex**

| | | | | | | | |
|---|---|---|---|---|---|---|---|
| Male | 64,485 | (62.4) | 40.3% | 0.6% | 3.7% | 54.9% | 0.5% |
| Female | 102,881 | (60.5) | 52.2% | 0.5% | 3.0% | 43.7% | 0.5% |

**Stroke subtype[5]**

| | | | | | | | |
|---|---|---|---|---|---|---|---|
| Subarachnoid hemorrhage | 6,489 | (2.4) | 13.7% | 1.1% | 7.8% | 76.8% | 0.6% |
| Intracerebral hemorrhage | 25,461 | (9.4) | 12.6% | 0.3% | 5.4% | 80.7% | 0.9% |
| Ischemic | 114,253 | (42.2) | 23.3% | 0.6% | 2.7% | 42.9% | 0.5% |
| Sequelae of stroke | 21,163 | (7.8) | 69.1% | 0.6% | 2.7% | 27.3% | 0.3% |

*Age-adjusted death rates (per 100,000 population) were calculated by using the 2000 U.S. standard population.

[1]International Classification of Disease, Tenth Revision (ICD-10) codes I60-I69.

[2]Dead on or before arrival at a hospital.

[3]Emergency department.

[4]Non-Hispanic includes 402 stroke deaths for which Hispanic origin was not stated.

[5]Stroke subtypes were categorized as subarachnoid hemorrhagic (ICD-10 code I60), intracerebral hemorrhagic (I61-I62), ischemic (I63-I67), and sequelae of stroke (I69).

**Table 2.7.** Number, Rate*, and Place of Stroke-Related Deaths,[1] by State[2]—United States, 1999

| State | No. | Rate | Place of death | | | | |
|---|---|---|---|---|---|---|---|
| | | | Pretransport | DOA[3] | ED[4] | In hospital | Data missing |
| Alabama | 3,066 | 70.5 | 39.9% | 0.1% | 3.7% | 55.6% | 0.6% |
| Alaska | 170 | 70.7 | 37.1% | 0.0% | 3.5% | 59.4% | 0.0% |
| Arizona | 2,649 | 57.0 | 59.7% | 0.1% | 2.1% | 38.0% | 0.1% |
| Arkansas | 2,183 | 77.3 | 42.2% | 0.2% | 3.4% | 54.2% | 0.0% |
| California | 17,964 | 63.3 | 49.2% | 0.0% | 3.1% | 47.3% | 0.3% |
| Colorado | 1,867 | 57.7 | 60.0% | 0.0% | 3.0% | 36.8% | 0.0% |
| Connecticut | 1,961 | 50.8 | 54.7% | 0.4% | 3.5% | 40.3% | 1.1% |
| Delaware | 359 | 49.6 | 44.3% | 0.0% | 3.1% | 52.6% | 0.0% |
| District of Columbia | 339 | 59.9 | 23.3% | 0.6% | 8.3% | 67.8% | 0.0% |
| Florida | 10,636 | 51.9 | 45.0% | 0.1% | 3.2% | 51.6% | 0.0% |
| Georgia | 4,453 | 74.3 | 35.5% | 4.6% | 4.5% | 54.2% | 0.0% |
| Hawaii | 760 | 63.0 | 33.0% | 1.6% | 2.5% | 59.5% | 0.4% |
| Idaho | 764 | 66.5 | 64.0% | 0.4% | 2.6% | 32.9% | 0.1% |
| Illinois | 7,487 | 62.0 | 45.4% | 2.2% | 4.0% | 48.4% | 0.0% |
| Indiana | 4,128 | 70.6 | 52.3% | 0.1% | 3.2% | 44.3% | 0.0% |
| Iowa | 2,300 | 62.2 | 52.8% | 0.1% | 2.1% | 45.0% | 0.0% |
| Kansas | 1,785 | 59.7 | 50.5% | 0.1% | 2.0% | 47.5% | 0.0% |
| Kentucky | 2,642 | 69.3 | 43.5% | 0.4% | 2.9% | 52.6% | 0.0% |
| Louisiana | 2,705 | 70.2 | 28.9% | 0.8% | 3.1% | 64.2% | 0.0% |
| Maine | 873 | 62.9 | 58.5% | 0.1% | 2.1% | 39.3% | 0.0% |
| Maryland | 2,879 | 62.9 | 53.9% | 0.6% | 4.0% | 41.5% | 0.0% |

| State | | | | | | | |
|---|---|---|---|---|---|---|---|
| Massachusetts | 3,563 | 50.5 | 54.6% | 0.2% | 2.0% | 42.7% | 0.4% |
| Michigan | 5,951 | 62.3 | 50.6% | 0.3% | 3.7% | 45.3% | 0.1% |
| Minnesota | 2,972 | 59.5 | 62.1% | 0.1% | 1.6% | 35.5% | 0.8% |
| Mississippi | 1,769 | 67.6 | 30.4% | 0.8% | 6.0% | 62.9% | 0.0% |
| Missouri | 4,106 | 68.7 | 48.4% | 0.1% | 2.5% | 48.7% | 0.2% |
| Montana | 599 | 62.7 | 57.4% | 0.0% | 2.0% | 40.6% | 0.0% |
| Nebraska | 1,187 | 61.2 | 56.2% | 0.0% | 2.9% | 40.5% | 0.0% |
| Nevada | 928 | 63.5 | 32.5% | 0.0% | 3.8% | 63.4% | 0.3% |
| New Hampshire | 690 | 33.0 | 54.5% | 0.3% | 2.6% | 42.5% | 0.1% |
| New Jersey | 4,073 | 46.9 | 37.2% | 0.2% | 3.2% | 59.4% | 0.1% |
| New Mexico | 789 | 52.8 | 51.8% | 0.2% | 3.4% | 44.5% | 0.0% |
| New York | 7,954 | 41.2 | 35.7% | 0.4% | 3.4% | 59.8% | 0.6% |
| North Carolina | 5,649 | 78.4 | 45.3% | 0.4% | 3.3% | 50.6% | 0.4% |
| North Dakota | 554 | 69.2 | 51.1% | 0.0% | 1.8% | 47.1% | 0.0% |
| Ohio | 7,199 | 61.8 | 54.4% | 0.5% | 3.4% | 40.6% | 1.1% |
| Oklahoma | 2,401 | 67.6 | 43.5% | 0.3% | 3.3% | 52.8% | 0.0% |
| Oregon | 2,803 | 78.7 | 67.3% | 0.0% | 2.1% | 30.6% | 0.0% |
| Pennsylvania | 8,655 | 58.5 | 50.7% | 0.4% | 2.9% | 46.0% | 0.0% |
| Rhode Island | 648 | 51.1 | 58.6% | 0.6% | 1.7% | 33.5% | 5.6% |
| South Carolina | 2,910 | 83.8 | 44.3% | 0.4% | 4.6% | 50.6% | 0.0% |
| South Dakota | 569 | 63.4 | 54.3% | 0.2% | 0.9% | 44.6% | 0.0% |
| Tennessee | 4,395 | 83.3 | 37.0% | 3.4% | 4.7% | 54.1% | 0.7% |
| Texas | 10,552 | 67.1 | 41.7% | 0.3% | 4.2% | 53.6% | 0.2% |
| Utah | 881 | 61.5 | 60.7% | 0.3% | 2.7% | 36.2% | 0.0% |

*Table continues on next page.*

17

**Table 2.7.** Number, Rate*, and Place of Stroke-Related Deaths,[1] by State[2]—United States, 1999. Continued from previous page.

|  |  |  | Place of death |  |  |  |  |
|---|---|---|---|---|---|---|---|
| State | No. | Rate | Pretransport | DOA[3] | ED[4] | In hospital | Data missing |
| Vermont | 335 | 56.0 | 67.2% | 0.6% | 1.5% | 30.7% | 0.0% |
| Virginia | 4,108 | 69.8 | 44.0% | 0.5% | 2.7% | 40.6% | 11.2% |
| Washington | 3,724 | 69.9 | 64.4% | 0.0% | 0.8% | 34.7% | 0.0% |
| West Virginia | 1,333 | 63.6 | 39.2% | 0.9% | 3.1% | 56.7% | 0.0% |
| Wisconsin | 3,841 | 67.3 | 60.7% | 0.1% | 1.9% | 37.2% | 0.0% |
| Wyoming | 255 | 59.5 | 55.1% | 0.0% | 2.4% | 42.5% | 0.0% |
| Total | 167,399 | 63.4 | 47.6% | 0.5% | 3.3% | 48.0% | 0.5% |

*Age-adjusted death rates (per 100,000 population) were calculated by using the 2000 U.S. standard population.

[1]International Classification of Disease, Tenth Revision (ICD-10) codes I60-I69.

[2]Percentages for place of death are based on state of occurrence.

[3]Dead on or before arrival at a hospital.

[4]Emergency department.

18

## State-Specific Mortality from Stroke and Distribution of Place of Death—United States, 1999

In the United States, stroke is the third leading cause of death and one of the major causes of serious, long-term disability among adults. Each year, approximately 500,000 persons suffer a first-time stroke, and approximately 167,000 deaths are stroke-related.[1] This report presents national and state-specific death rates for stroke in 1999, which indicate state-by-state variations in both stroke-related death rates and the proportions of stroke decedents who die before transport to an emergency department (ED). Prevention through public and medical education remains a key strategy for reducing stroke-related deaths and disability.

CDC compiled national and state mortality data based on death certificates from state vital statistics offices.[2] Demographic data were reported by funeral directors or provided by family members of the decedent. Stroke-related deaths are those for which the underlying cause listed on the death certificate by a physician or a coroner is classified according to the International Classification of Diseases, Tenth Revision (ICD-10) codes I60-I69. Stroke subtypes are defined as subarachnoid hemorrhagic stroke (I60), intracerebral hemorrhagic stroke (I61-I62), ischemic stroke (I63-I67), and sequelae of stroke (I69). Place of death was defined as either pretransport, dead on arrival (DOA), in the ED, or in the hospital after admission. Pretransport deaths occurred at the decedent's residence, in a nursing home, or in an extended-care facility before transport to a hospital or ED. Stroke-related death rates for groups defined by age, sex, race/ethnicity, stroke subtype, and state were determined by dividing the number of deaths by the population at risk in that group. Estimates of resident populations and age-adjusted death rates were calculated by using the 2000 U.S. standard population.[3]

Among U.S. residents, 167,366 stroke-related deaths occurred in 1999, with an age-adjusted rate of 63.4 per 100,000 population. The greatest proportion of deaths occurred among persons aged >85 years (40.1%) followed by those aged 75-84 years (34.3%), those aged 65-74 years (14.4%), and those aged <65 years (11.2%). Age-specific death rates increased for successive age groups (Table 2.6). By race/ethnicity, the highest age-adjusted death rates for stroke occurred among blacks followed by whites (225.2 and 166.7 per 100,000 population, respectively). Age-adjusted death rates for stroke were slightly higher among men (62.4) than among women (60.5). Ischemic strokes accounted for 68.3% of all stroke-related deaths; age-adjusted death rates were higher for ischemic stroke than for all other stroke subtypes.

19

In 1999, a total of 79,663 (47.6%) stroke-related deaths occurred pretransport, 926 (0.7%) occurred as DOA, 5,519 (3.3%) occurred in the ED, and 80,369 (48.0%) occurred after admission to the hospital; for 889 (0.5%) deaths, place-of-death data were not available. The proportion of pretransport deaths increased with age, and the proportion of deaths that occurred as DOA or in the ED decreased with age. The proportion of pretransport deaths was higher among women (52.2%) than among men (40.3%) and higher among whites (50.1%) than among other racial/ethnic populations. Conversely, the proportion of stroke-related deaths that occurred in the ED was higher among blacks (5.8%) than among other racial/ethnic populations, and higher among Hispanics (4.8%) than among non-Hispanics (3.2%). Compared with other stroke subtypes, the highest proportion of pretransport deaths was among persons who died of sequelae of stroke or other cerebrovascular disease (69.1%), followed by ischemic stroke (23.3%), subarachnoid hemorrhagic stroke (13.7%), and intracerebral hemorrhagic stroke (12.6%). Persons who died of subarachnoid hemorrhagic stroke accounted for the highest proportion of deaths that occurred as DOA or in the ED (1.1% and 7.8%, respectively).

The state-specific, age-adjusted death rates for stroke ranged from 33.0 per 100,000 population in New Hampshire to 83.8 in South Carolina (Table 2.7). The proportion of pretransport deaths ranged from 23.3% in the District of Columbia to 67.3% in Oregon. States with >60% of stroke deaths reported as occurring pretransport were Colorado (60.0%), Wisconsin (60.7%), Utah (60.7%), Minnesota (62.1%), Idaho (64.0%), Washington (64.4%), Vermont (67.2%), and Oregon (67.3%). The proportion of stroke-related deaths reported as DOA ranged from zero to 4.6%; those having occurred in the ED ranged from 0.8% to 8.3%. The proportion of stroke-related deaths for which place-of-death data were missing ranged from zero to 11.2%.

Reported by: JE Williams, PhD, CS Ayala, PhD, JB Croft, PhD, KJ Greenlund, PhD, NL Keenan, PhD, LJ Neff, PhD, WA Wattigney, MStat, ZJ Zheng, MD, GA Mensah, MD, Div of Adult and Community Health, National Center for Chronic Disease Prevention and Health Promotion, CDC.

Editorial Note: The findings in this report indicate that ischemic strokes account for most stroke-related deaths and that state-by-state variations exist in the proportion of stroke-related deaths that occur pretransport. These findings are consistent with other evidence that many acute ischemic stroke patients cannot benefit from thrombolytic therapy because they do not reach medical treatment in time.[4-6] Thrombolytic therapy is a time-dependent therapy with a window of efficacy of <3 hours after the onset of symptoms.[4] The reported pre-hospital delay ranges from 1 to 14 hours, with 3-6 hours as the typical time range.[6] Because the advent of thrombolytic therapy has made the early recognition of stroke symptoms and rapid medical response imperative, educational programs are needed for both health care providers and the public to reduce stroke-related deaths and disability.

Educating the public about signs and symptoms of stroke, the need for emergency response (i.e., calling 911), and the importance of immediate transport to an ED might help promote prompt and effective treatment. State-by-state variations in the proportion of stroke-related deaths that occurred pretransport might reflect differences in public awareness of stroke symptoms. Results from population-based surveys suggest that many persons are unaware of the five most common signs and symptoms of stroke: sudden numbness or weakness, sudden dimness or loss of vision, sudden dizziness or loss of balance, sudden severe headache, and confusion or difficulty speaking. Only 57% of survey respondents in the Greater Cincinnati area and 39% in Georgia could identify at least one of these symptoms.[7,8]

The accurate identification and rapid transport of stroke patients by emergency medical system (EMS) personnel are crucial to the successful early treatment of stroke.[9] To assess whether a patient is having a stroke, EMS personnel should be trained properly and equipped with the appropriate technology. In addition, triage nurses and physicians in the ED should be educated to treat stroke as a medical emergency. State-by-state variations in the proportions of stroke-related deaths by place of death might reflect different EMS policies about the need to transport persons who have already died. The high proportion (63.9%) of stroke-related deaths that occurred pretransport among adults aged >85 years might be explained, at least in part, by do-not-resuscitate orders in nursing homes and long-term care facilities, especially for older persons disabled by the sequelae of previous strokes. However, approximately 25% of stroke-related deaths among persons aged <65 years occurred pretransport, as DOA, or in the ED, suggesting that persons in this age group might dismiss stroke as a problem of the elderly and therefore delay their response to symptoms.

The findings in this report are subject to at least two limitations. First, data are subject to misclassification of race/ethnicity both in the population census and on death certificates, which might result in over-reporting of deaths among blacks and whites and underreporting deaths among other racial/ethnic groups.[10] Second, data on underlying

21

cause and place of death are subject to error because they originate from the physicians or coroners who certify each death.

Because high blood pressure, diabetes, high cholesterol, and smoking remain the major risk factors for stroke, prevention through public and medical education and through risk-factor reduction should continue to be the focus of public health efforts to reduce the number of stroke-related deaths. Prevention efforts also must include broad-based public health efforts to increase awareness of stroke symptoms and to foster an appropriate and timely response from health care providers and the public.

## *References*

1.  American Heart Association. 2002 heart and stroke statistical update. Dallas, Texas: American Heart Association, 2001. Available at http://www.americanheart.org/statistics/index.html.

2.  Hoyert DL, Arias E, Smith BL, Murphy SL, Kochanek KD. Deaths: final data for 1999. *Natl Vital Stat Rep*, vol. 49, no. 8. Hyattsville, Maryland: U.S. Department of Health and Human Services, CDC, National Center for Health Statistics, 2001.

3.  Anderson RN, Rosenberg HM. Age standardization of death rates: implementation of the year 2000 standard. *Natl Vital Stat Rep*, vol. 47, no. 3. Hyattsville, Maryland: U.S. Department of Health and Human Services, CDC, National Center for Health Statistics, 1998.

4.  O'Connor RE, McGraw P, Edelsohn L. Thrombolytic therapy for acute ischemic stroke: why the majority of patients remain ineligible for treatment. *Ann Emerg Med* 1999;33:9-14.

5.  The National Institute for Neurological Disorders and Strokert-PA Stroke Study Group. Tissue plasminogen activator for acute ischemic stroke. *N Engl J Med* 1995:333:1581-7.

6.  Evenson KR, Rosamond WD, Morris DL. Prehospital and in-hospital delays in acute stroke. *Neuroepidemiology* 2001;20:65-76.

7.  Pancioli AM, Broderick J, Kothari R, et al. Public perception of stroke warning signs and knowledge of potential risk factors. *JAMA* 1998;279:1288-92.

8.  Rowe AK, Frankel MR, Sanders KA. Stroke awareness among Georgia adults: epidemiology and considerations regarding measurement. *South Med J* 2001;94:613-8.

9.  Porteus GH, Corry MD, Smith WS. Emergency medical services dispatcher identification of stroke and transient ischemic attack. *Prehosp Emerg Care* 1999:3;211-6.

10. Rosenberg HM, Maurer JD, Sorlie PD, et al. Quality of death rates by race and Hispanic origin: a summary of current research, 1999. *Vital Health Stat* 1999;2:1-13.

# Chapter 3

# *The Cost of Stroke to All Americans*

- Stroke, or brain attack, is our nation's third leading cause of death, killing nearly 160,000 Americans every year.

- Every year approximately 750,000 Americans have a new or recurrent stroke.

- Every forty-five seconds in the United States, someone experiences a stroke.

- Over the course of a lifetime, four out of every five American families will be touched by stroke.

- Approximately one-third of all stroke survivors will have another stroke within five years.

- Of the 590,000 Americans who survive a stroke each year, approximately 5 to 14 percent will have another stroke within one year. The rate of having another stroke is about 10 percent per year thereafter.

- Stroke is one of the leading causes of adult disability. Four million Americans are living with the effects of stroke. About one-third have mild impairments, another third are moderately impaired, and the remainder are severely impaired.

---

"The Cost of Stroke to All Americans," © 2002 National Stroke Association (www.stroke.org); reprinted with permission.

- Stroke costs the United States $30 billion annually. Direct costs, such as hospitals, physicians, and rehabilitation add up to $17 billion; indirect costs, such as lost productivity, total $13 billion. The average cost per patient for the first 90 days post-stroke is $15,000, although 10 percent of the cases exceed $35,000. (PORT Study)

**Table 3.1.** Recurrent Stroke Rates

| Time after Completed Stroke | Cumulative Risk of Subsequent Stroke |
|---|---|
| 30 days | 3% to 10% |
| 1 year | 5% to 14% |
| 5 years | 25% to 40% |

## The Rise in Stroke Mortality

In 1993, the U.S. stroke mortality rate increased for the first time in four decades from 26.2 deaths per 100,000 to 26.5 deaths per 100,000. The mortality rate inched up again in 1995 to 26.7. Statistics for 1997 show that the stroke death rate has declined slightly to 25.9 with a total of 159,791 deaths. Stroke remains the third leading cause of death in the United States. Death rates for the other two leading killers, heart disease and cancer are decreasing at a higher rate. In addition, from the 1960s to 1992, the dramatic decrease in stroke mortality paralleled the decrease in high blood pressure attributed to antihypertensive medication, and may now be paralleling increasing noncompliance to high blood pressure medication.

## The Poor Public Awareness of Stroke

A 1996 National Stroke Association (NSA)/Gallup Survey on stroke awareness in the United States revealed the following:

- Among adults age 50 or older, 38 percent did not know where in the body a stroke occurs.

- 19 percent were unaware that there are things you can do to help prevent a stroke.

- Only 40 percent would call 911 immediately if they were having a stroke.

26

- Two-thirds were unaware of the short time frame in which a person must seek treatment.

- Only 3 percent correctly defined a TIA as a small stroke. The survey also showed that older Americans could not identify the following stroke symptoms:
    - Sudden blurred or decreased vision in one or both eyes—91 percent
    - Loss of balance or coordination (a major sign when accompanied by another symptom)—85 percent
    - Difficulty speaking or understanding simple statements—68 percent
    - Weakness/numbness/paralysis in the face, arm, or leg—42 percent

## The Toll on Older Adults

- Stroke risk increases with age. For each decade after age 55, the risk of stroke doubles.

- For adults over age 65, the risk of dying from stroke is seven times that of the general population.

- Two-thirds of all strokes occur in people over age 65. The over-50 population is expected to rise by 19 percent from 1994 to 2000, making it the fastest growing U.S. age group. This puts more people at higher risk for stroke every day.

- Stroke is a major and increasing factor in the late-life dementia that affects more than 40 percent of Americans over age 80.

## The Toll on Women

- Stroke kills more than twice as many American women every year as breast cancer.

- Stroke has a disproportionate effect on women. Women account for approximately 43 percent of the strokes that occur each year, yet they account for 62 percent of stroke deaths (97,467 of the 159,942 annual deaths). The explanation may be that stroke risk increases with age, and women generally live longer than men. In addition, women may on average be older than men at the time of stroke.

27

- Women over age 30 who smoke and take high-estrogen oral contraceptives have a stroke risk 22 times higher than average.

## The Toll on African-Americans

- Incidence rate for first stroke among African-Americans is almost double that of white Americans, 288 per 100,000 African-Americans, compared to 179 per 100,000 whites.

- African-Americans not only have a higher incidence of strokes than whites and Hispanics, but they also suffer more extensive physical impairments that last longer than those of other racial groups in the United States.

- Not only are African-Americans twice as likely as whites to have a stroke, they're also twice as likely to die from a stroke. Stroke mortality for this group is nearly double the rate for whites.

- African-Americans have a disproportionately high incidence of risk factors for stroke, particularly hypertension, diabetes, obesity, smoking, and sickle cell anemia.

## The "Stroke Belt"

- Twelve contiguous states and the District of Columbia have stroke death rates that are consistently more than 10 percent higher than the rest of the country. These states (Virginia, North Carolina, South Carolina, Georgia, Florida, Alabama, Mississippi, Louisiana, Arkansas, Tennessee, Kentucky, and Indiana), along with Washington, DC, are often referred to as the "stroke belt." Their higher incidence and mortality may be linked to a number of factors, including:
    - A higher than average population of African-Americans
    - A higher than average population of older adults
    - Dietary factors

# Chapter 4

# *Types of Stroke*

## Contents

# Section 4.1

## *Ischemic Stroke*

Excerpted from "Stroke: Hope Through Research," National Institute of Neurological Disorders and Stroke (NINDS), NIH Publication No. 99-2222, May 1999, reviewed July 1, 2001.

### *Introduction*

More than 2,400 years ago the father of medicine, Hippocrates, recognized and described stroke—the sudden onset of paralysis. Until recently, modern medicine has had very little power over this disease, but the world of stroke medicine is changing and new and better therapies are being developed every day. Today, some people who have a stroke can walk away from the attack with no or few disabilities if they are treated promptly. Doctors can finally offer stroke patients and their families the one thing that until now has been so hard to give—hope.

In ancient times stroke was called apoplexy, a general term that physicians applied to anyone suddenly struck down with paralysis. Because many conditions can lead to sudden paralysis, the term apoplexy did not indicate a specific diagnosis or cause. Physicians knew very little about the cause of stroke and the only established therapy was to feed and care for the patient until the attack ran its course.

The first person to investigate the pathological signs of apoplexy was Johann Jacob Wepfer. Born in Schaffhausen, Switzerland in 1620, Wepfer studied medicine and was the first to identify postmortem signs of bleeding in the brains of patients who died of apoplexy. From autopsy studies he gained knowledge of the carotid and vertebral arteries that supply the brain with blood. He also was the first person to suggest that apoplexy, in addition to being caused by bleeding in the brain, could be caused by a blockage of one of the main arteries supplying blood to the brain; thus stroke became known as a cerebrovascular disease (cerebro refers to a part of the brain; vascular refers to the blood vessels and arteries).

Medical science would eventually confirm Wepfer's hypotheses, but until very recently doctors could offer little in the area of therapy. Over the last two decades basic and clinical investigators, many of them sponsored and funded in part by the National Institute of Neurological Disorders and Stroke (NINDS), have learned a great deal about stroke. They have identified major risk factors for the disease and have developed surgical techniques and drug treatments for the prevention of stroke. But perhaps the most exciting new development in the field of stroke research is the recent approval of a drug treatment that can reverse the course of stroke if given during the first few hours after the onset of symptoms.

Studies with animals have shown that brain injury occurs within minutes of a stroke and can become irreversible within as little as an hour. In humans, brain damage begins from the moment the stroke starts and often continues for days afterward. Scientists now know that there is a very short window of opportunity for treatment of the most common form of stroke. Because of these and other advances in the field of cerebrovascular disease stroke patients now have a chance for survival and recovery.

## What Is Stroke?

A stroke occurs when the blood supply to part of the brain is suddenly interrupted or when a blood vessel in the brain bursts, spilling blood into the spaces surrounding brain cells. In the same way that a person suffering a loss of blood flow to the heart is said to be having a heart attack, a person with a loss of blood flow to the brain or sudden bleeding in the brain can be said to be having a brain attack.

Brain cells die when they no longer receive oxygen and nutrients from the blood or when they are damaged by sudden bleeding into or around the brain. Ischemia is the term used to describe the loss of oxygen and nutrients for brain cells when there is inadequate blood flow. Ischemia ultimately leads to infarction, the death of brain cells which are eventually replaced by a fluid-filled cavity (or infarct) in the injured brain.

When blood flow to the brain is interrupted, some brain cells die immediately, while others remain at risk for death. These damaged cells make up the ischemic penumbra and can linger in a compromised state for several hours. With timely treatment these cells can be saved.

Even though a stroke occurs in the unseen reaches of the brain, the symptoms of a stroke are easy to spot. They include sudden numbness or weakness, especially on one side of the body; sudden confusion or trouble speaking or understanding speech; sudden trouble seeing in one or both eyes; sudden trouble walking, dizziness, or loss of balance or coordination; or sudden severe headache with no known cause. All of the symptoms of stroke appear suddenly, and often there is more than one symptom at the same time. Therefore stroke can usually be distinguished from other causes of dizziness or headache. These symptoms may indicate that a stroke has occurred and that medical attention is needed immediately.

There are two forms of stroke: ischemic—blockage of a blood vessel supplying the brain, and hemorrhagic—bleeding into or around the brain. The following sections describe these forms in detail.

## Ischemic Stroke

An ischemic stroke occurs when an artery supplying the brain with blood becomes blocked, suddenly decreasing or stopping blood flow and ultimately causing a brain infarction. This type of stroke accounts for approximately 80 percent of all strokes. Blood clots are the most common cause of artery blockage and brain infarction. The process of clotting is necessary and beneficial throughout the body because it stops bleeding and allows repair of damaged areas of arteries or veins. However, when blood clots develop in the wrong place within an artery they can cause devastating injury by interfering with the normal flow of blood. Problems with clotting become more frequent as people age.

Blood clots can cause ischemia and infarction in two ways. A clot that forms in a part of the body other than the brain can travel through blood vessels and become wedged in a brain artery. This free-roaming clot is called an embolus and often forms in the heart. A stroke caused by an embolus is called an *embolic stroke*. The second kind of ischemic stroke, called a *thrombotic stroke*, is caused by thrombosis, the formation of a blood clot in one of the cerebral arteries that stays attached to the artery wall until it grows large enough to block blood flow.

Ischemic strokes can also be caused by stenosis, or a narrowing of the artery due to the buildup of plaque (a mixture of fatty substances, including cholesterol and other lipids) and blood clots along the artery wall. Stenosis can occur in large arteries and small arteries and is therefore called large vessel disease or small vessel disease, respectively. When a stroke occurs due to small vessel disease, a very small infarction results, sometimes called a lacunar infarction, from the French word *lacune* meaning gap or cavity.

The most common blood vessel disease that causes stenosis is atherosclerosis. In atherosclerosis, deposits of plaque build up along the inner walls of large and medium-sized arteries, causing thickening, hardening, and loss of elasticity of artery walls and decreased blood flow.

## The Ischemic Cascade

The brain is the most complex organ in the human body. It contains hundreds of billions of cells that interconnect to form a complex network of communication. The brain has several different types of cells, the most important of which are neurons. The organization of neurons in the brain and the communication that occurs among them lead to thought, memory, cognition, and awareness. Other types of brain cells are generally called glia (from the Greek word meaning glue). These supportive cells of the nervous system provide scaffolding and support for the vital neurons, protecting them from infection, toxins, and trauma. Glia make up the blood-brain barrier between blood vessels and the substance of the brain.

Stroke is the sudden onset of paralysis caused by injury to brain cells from disruption in blood flow. The injury caused by a blocked blood vessel can occur within several minutes and progress for hours as the result of a chain of chemical reactions that is set off after the start of stroke symptoms. Physicians and researchers often call this chain of chemical reactions that lead to the permanent brain injury of stroke the ischemic cascade.

### Primary Cell Death

In the first stage of the ischemic cascade, blood flow is cut off from a part of the brain (ischemia). This leads to a lack of oxygen (anoxia) and lack of nutrients in the cells of this core area. When the lack of oxygen becomes extreme, the mitochondria, the energy-producing structures within the cell, can no longer produce enough energy to keep the cell functioning. The mitochondria break down, releasing toxic chemicals called oxygen-free radicals into the cytoplasm of the cell. These toxins poison the cell from the inside-out, causing destruction of other cell structures, including the nucleus.

The lack of energy in the cell causes the gated channels of the cell membrane that normally maintain homeostasis to open and allow toxic amounts of calcium, sodium, and potassium ions to flow into the cell. At the same time, the injured ischemic cell releases excitatory amino acids, such as glutamate, into the space between neurons, leading to over-excitation and injury to nearby cells. With the loss of

33

homeostasis, water rushes into the cell making it swell (called cyto-toxic edema) until the cell membrane bursts under the internal pressure. At this point the nerve cell is essentially permanently injured and for all purposes dead (necrosis and infarction). After a stroke starts, the first cells that are going to die may die within 4 to 5 minutes. The response to the treatment that restores blood flow as late as 2 hours after stroke onset would suggest that, in most cases, the process is not over for at least 2 to 3 hours. After that, with rare exceptions, most of the injury that has occurred is essentially permanent.

### Secondary Cell Death

Due to exposure to excessive amounts of glutamate, nitric oxide, free radicals, and excitatory amino acids released into the intercellular space by necrotic cells, nearby cells have a more difficult time surviving. They are receiving just enough oxygen from cerebral blood flow (CBF) to stay alive. A compromised cell can survive for several hours in a low-energy state. If blood flow is restored within this narrow window of opportunity, at present thought to be about 2 hours, then some of these cells can be salvaged and become functional again. Researchers funded by the NINDS have learned that restoring blood flow to these cells can be achieved by administrating the clot-dissolving thrombolytic agent tPA within 3 hours of the start of the stroke.

### Inflammation and the Immune Response

While anoxic and necrotic brain cells are doing damage to still viable brain tissue the immune system of the body is injuring the brain through an inflammatory reaction mediated by the vascular system. Damage to the blood vessel at the site of a blood clot or hemorrhage attracts inflammatory blood elements to that site. Among the first blood elements to arrive are leukocytes, white blood cells that are covered with immune system proteins that attach to the blood vessel wall at the site of the injury. After they attach, the leukocytes penetrate the endothelial wall, move through the blood-brain barrier, and invade the substance of the brain causing further injury and brain cell death. Leukocytes called monocytes and macrophages release inflammatory chemicals (cytokines, interleukins, and tissue necrosis factors) at the site of the injury. These chemicals make it harder for the body to naturally dissolve a clot that has caused a stroke by inactivating anti-clotting factors and inhibiting the release of natural tissue plasminogen activator. NINDS researchers are currently working to create interventional therapies that will inhibit the effects of cytokines and other chemicals in the inflammatory process during stroke.

These brain cells that survive the loss of blood flow (ischemia) but are not able to function make up the ischemic penumbra. These areas of still-viable brain cells exist in a patchwork pattern within and around the area of dead brain tissue (also called an infarct).

# Section 4.2.

# *Hemorrhagic Stroke*

"Hemorrhagic Stroke," © 2002, A.D.A.M., Inc. Reprinted with permission.

Alternative names: Stroke-hemorrhagic

## Definition

A hemorrhagic stroke is bleeding that occurs within ischemic brain tissue.

## Causes and Risks

Hemorrhagic stroke occurs when a blood vessel that is damaged or dead from lack of blood supply (infarcted)—located within an area of infarcted brain tissue—ruptures. This transforms the previously *ischemic* stroke into a *hemorrhagic* stroke. (Note: ischemia is inadequate tissue oxygenation caused by reduced blood flow; infarction is tissue death resulting from ischemia.)

Bleeding irritates the brain tissues, causing swelling (cerebral edema). Blood collects into a mass (hematoma). Both swelling and hematoma will compress and displace brain tissue.

Risks for hemorrhagic stroke include hemophilia, decreased platelet count, sickle cell anemia, DIC, and anticoagulant medications. Hypertension and embolic strokes may also increase the risk of hemorrhagic stroke.

The initial effects of hemorrhagic stroke may be more severe than "simple" ischemic-type stroke, but long-term effects are essentially the same.

Subarachnoid hemorrhage, intracerebral hemorrhage, or other forms of intracranial hemorrhage may rarely cause stroke-like symptoms.

## Prevention

Most cases of hemorrhagic stroke are associated with cardiac embolism, which is associated with atrial fibrillation. Prevention includes treatment of atrial fibrillation.

## Symptoms

Stroke symptoms include:

- Weakness or total inability to move a body part
- Numbness, loss of sensation
- Tingling or other abnormal sensations
- Decreased or lost vision, (may be partial, may be temporary)
- Eyes (pupils different sizes)
- Eyelid drooping (ptosis)
- Language difficulties (aphasia)
- Inability to recognize or identify sensory stimuli (agnosia)
- Loss of memory
- Vertigo (abnormal sensation of movement)
- Dizziness
- Loss of coordination
- Swallowing difficulties
- Personality changes
- Mood and emotion changes
- Urinary incontinence (lack of control over bladder)
- Lack of control over the bowels
- Consciousness changes:
  - Sleepy
  - Stuporous/somnolent/lethargic
  - Comatose or unconscious

## Signs and Tests

Examination may indicate increased intracranial pressure. Eye examination may show abnormalities of movement, or changes may be seen in the retinal examination (examination of the back of the eye). Reflexes may be abnormal in extent, or abnormal reflexes may be present.

Tests may include:

- CBC (complete blood count)
- Platelet count
- Bleeding time
- Prothrombin/partial thromboplastin time (PT/PTT)
- Liver function tests
- Kidney function tests
- CSF (cerebrospinal fluid) examination (may show evidence of blood)

Hemorrhagic stroke may be confirmed, and the location and amount of bleeding and brain tissue damage determined, by:

- Head CT scan
- Head MRI

## Treatment

Treatment includes lifesaving measures, relief of symptoms, repair of the cause of the bleeding, prevention of complications, and maximizing the ability of the person to function.

There is no known cure for stroke. Treatment is essentially based on controlling the symptoms. Recovery may occur as other areas of the brain take over functioning for the damaged areas.

## Immediate Treatment

Treatment for coma or decreased mental status may be required, including positioning, airway protection (to prevent aspiration pneumonia), and life support as needed. Strict bed rest may be advised to avoid increasing the pressure in the head (intracranial pressure). This may include avoiding activities such as bending over, straining, lying flat, sudden position changes, or similar activities. Stool softeners or laxatives may prevent straining during bowel excretion (straining also causes increased intracranial pressure).

Analgesics and antianxiety medications may relieve headache and reduce intracranial pressure. Antihypertensive medications may be prescribed to moderately reduce high blood pressure. Phenytoin or other medications may be needed to prevent or treat seizures.

Nutrients and fluids may need to be supplemented if swallowing difficulties are present. This can be intravenous or through a tube in the stomach (feeding tube or gastrostomy tube). Swallowing difficulties may be temporary or permanent.

Positioning, range-of-motion exercises, speech therapy, occupational therapy, physical therapy, and other interventions may be advised to prevent complications and promote maximum recovery of function.

## Long-Term Treatment

Recovery time and the need for long-term treatment are highly variable in each case. Physical therapy may benefit some persons. Activity should be encouraged within the physical limitations. Alternative forms of communication, such as pictures, verbal cues, demonstration, or others, may be needed depending on the type and extent of language deficit. Speech therapy, occupational therapy, or other interventions may increase the ability of some persons to function. Alternative forms of communication, such as pictures, verbal cues, and demonstration, may be needed depending on the type and extent of language deficit.

Urinary catheterization or bladder (or bowel) control programs may be required to control incontinence.

A safe environment must be considered. Some people with stroke appear to have no awareness of their surroundings on the affected side. Others show a marked indifference or lack of judgment, which increases the need for safety precautions.

In-home care, boarding homes, adult day care, or convalescent homes may be required to provide a safe environment, control aggressive or agitated behavior, and meet physiologic needs.

Behavior modification may be helpful for some persons in controlling unacceptable or dangerous behaviors. This consists of rewarding appropriate or positive behaviors and ignoring inappropriate behaviors (within the bounds of safety). Reality orientation, with repeated reinforcement of environmental and other cues, may help reduce disorientation.

Family counseling may help in coping with the changes required for home care. Visiting nurses or aides, volunteer services, homemakers, adult protective services, and other community resources may be helpful.

Legal advice may be appropriate early in the course of the disorder. Advance directives, power of attorney, and other legal actions may make it easier to make ethical decisions regarding the care of the person with hemorrhagic stroke.

## Prognosis

Stroke is the third leading cause of death in developed countries. About one-fourth of the sufferers die as a result of the stroke or its complications, about one-half have long-term disabilities, and about one-forth recover most or all function. Hemorrhagic stroke is the most frequently fatal form of stroke.

## Complications

* Pressure sores
* Permanent loss of movement or sensation of a part of the body
* Bone fractures
* Joint contractures
* Muscle spasticity
* Permanent loss of cognitive or other brain functions
* Disruption of communication, decreased social interaction
* Decreased ability to function or care for self
* Decreased life span
* Multi-infarct dementia

## Call Your Health Care Provider If

Go to the emergency room or call the local emergency number (such as 911) if symptoms of hemorrhagic stroke are present. Emergency symptoms include seizures or breathing difficulties, loss of consciousness, difficulties with movement/sensation, eating or swallowing difficulties, sudden vision change or loss of vision in one or both eyes, rapid onset of speech changes, and sudden (severe) headache.

Call your health care provider if the condition of a family member with stroke deteriorates to the point that the person cannot be cared for at home.

# Section 4.3

# *Transient Ischemic Attack (TIA)*

This section includes, "Transient Ischemic Attack (TIA)," © 2002, A.D.A.M., Inc. Reprinted with permission. Also, "Researchers Question Conventional Wisdom on 'Mini-Strokes'," Reprinted with permission from the American Heart Association World Wide Web Site, www.americanheart.org. © 2002, Copyright American Heart Association; and "Clinical Decision-Making: Outpatient Management of New TIA or Minor Stroke Could Be Improved," Agency for Healthcare Research and Quality (AHRQ), 2000.

## *Transient Ischemic Attack (TIA)*

Alternative names: Mini stroke; TIA; Little stroke

### *Definition*

A brain disorder caused by temporary disturbance of blood supply to an area of the brain, resulting in a sudden, brief (less than 24 hours, usually less than 1 hour) decrease in brain functions.

### *Causes and Risks*

The brain requires about 20% of the circulation of blood in the body. A primary blood supply to the brain is through two arteries in the neck (the carotid arteries) that branch off within the brain to multiple arteries that supply specific areas of the brain.

The vertebral arteries supply the posterior part of the brain and brainstem. Even a brief interruption to the blood flow can cause a decrease in brain function (neurologic deficit). Symptoms vary with the area of the brain affected and commonly include such problems as changes in vision, speech or comprehension changes, vertigo, decreased movement or sensation in a part of the body, and changes in the level of consciousness. If the blood flow is decreased for longer than a few seconds, brain cells in the area die (infarct), causing permanent damage to that area of the brain or even death. The major causes of loss of blood circulation to areas of the brain are reduced blood flow (ischemia) and bleeding (hemorrhage).

Transient ischemic attack (TIA, "little stroke") is a warning that the body's safety mechanisms are overloaded and indicates that a stroke may be pending.

About one-third of the people with TIA will later have a stroke. However, about 80 to 90% of people who have a stroke secondary to atherosclerosis had TIA episodes before their stroke. Approximately one-third of the people with TIA will have recurrent TIAs, and one-third will have only a single episode of TIA. The age of onset varies, but incidence rises dramatically after age 50. TIA is more common among men and African-Americans.

A TIA is caused by a temporary state of reduced blood flow (ischemia) in a portion of the brain. This is most frequently caused by tiny blood clots (microemboli) that temporarily occlude a portion of the brain. The microemboli are caused by atherosclerotic plaque in the arteries that supply the brain. Atherosclerosis ("hardening of the arteries") is a condition where fatty deposits occur on the inner lining of the arteries. Atherosclerotic plaque is formed when damage occurs to the lining of an artery. Platelets clump around the area of injury as a normal part of the clotting and healing process. Cholesterol and other fats also collect at this site, forming a mass within the lining of the artery. Clots (thrombus) may form at the site of the plaque, triggered by irregular blood flow in this location, and the thrombus may occlude the blood vessels in the brain. Pieces of plaque or clots may break off and travel through the bloodstream from distant locations, forming an embolus that can occlude the small arteries, causing TIAs. Occlusions that last for more than a few minutes more commonly cause stroke.

Less common causes of TIA include blood disorders (including polycythemia, sickle cell anemia, and hyperviscosity syndromes where the blood is very thick), spasm of the small arteries in the brain, abnormalities of blood vessels caused by disorders such as fibromuscular dysplasia, inflammation of the arteries (arteritis, polyarteritis, granulomatous angiitis), systemic lupus erythematosus, and syphilis. Hypotension (low blood pressure) may precipitate symptoms in an individual with a pre-existing vascular lesion.

Risks for TIA include high blood pressure (hypertension), heart disease, migraine headaches, smoking, diabetes mellitus, and increasing age.

### Prevention

Prevention of TIA includes control of risk factors. Hypertension, diabetes, heart disease, and other associated disorders should be treated as appropriate. Smoking should be stopped or minimized.

## *Symptoms*

- numbness, tingling, changes in sensation
- weakness, heavy feeling of extremities
- speech difficulty
  - garbled speech
  - slurred speech
  - thick speech
- vision changes
  - loss of vision in one eye
  - decreased vision
  - double vision
- sensation that the person or the room is moving (vertigo)
- loss of balance
- lack of coordination
- gait changes, staggering
- falling (caused by weakness in the legs)

Symptoms that may be confused with TIA but are not usually part of the disorder may include:

- simple changes in consciousness (may be caused by medications or other disorders)
- fainting
- lightheadedness or dizziness by itself
- vertigo by itself
- seizures
- nausea and vomiting (without other symptoms)
- transient amnesia

Additional symptoms that may be associated with this disease:

- facial paralysis
- eye pain
- confusion

Note: Symptoms begin suddenly, last only a short time (from a few minutes to 24 hours) and disappear completely. Symptoms may occur again at a later time. Specific symptoms vary depending on the location (which vessel is involved), the degree of vessel involvement, and the extent of collateral circulation. Symptoms usually occur on the same side of the body if more than one body part is involved.

### Signs and Tests

A detailed and complete history is vital to the diagnosis, because the specific deficits demonstrated correspond well with the specific lesion or affected area of the brain. For example, involvement of one arm or leg may indicate damage to one brain artery, while loss of vision or difficulty talking may suggest a different location.

Physical examination may include neurologic examination, which may be abnormal during an episode but normal after the episode has passed. It may also be used to rule out a stroke in evolution rather than TIA. The eyes may be examined, including a check of the pressures within the eye. Blood pressure may be high. Auscultation with a stethoscope over the carotid or other artery may show a bruit, an abnormal sound caused by irregular blood flow, which may indicate atherosclerotic plaque or a thrombus in the area.

Tests for TIA may include tests to determine the cause, extent of blood vessel involvement, and to rule out stroke or other disorder that may cause the symptoms.

- CBC (complete blood count) and PT (prothrombin time) tests are used to rule out hematologic disease.

- Head CT scan or cranial MRI are used to rule out focal lesions as the cause of symptoms.

- A carotid duplex (ultrasound) may be performed if there is suspected carotid stenosis.

- An echocardiogram may be performed to look for a source of embolism.

- A cerebral arteriogram may be performed if there is suspected localized vascular (blood vessel) disease, such as carotid artery stenosis ("hardening") or vasculitis (inflammation of the blood vessels in the brain).

Other tests and procedures may be performed to determine underlying disorders and to rule out other disorders that may cause the symptoms. This may include examination for hypertension, heart disease, diabetes, high blood lipids, and peripheral vascular disease. These tests and procedures may include:

- blood glucose
- blood chemistry
- serum lipids
- tests for syphilis
- ECG
- chest x-ray
- echocardiography (if heart disorder is suspected)

### Treatment

The goal of treatment is to improve the arterial blood supply to the brain and prevent development of stroke.

Treatment of recent TIA (within the prior 48 hours) usually requires admission to the hospital for evaluation of the specific cause and determination of long-term treatment. Underlying disorders should be treated appropriately, including such disorders as hypertension, heart disease, diabetes, arteritis, blood disorders, etc.

Smoking should be stopped.

Treatment of symptoms of blood disorders (such as erythrocytosis, thrombocytosis, or polycythemia vera, which include increase in the number of some of the cellular components of blood) may include phlebotomy, hydration, and treatment of the underlying (causative) blood disorder. Antihypertensive medications may be used to control high blood pressure. Medications to lower cholesterol may be useful in reducing high blood cholesterol levels.

Platelet inhibitors and anticoagulant medications ("blood thinners") may be used to reduce clotting. Aspirin is the most commonly used medication; others include dipyridamole, clopidogrel, Aggrenox or heparin, coumadin, or other similar medications. Treatment may be continued for an indefinite time period.

A reduced amount of sodium (salt) in diet to help control high blood pressure; diet for diabetics; reduced dietary fat, or other dietary changes may be recommended.

Surgery (carotid endarterectomy, removal of atherosclerotic plaque from the carotid arteries in the neck) may be appropriate for some people, particularly those with carotid artery stenosis of greater than 70% of the artery and without coexisting terminal disease or dementia.

## *Prognosis*

Each episode of TIA is brief and recovery is complete. It may recur later that same day or at a later time. Some people have only a single episode, some have recurrent episodes, and some will have a stroke.

## *Complications*

- stroke
- TIA recurrence
- injury that occurs from falls
- bleeding as a result of anti-coagulant medications

## *Call Your Health Care Provider If*

Call your health care provider if symptoms indicate TIA. Do not ignore symptoms just because they resolve! They may be a warning of an impending stroke.

Go to the emergency room or call the local emergency number (such as 911) if symptoms worsen or new symptoms develop. Emergency symptoms include loss of consciousness, sudden development of partial or complete paralysis or numbness, sudden vision change or loss of vision in one or both eyes, and rapid onset of speech changes.

## *Researchers Question Conventional Wisdom on "Mini-Strokes"*

People who experience transient ischemic attacks (TIAs) have different risk profiles from those who suffer mild strokes, which may indicate a different underlying cause and treatment, researchers reported February 8, 2002 at the American Stroke Association's 27th International Stroke Conference. The American Stroke Association is a division of the American Heart Association.

The assumption that TIAs are simply mild ischemic strokes is widespread and thus, they are often referred to as mini-strokes. TIAs are thought to occur when a blood clot temporarily clogs an artery, blocking blood flow to the brain. The symptoms are the same as for stroke but are temporary. Most of them last less than five minutes. Unlike stroke, TIA doesn't permanently injure the brain.

Although most strokes are not preceded by TIAs, more than one-third of people who have had one or more TIAs will later have a stroke, according to American Stroke Association statistics.

A team of Danish researchers noticed that some patients seemed to experience a cluster of TIAs with the same symptoms—indicating that the same part of the brain is affected. In addition, the deficits in speech and motor ability that were observed sometimes reflected that large areas of the brain were involved. However, because they were TIAs, the events left no permanent disability. So, they began looking for possible differences in the causes of TIAs and stroke.

"It was hard for us to believe that those events were caused by blood clots forming and dissolving in the same part of the brain again and again," explains lead researcher Tom S. Olsen, M.D., Ph.D., chairman of the department of neurology, Gentofte University Hospital in Hellerup, Denmark.

They used data from the community-based prospective Copenhagen Stroke Study to compare the risk factor profiles and short- and long-term outcomes of 154 individuals who had TIAs with 482 who had experienced mild strokes.

"If TIAs are *just* small strokes, one might expect similarities in the risk-factor profile and the outcome of patients with TIAs and mild stroke," he notes.

Instead, they found differences. TIA patients were half as likely to have diabetes (9 percent vs. 18 percent) and half as likely to have claudication—narrowing of the leg arteries, which indicates atherosclerosis throughout the body (7 percent vs. 15 percent).

"A different risk-factor profile may indicate that some TIAs have a different cause than strokes," he says. "It is clear that many transient ischemic attacks are due to blood clots. But it could be that some of them are due to spasm of brain arteries instead of a clot."

If some TIAs are not caused by blood clots, then aspirin therapy, which makes the blood less likely to clot, cannot be expected to prevent them, he notes.

"In addition, our results may mean that patients with TIAs should not be included in randomized trials of drugs to prevent stroke," Olsen says. "This is important because it raises the question: Does spontaneous vasospasm (the sudden constriction of a blood vessel that reduces blood flow) play a role in TIAs and maybe even stroke?"

Even though risk factors are different, both events can be deadly. Short-term mortality rates indicated that 1.3 percent of TIA patients died, as did 2.3 percent of the minor stroke patients. After five years the survival rates were virtually the same for both conditions—57.9 percent of TIA patients and 56.8 percent of those who had a minor stroke were alive five years later. Symptoms of stroke are:

- Sudden numbness or weakness of the face, arm or leg, especially on one side of the body.

- Sudden confusion, trouble speaking or understanding.

- Sudden trouble seeing in one or both eyes.

- Sudden trouble walking, dizziness, loss of balance or coordination.

- Sudden, severe headache with no known cause.

The symptoms are the same for TIA, but are temporary.

## Outpatient Management of New TIA or Minor Stroke Could Be Improved

About 750,000 Americans have strokes each year, and many die or are disabled as a result. Patients who have suffered a recent transient ischemic attack (TIA or mini stroke) are at highest risk of stroke soon after the TIA. Thus, even in those not admitted to a hospital, a rapid and complete diagnostic evaluation is warranted.

Yet in a recent study, one-third (32 percent) of patients with a first TIA or stroke initially evaluated in the office by their primary care physician (PCP) were not hospitalized and had no further diagnostic evaluations over the next 30 days. The study was carried out by the Stroke Prevention Patient Outcomes Research Team (PORT) and supported by the Agency for Healthcare Research and Quality (PORT contract 290-91-0028). In fact, diagnostic studies necessary for rational therapeutic decisions, for example, brain imaging and vascular imaging, frequently were not performed.

Some PCPs also appeared to underuse anticoagulants to prevent stroke in patients who had atrial fibrillation and additional cardioembolic risk factors, notes PORT principal investigator David B. Matchar, M.D., of Duke University. The researchers retrospectively audited medical records from 27 primary care practices of 95 patients with a first-ever TIA and 81 patients with a first stroke.

Only 6 percent of these patients were admitted to a hospital for further diagnostic testing and management on the day of their initial office evaluation (2 percent of TIA patients and 10 percent of stroke patients). An additional 3 percent of patients were admitted to a hospital during the subsequent 30 days. PCPs ordered a brain computerized tomography scan or magnetic resonance imaging on the day of the initial visit in only 30 percent of patients (23 percent TIA, 37 percent stroke), regardless of whether the patient was referred to a specialist. They obtained carotid ultrasound studies in 28 percent, electrocardiograms in 19 percent, and echocardiograms in 16 percent of patients. Fewer than half of patients with a prior history of atrial fibrillation were anticoagulated. Larry B. Goldstein, M.D., the study's lead author, cautions that the patients in this study represent a biased sample of stroke patients, many of whom were evaluated primarily in hospital settings, and the data used for the study were limited to those documented in the patients' records.

## Reference

"New transient ischemic attack and stroke: Outpatient management by primary care physicians," by Dr. Goldstein, John Bian, M.S., Gregory P. Samsa, Ph.D., and others, in the October 23, 2000 *Archives of Internal Medicine* 160, pp. 2941-2946.

## Section 4.4.

# *Stroke Secondary to Carotid Dissection*

"Stroke Secondary to Carotid Dissection," © 2002, A.D.A.M., Inc.
Reprinted with permission.

## Definition

Loss of brain function due to stroke caused by bleeding within the lining of the carotid artery of the neck.

## Causes and Risks

Stroke secondary to carotid dissection, unlike many other forms of stroke, may occur in young people, usually under 40 years old.

Stroke involves loss of brain functions (neurologic deficits) caused by a loss of blood circulation to areas of the brain. The specific neurologic deficits may vary depending on the location, extent of the damage, and cause of the disorder. Stroke is caused by reduced blood flow (ischemia) that results in deficient blood supply and death of tissues in that area (infarction).

The carotid arteries are two arteries in the neck that supply blood to the anterior part of the brain. "Carotid dissection" means that there is an injury to the artery or a weakened area in the lining of the artery. Blood leaks into the lining of the artery, possibly causing a clot in the wall of the artery and therefore reducing blood flow to the brain.

Risks for stroke secondary to carotid dissection include a history of Marfan's syndrome, fibromuscular dysplasia, or other disorders that may involve weakness of the blood vessels. Risks also include a history of injury or trauma involving the neck. Rarely, cases of carotid dissection have occurred as a result of massage of the neck.

## Prevention

Stroke secondary to carotid dissection may not be preventable in some instances. Care should be taken to protect the neck from injury, especially if diseases associated with increased risk of this disorder are present.

## Symptoms

- facial pain occurring prior to other neurologic deficits
- neck pain occurring prior to other neurologic deficits
- pulsating noises may be present in the ear (pulsatile tinnitus)
- weakness or total inability to move a body part
- numbness, loss of sensation
- tingling or other abnormal sensations
- decreased or lost vision, partial or temporary
- language difficulties (aphasia)
- inability to recognize or identify sensory stimuli (agnosia)
- loss of memory
- vertigo (abnormal sensation of movement)
- loss of coordination
- swallowing difficulties
- personality changes
- mood and emotion changes

- urinary incontinence (lack of control over bladder)
- lack of control over the bowels
- eyelid drooping
- consciousness changes
  - sleepy
  - stuporous, somnolent, lethargic
  - comatose, unconscious

## Signs and Tests

Maximum neurologic deficits may be present at the beginning (onset) of the stroke, or symptoms may progress or fluctuate for the first day or two (stroke in evolution). Once there is no further deterioration, the stroke is considered a complete stroke.

An examination may include neurologic, motor, and sensory testing to determine the specific deficits present. The examination may show changes in vision or visual fields, changes in reflexes including abnormal reflexes or abnormal extent of "normal" reflexes, abnormal eye movements, muscle weakness, decreased sensation, and other changes. A bruit, an abnormal sound heard with the stethoscope, may be heard over the carotid arteries of the neck. The blood pressure may be high. Horner's syndrome may occur, which involves a small pupil, drooping of one eyelid, lack of sweating on one side of the forehead, and a sunken appearance to one eye.

## Tests

- a cerebral angiography reveals changes indicating carotid dissection
- a duplex/Doppler ultrasound can also detect dissection
- MRI or CT of the head to determine extent and location of stroke

## Treatment

See "Treatment" in Section 4.2.

**Additional treatment:** Antihypertensive medication may be needed to control high blood pressure. Anti-coagulation with coumadin or aspirin may be indicated for a period of 3-6 months. Surgical repair of the carotid dissection may be indicated.

## Prognosis

The outcome for stroke secondary to carotid dissection may be better than for stroke from many other causes, especially if the dissection is discovered and treated promptly.

## Complications

See "Complications" in Section 4.2.

## Call Your Health Care Provider If

Go to the emergency room or call the local emergency number (such as 911) if symptoms occur.

Note: Stroke requires immediate treatment.

# Chapter 5

# *Stroke in Children*

## *Understanding Stroke in Children*

Chickenpox, croup, ear infections—these are the things we associate with sick children. Not stroke. Yet a small percentage of children do have strokes, and the causes are dramatically different from those in adults. Strokes in adults often can be blamed on a history of smoking, atherosclerosis (plaque buildup in the arteries), high blood pressure, or high cholesterol. Children's strokes more often are related to birth defects, infections, trauma, and blood disorders such as sickle cell disease.

The incidence of stroke in children is relatively low, about three cases in every 100,000 children per year, compared to 100 cases in adults per 100,000, according to figures from the United Cerebral Palsy Research Foundation. Children under age two suffer strokes more frequently than older children. While the numbers are small, childhood stroke may be rising, according to Dr. Lidia Gabis, a child neurologist and developmental disabilities fellow with the State

This chapter includes, "Understanding Stroke in Children," by Verna Noel Jones, *Stroke Smart Magazine*, September/October 2001 © National Stroke Association, reprinted with permission; and "Childhood Stroke Deaths Drop, but Still Higher among Blacks," reprinted with permission from the American Heart Association World Wide Web Site, www.americanheart.org. © 2002, Copyright American Heart Association. Also, "Recognition and Treatment of Stroke in Children," National Institute of Neurological Disorders and Stroke (NINDS), reviewed July 1, 2001.

University of New York (SUNY) at Stony Brook. This is particularly true for children with developmental heart defects.

"In the past, babies would die from heart anomalies to the valves or blood vessels," she says. "Now, some of the heart anomalies are surgically repaired, but the babies have a lifelong increased risk of stroke. Children with leukemia also are treated with good results, but these children have a higher risk of stroke due to the disorder itself and the treatment—chemotherapy or radiation to the brain."

### Signs of Stroke in Children

It is important to quickly recognize signs of stroke in children so that effective treatments can be given.

- Headaches
- Speech difficulties
- Eye movement problems
- Numbness

Some strokes occur in utero or just after birth. Dr. John Kylan Lynch and Karin Nelson, of the National Institutes of Health, recently reviewed discharge data from hospitals across the United States and found about 19,000 cases of neonatal stroke in the last 20 years. The strokes in the newborns were most often linked with blood disorders, heart disorders, and infections.

Blood disorders, such as sickle cell disease or blood clotting defects, are the next most common cause of childhood strokes. Dr. Cynthia Curry and colleagues from the University of California, San Francisco, recently tested 27 pairs of mothers and children with a history of neonatal stroke and found that 53% had one or more abnormal blood clotting factors. The study suggested that blood-clotting abnormalities in mothers or children may lead to neonatal strokes.

Some childhood strokes are connected to cerebral palsy, a movement disorder, says Dr. Murray Goldstein, DO, a neurology specialist and medical director of the United Cerebral Palsy Research and Educational Foundation. Nearly three infants for every 1,000 live births have cerebral palsy.

"More than 50% of cerebral palsy is caused by stroke," says Goldstein, a National Stroke Association board member. "About 20% of cases are caused by a hemorrhage or lack of oxygen to the brain after a difficult labor."

Older children have a risk of stroke due to head injuries, says Goldstein. "A child's head is larger in proportion to his body, so he's top-heavy. If he falls off his tricycle, the first thing he hits is his head."

Infections such as encephalitis and meningitis are another source of childhood strokes. And a recent study by Rand Askalan, PhD and colleagues at the University of Toronto, Canada, found a higher incidence of stroke in children who previously had measles.

It is important to recognize signs of stroke in children quickly so that effective treatments can be given. Gabis and her colleagues at SUNY recently looked into delays in diagnosis of childhood stroke and reported the results at a meeting of the American Academy of Neurology. "We looked at how long it takes from a child's initial complaint until they get a stroke diagnosis," she says. "It took as long as one or two days."

The first complaint made by one-third of the children whose records were analyzed was a headache. Then, other signs of stroke were recognized, such as speech difficulties, eye movement problems, and numbness.

One of Gabis' patients, a 14-year-old boy, experienced a pressing headache while taking a test in school. He also had blurred and double vision. He went to a school nurse who called his mom. The mother thought he was stressed and dehydrated. The boy went to sleep and the next morning reported double vision, so his mother took him to a primary care physician who sent him to the emergency room. A CT and MRI pinpointed a small stroke in the midbrain, though no cause could be found. He was given aspirin and recovered completely.

Surprisingly, the cause of stroke is unknown in about one-third of childhood strokes. The good news is that, while strokes in children can be devastating, children have a better ability to heal. "This is called plasticity," says Gabis. "The brain's healing possibilities are higher when the child is younger. While 75% of children who have stroke will have some problems, such as cognitive difficulties or cerebral palsy, another 25% will have no deficit."

"The outcome of babies who have a stroke in utero is better. Sometimes an image study is done for a child with headaches and it is found that he's had a stroke in utero, yet he was unaffected. He's a completely healthy child."

### Ask The Expert: Dr. Lidia Gabis, Pediatric Neurologist, State University of New York

**Q:** My one-year-old daughter was diagnosed with a blood clotting disorder. It was determined that she had a stroke at birth. I am still investigating the cause of her first stroke. Is there something I can do to prevent her from having a second stroke?

**A:** Blood clotting disorders are one of the causes of stroke in children. The treatments available for children are similar to those used for secondary stroke prevention in adults: anti-platelet agents.

The most common anti-platelet agent is aspirin. It is efficient with many blood-clotting disorders. The main problem in children is the rare risk of Reye's Syndrome (a severe liver dysfunction) with aspirin. That's why aspirin should not be used for fever or pain in children. Anti-coagulant agents, such as warfarin, also may be used in children in some cases. Because of the low incidence of stroke in children, there isn't enough information to answer all the questions about stroke prevention in children. More research is needed in this area. Parents should discuss treatment options with their children's health care providers. With any treatment, the overall stroke prevention benefits must be weighed against the risks and side effects.

## Childhood Stroke Deaths Drop, but Still Higher among Blacks

Stroke deaths for children have declined sharply, but black children have higher stroke death rates than other youngsters, according to research presented February 8, 2002 at the American Stroke Association's 27th annual meeting. The American Stroke Association is a division of the American Heart Association.

Recent declines in adult stroke deaths have been attributed to more people controlling well-known risk factors such as hypertension and cigarette smoking. But these factors are irrelevant in children.

"Childhood stroke deaths are poorly understood," says Heather Fullerton, M.D., the study's lead author. "You can't turn to the risk factors important for strokes in adults, such as hypertension, a poor diet, or diabetes, and apply them to kids."

Although childhood strokes are far less common than adult strokes, they, too, can kill or leave survivors disabled. Only a few small studies have examined childhood stroke deaths, according to Fullerton, a child neurology fellow at the University of California San Francisco. Known risk factors for childhood hemorrhagic strokes (caused by bleeding) include brain tumors or vascular malformations, hemophilia, cancer, and sickle cell disease. Childhood ischemic strokes (caused by blockages) have also been linked to sickle cell disease and cancer. Risk factors that contribute to ischemic strokes alone include meningitis, encephalitis, congenital heart disease, and certain blood clotting disorders.

In this study, researchers analyzed data from the National Center for Health Statistics mortality database, which compiles death certificate data across the country. They examined childhood stroke deaths in people age 20 and under who died from a stroke, as specified on death certificates, between 1979-98. They found an average of 244 deaths per year due to childhood stroke in the United States. Overall, the study found stroke deaths declined by 58 percent in the 20-year period. However, the reduction in deaths varied by type of stroke. Hemorrhagic strokes showed the steepest fall: childhood stroke deaths from subarachnoid hemorrhagic strokes (bleeding into the space between the brain and the skull) dropped by 79 percent, while strokes from intracerebral hemorrhages (bursting of a defective brain vessel) declined by 54 percent.

The declines were not as marked for deaths from ischemic stroke, which results from a blood clot that blocks blood flow to the brain. Ischemic stroke deaths declined 19 percent in the same time period.

These declines were tempered by the finding that black children and boys had higher risks for dying of strokes, says Fullerton. Black children were more than twice as likely to die from strokes caused by intracerebral hemorrhage, and approximately 75 percent more likely to die from both ischemic strokes and subarachnoid hemorrhage. Black adults are also at greater risk from stroke than other adults.

No factors, such as sickle cell disease—which is more prevalent in blacks than whites—fully accounted for excess stroke deaths, Fullerton notes. Boys were 30 percent more likely to die from subarachnoid hemorrhage and 21 percent more likely to die from intracerebral hemorrhage than girls. Stroke is also more common in adult men than women.

"With further research, we may be able to uncover other risk factors that we are not recognizing and find effective ways of preventing strokes in these kids," Fullerton says.

She suspects an unknown genetic predisposition may play a role in these deaths. As for the higher stroke rates in boys, Fullerton suspects that hormonal differences may be a factor.

The study found no stroke belt for children like there is in adults, where deaths are disproportionally higher in the southeastern United States.

Next, the research team plans to examine a California-wide database, exploring the impact of socioeconomic status, insurance coverage or lack thereof, and geographic factors, such as urban and rural residence on childhood stroke deaths.

## *Recognition and Treatment of Stroke in Children*

Despite growing appreciation by neurologists that cerebrovascular disorders occur more often in children than once suspected, the study of stroke in children and adolescents has remained largely descriptive. Child neurologists often encounter children with a cerebrovascular lesion, yet large-scale clinical research is difficult because these disorders are less common than in adults and arise from diverse causes. Three fundamental problems hinder both clinical research and the routine clinical care of children with cerebrovascular disease:

1. The infrequency of cerebrovascular disorders in children makes it difficult to organize multi-center controlled clinical trials of the sort done in adults in recent years. The relative rarity of stroke in children also contributes to the still remaining reluctance of some clinicians to consider the diagnosis in individual children.

2. The causes of cerebrovascular disease in children are legion, and no one risk factor predominates. Thus, not only is stroke less common in children, but the diversity of risk factors creates a heterogeneous patient population which hinders clinical research.

3. Despite improved diagnostic techniques which make rapid, noninvasive diagnosis of cerebrovascular disease possible, many physicians still know very little about cerebrovascular disorders in children. This lack of awareness contributes to delayed diagnosis and in the near future will make it more difficult to use thrombolytic agents or other treatments which require early diagnosis and treatment.

### *Frequency of Pediatric Cerebrovascular Disease*

Although cerebrovascular disorders occur less often in children than in adults, recognition of stroke in children has probably increased because of the widespread application of noninvasive diagnostic studies such as magnetic resonance imaging (MRI), magnetic resonance angiography (MRA), computed tomography (CT), and, in the neonate, cranial ultrasound studies.[1-3] These studies allow confirmation of a diagnosis that in previous years would not have been suspected or at least not recognized as a vascular lesion. Also, the number of patients with cerebrovascular lesions from certain risk factors may have increased as more effective treatments for some causes of stroke have allowed patients to survive long enough to develop vascular complications. Patients with sickle cell disease or with leukemia, for example, now have a longer life expectancy, and during this time they may have a stroke.

Most of the pediatric cerebrovascular literature consists of single case reports or small groups of children with a common etiology. These reports offer some insight into the relative frequency of various causes of stroke and draw attention to individual risk factors, but their usefulness is otherwise limited. Larger series of children selected for a common anatomic lesion or a single cause offer additional insight into the unique features of cerebrovascular lesions in children,[4] but patients collected from large medical centers may not be representative of all children with stroke. None of these studies can accurately judge the incidence of cerebrovascular disease in children.

Schoenberg and colleagues studied cerebrovascular disease in children of Rochester, Minnesota from 1965 through 1974.[5] Excluding strokes related to intracranial infection, trauma, or birth, they found three hemorrhagic strokes and one ischemic stroke in an average at-risk population of 15,834, for an estimated average annual incidence rate of 1.89/100,000/year and 0.63/100,000/year for hemorrhagic and ischemic strokes respectively. Their overall average annual incidence rate for children through fourteen years of age was 2.52/100,000/year. In this population, hemorrhagic strokes occurred more often than ischemic strokes, while in the Mayo Clinic referral population, ischemic strokes were more common. The risk of childhood cerebrovascular disease in this study is about half the risk for neoplasms of the central nervous system of children, but neonates and children with traumatic lesions are excluded. Despite our impression that cerebrovascular disorders are recognized more often in children than in previous years, Broderick and colleagues[6] found an incidence of 2.7 cases/100,000/year, similar to the figure reported by Schoenberg and colleagues.[5] In the Canadian Pediatric Ischemic Stroke Registry incidence of arterial and venous occlusion is estimated to be 1.2/100,000 children/year.

The frequency of several individual risk factors for stroke in children is known, but in most instances, the occurrence of secondary cerebrovascular disease is so variable that it is difficult to assess the relative contribution of each risk factor to the problem of cerebrovascular disease as a whole. In one report which included both children and young adults, children were less likely than young adult stroke patients to have identifiable risk factors and more often fall victim to infectious or inflammatory disorders.[7] The implication is that children may have additional, as yet unknown, risk factors.

## Etiology of Stroke in Children

Probably the most fundamental difference between cerebrovascular diseases in children and adults is the wide array of risk factors seen in children versus adults (see section "Risk Factors for Pediatric Cerebrovascular Disease," in this chapter).[8] Congenital heart disease and sickle cell disease, for example, are common causes of stroke in children, while atherosclerosis is rare in children. No cause can be detected in about a fifth of the children with ischemic infarction, yet many of these children seem to do well. The recognized causes of cerebrovascular disorders in children are numerous, and the probability of identifying the cause depends on the thoroughness of the evaluation. A probable cause of cerebral infarction was identified in 184 of 228 (79%) children in the Canadian Pediatric Ischemic Stroke Registry. The source of an intracranial hemorrhage is even more likely to be found.[8]

The most common cause of stroke in children is probably congenital or acquired heart disease. In the Canadian Pediatric Ischemic Stroke Registry, heart disease was found in 40 of 228 (19%) of the children with arterial thrombosis. Many of these children are already known to have heart disease prior to their stroke, but in other instances a less obvious cardiac lesion is discovered only after a stroke. Complex cardiac anomalies involving both the valves and chambers are collectively the biggest problem, but virtually any cardiac lesion can sometimes lead to a stroke. Of particular concern are cyanotic lesions with polycythemia, which increase the risk of both thrombosis and embolism.

Both the frequency and the cause of pediatric stroke may depend somewhat on both the geographic location and the specific hospital setting. The Canadian Pediatric Ischemic Stroke Registry, for example, lists only 5 children (2%) with cerebral infarction due to sickle cell anemia. A large metropolitan hospital in the United States might care for this many patients in a year, but early estimates[9] that cerebral infarction occurred in 17% of people with sickle cell disease proved far higher than the 4-5% figure derived from more representative samples in Jamaica and in Africa.[10, 11]

## Prehospital Emergency Care

Lack of general awareness of cerebrovascular disorders in children probably delays medical attention for children with cerebrovascular disorders. It is not unusual, for example, for children with a cerebral infarction to be brought to a physician several days after the onset of symptoms. In contrast, family members are usually well aware of the significance of an acute neurological impairment in older individuals, and these patients are typically seen by a physician earlier than children with a similar lesion.

Data from the Canadian Pediatric Ischemic Stroke Registry indicate that 48-72 hours often elapse between the onset of symptoms of arterial occlusion and a child's diagnosis.[12] Venous occlusion was discovered a bit more quickly than arterial occlusion, at least in younger children, perhaps because of the common occurrence of epileptic seizures in children with venous thrombosis. This seems to be fairly typical of the pattern seen in the United States as well. The typical adult with a new onset neurological deficit from cerebrovascular disease undoubtedly sees a physician much sooner. It is likely that this delay in the diagnosis of children reflects a lack of awareness by both physicians and families that cerebrovascular disease occurs in children. To the extent that treatment might be improved by earlier evaluation and treatment, prompt recognition and treatment could improve management.

## Treatment and Rehabilitation

No randomized controlled treatment trials have been completed in children with stroke; many of the procedures increasingly used in children with cerebrovascular disease have been adapted from studies in adults. Accumulating experience with antithrombotic and anticoagulant treatment in children suggests that these agents can be safely used in children, though their efficacy and proper dose still need to be established by controlled trials. Thrombolytic agents should be as effective in children as in adults, but the safety data are inadequate for children and the timing and dosage need to be determined for children and adolescents.

*Aspirin*

1. Background: There are no controlled trials on the use of aspirin or other antiplatelet agents in children with ischemic cerebral infarction. Nevertheless, aspirin is being used more and more in the routine clinical care of children with cerebral ischemic disorders.

2. Safety: In addition to the potential complications of chronic aspirin use seen in adults, children taking daily aspirin could

have an increased risk of developing Reye's syndrome. Evidently the risk of Reye's syndrome is fairly small, due perhaps to the low aspirin dose typically used in children. Despite the increasingly common use of aspirin in children with stroke, we were unable to find in the literature even one child who developed Reye's syndrome while taking prophylactic aspirin. One 65 year-old, however, developed Reye's syndrome while taking aspirin for stroke prophylaxis, but he also took additional aspirin for influenza.[13]

3.  Efficacy: A daily aspirin dose of 2-3 mg/Kg/day causes an antiplatelet effect, though it remains to be seen whether this dose of aspirin is clinically effective in children.

*Heparin and Low Molecular Weight Heparins*

1.  Background: A decision to use heparin in a child rests on two questions: What is the likelihood of either extension of an infarction or of a second infarction from an embolus which might be prevented by treatment, and what is the risk of inducing a hemorrhage because of anticoagulation? Much like the situation in adults, heparin should be used in children thought to have a high risk of recurrence and a low risk of secondary hemorrhage.

2.  Safety: There are no large scale trials of heparin in children with ischemic stroke, but increasing clinical experience suggests that children can be treated along the same lines as adult patients with reasonable safety.[8, 14, 15] Combined experience with over 100 pediatric patients treated for systemic clots with low molecular weight heparin indicates a good safety profile and dose finding feasibility.[16] No significant hemorrhagic complications occurred in these initial 100 children.[18]

3.  Efficacy: The value of anticoagulation in children is difficult to assess without more information. Anticoagulation is commonly used in children with arterial dissection, dural sinus thrombosis, coagulation disorders, or a high risk of embolism.[8, 15] It also seems reasonable to anticoagulate a child with progressive deterioration or during the initial evaluation of a new cerebral infarction.[8] The loading dose of heparin is 75 units/Kg intravenously followed by 20 units/Kg/hour for children over

one year of age (or 28 units/Kg/hour below one year of age). The target APTT to 60-85 is seconds.[14]

Adult stroke patients who receive low molecular weight heparin for ten days starting within 48 hours of diagnosis have a better outcome,[17] and it may be possible to adapt this approach for children. Low molecular weight heparin (Lovenox, Rhone-Poulenc) can be given to children subcutaneously in two divided doses of 1 mg/Kg/dose (or in neonates, 1.5 mg/Kg every 12 hours).

*Warfarin*

1. Background: Experience in children with long-term anti-coagulation to prevent cerebral infarction is limited, and there is additional concern about anticoagulating an active child who may be prone to minor injuries through normal activities. Nevertheless, warfarin is the most effective means of prolonged anticoagulation in children.

2. Safety: Clinical experience suggests that warfarin can be used in children and adolescents with reasonable safety. The concern that active children could have an increased risk of hemorrhage due to trauma seems to be largely unfounded, though it is recommended that they avoid activities that carry an especially high risk of injury (e.g., contact sports).

3. Efficacy: The rationale for using warfarin in children with cerebrovascular disorders follows closely the approach used in adults. Thus, major uses of warfarin treatment in children include congenital or acquired heart disease, hypercoagulable states, arterial dissection, and dural sinus thrombosis. An INR of 2.0 to 3.0 is appropriate for most children on warfarin; for children with mechanical heart valves the INR should be 2.5 to 3.5.

*Thrombolytic Agents*

1. Background: There is ample reason to seek new treatments for children with ischemic cerebral infarction, because 75% of the children have serious sequelae including neurologic deficit, epilepsy, or death. While there is little information about the use of thrombolytic agents in children with stroke, enough work has been done with adult patients that the technique could possibly be adapted for selected children.

2. Safety: Urokinase and streptokinase are used infrequently in children with cerebrovascular disease, but no serious complications occurred in the few children treated for dural sinus thrombosis. Thrombolytic therapy for children with non-cerebral thrombotic complications has recently been evaluated. Pooled literature analysis of 203 children treated with thrombolytic agents (including 39 patients who received tPA) indicated that the thrombus was cleared in 80% of the children, but 54% had minor bleeding (not requiring transfusion) and one child suffered an intracranial hemorrhage. In 29 consecutive children treated with tPA (0.5 mg/Kg) at Toronto's Hospital for Sick Children, the clot was dissolved in 79%, but almost a fourth of these children had bleeding which required transfusion.[19, 20] Given this high rate of serious bleeding after systemic tPA and the lack of studies demonstrating improved outcome, we cannot recommend tPA except in the setting of a controlled clinical trial.

3. Efficacy: The delayed diagnosis which so often occurs in children with ischemic stroke reduces the likelihood that a child with an ischemic stroke will be seen early enough to benefit from thrombolytic agents. Intravascular urokinase or streptokinase have been used with apparent success in a few children with dural sinus thrombosis, [8, 21-23] but there is even less experience with these agents in children with arterial thrombosis. The available data are insufficient to comment on the effectiveness of any of the thrombolytic agents in children with ischemic stroke. Certainly they would be expected to produce unacceptable roles of bleeding as seen in adults if given more than 4-6 hours after onset of stroke.

*Transfusion*

1. Background: About half of the patients with a stroke due to sickle cell disease will have another stroke,[11] and this increased risk can be reduced by repeated transfusions to suppress the level of circulating sickle hemoglobin to 30% or less. The risk of stroke increases again if the transfusions are discontinued even after a prolonged stroke-free interval, so most patients who begin transfusions must continue them.

2. Safety: Although the risk can be reduced by iron chelation, iron toxicity from repeated blood transfusions remains a major

problem. Cohen and colleagues[24] proposed a less aggressive transfusion program to maintain the hemoglobin S near 50%; this regimen required an average of 31% less transfused blood and still no infarctions occurred. Miller and colleague had similar results, although their follow-up period was shorter. This new approach needs to be studied further.

3. Efficacy: Although no randomized clinical trials were ever done, years of clinical experience have produced general agreement that periodic transfusion greatly reduces the risk of ischemic cerebral infarction due to sickle cell disease. A patient who has had one stroke has about a 90% risk of having additional infarctions. The Stroke Prevention Trial in Sickle Cell Anemia (STOP) is now investigating the use of transcranial Doppler (TCD) to identify children at greatest risk for their first cerebral infarction due to sickle cell disease. This study could prove that periodic transfusions reduce the risk of ischemic infarction in children with sickle cell disease and that TCD can be used to identify those at greatest risk.

## *Directions for Research*

Given the paucity of information about many aspects of childhood stroke, what is the best approach to the diagnosis and management of stroke in children? How should our methods in children differ from those used in adults? Until more information on childhood stroke is available, we must of necessity continue to adapt the knowledge obtained from adult stroke patients. It should not be necessary to repeat in children all the work already done in adults, but we do need to identify areas which are age specific.

In some respects, our study of stroke in children recapitulates some of the early work in adult stroke patients. Databases such as the Canadian Pediatric Ischemic Stroke Registry will continue to provide data on the causes of childhood stroke as well as the patients' treatment and outcome. Under the best of circumstances, such databases are limited by the fact that the correct diagnosis may not be recognized or reported to the registry. Larger case series which concentrate on one cause of stroke or one anatomic lesion need to be published. Epidemiologic studies need to be reassessed to reflect better diagnostic techniques and the increased recognition of stroke in children by physicians.

Several specific causes of cerebrovascular disease are relatively common in children and have a high enough risk of stroke to make collaborative trials feasible. There are several potentially productive areas to study. Research should initially focus on the more common disorders or on children with risk factors which are usually identified before a stroke occurs:

- The Stroke Prevention Trial in Sickle Cell Anemia (STOP) trial now underway could serve as a model for studies of childhood stroke from other causes. Sickle cell disease is common in some medical centers, and cerebral infarction frequent enough to make a study feasible. Early diagnosis and treatment probably improve the patient's outlook. Additional multi-center trials for patients with sickle cell disease could also address the use of hydroxyurea or other drugs in stroke prevention.

- Sinovenous thrombosis seems to occur relatively more often in children than other cerebrovascular lesions and can now be identified quickly and noninvasively with MRI/MRA. Collaborative studies to evaluate systemic anticoagulation and/or thrombolysis should be feasible, particularly if similar trials in adults continue to show promise.

- Cardiac disease remains the most common cause of ischemic cerebral infarction in children. Most of these children have congenital heart lesions which are identified well before an infarction occurs, and ischemic infarction may occur frequently enough to warrant controlled trials of prophylactic agents or of neuroprotective agents during surgery when the risk of stroke is higher. Thrombolytic agents could play a greater role in children with heart disease because their families could be taught to recognize the significance of an acute neurologic deficit.

- Moyamoya is an uncommon condition but it could be studied via a collaborative approach. Most patients in the recent literature have had various surgical procedures designed to increase blood flow to the brain. But no controlled trials have ever been done to assess these operations, and there is some evidence that the natural history of untreated moyamoya may be less devastating than sometimes suggested. In one group of 27 children, 5 patients had no sequelae, 9 had only headache or transient ischemic symptoms, and 7 had mild intellectual or motor impairment. Only 6 of the 27 had a poor outcome: 1 death, 2 who required continuous care, and 3 who required special schooling or institutionalization. Only 11 of these 27 patients had surgery.[26]

The fact that so many patients do well without intervention makes it difficult to evaluate treatment in the absence of controlled trials.

- Several pediatric hospitals offer extracorporeal membrane oxygenation (ECMO), a technique which requires ligation of the right carotid artery. In some centers, the carotid artery is eventually reconstructed once ECMO is no longer needed.[27] These children provide an opportunity to study the long-term effects of altered cerebral circulation and, for the children whose carotid is reopened, to explore the effects of carotid artery trauma on the development of atherosclerosis.

### Summary

Increased awareness of these disorders by the public, and by medical personnel will potentially improve accessibility of pediatric stroke patients to newer forms of thrombolytic and neuroprotective agents. Increased awareness by research teams and research funding agencies will provide the means for the intervention trials critically necessary to realize that potential.

## Risk Factors for Pediatric Cerebrovascular Disease

### Congenital Heart Disease

- Ventricular septal defect
- Atrial septal defect
- Patent ductus arteriosus
- Aortic stenosis
- Mitral stenosis
- Coarctation
- Cardiac rhabdomyoma
- Complex congenital heart defects

### Acquired Heart Disease

- Rheumatic heart disease
- Prosthetic heart valve
- Libman-Sacks endocarditis
- Bacterial endocarditis

- Cardiomyopathy
- Myocarditis
- Atrial myxoma
- Arrhythmia

## Systemic Vascular Disease

- Systemic hypertension
- Volume depletion or systemic hypotension
- Hypernatremia
- Superior vena cava syndrome
- Diabetes

## Vasculitis

- Meningitis
- Systemic infection
- Systemic lupus erythematosus
- Polyarteritis nodosa
- Granulomatous angiitis
- Takayasu's arteritis
- Rheumatoid arthritis
- Dermatomyositis
- Inflammatory bowel disease
- Drug abuse (cocaine, amphetamines)
- Hemolytic-uremic syndrome

## Vasculopathies

- Ehlers-Danlos syndrome
- Homocystinuria
- Moyamoya syndrome
- Fabry's disease
- Malignant atrophic papulosis
- Pseudoxanthoma elasticurn
- NADH-CoQ reductase deficiency

### Vasospastic Disorders

- Migraine
- Ergot poisoning
- Vasospasm with subarachnoid hemorrhage

### Hematologic Disorders and Coagulopathies

- Hemoglobinopathies (sickle cell anemia, sickle cell-hemoglobin C)
- Immune thrombocytopenic purpura
- Thrombotic thrombocytopenic purpura
- Thrombocytosis
- Polycythemia
- Disseminated intravascular coagulation (DIC)
- Leukemia or other neoplasm
- Congenital coagulation defects
- Oral contraceptive use
- Pregnancy and the postpartum period
- Antithrombin IR deficiency
- Protein S deficiency
- Protein C deficiency
- Congenital serum C2 deficiency
- Liver dysfunction with coagulation defect
- Vitamin K deficiency
- Lupus anticoagulant
- Anticardiolipin antibodies

### Structural Anomalies of the Cerebrovascular System

- Arterial fibromuscular dysplasia
- Agenesis or hypoplasia of the internal carotid or vertebral arteries
- Arteriovenous malformation
- Hereditary hemorrhagic telangiectasia
- Sturge-Weber syndrome
- Intracranial aneurysm

## *Trauma*

- Child abuse
- Fat or air embolism
- Foreign body embolism
- Carotid ligation (eg, ECMO)
- Vertebral occlusion following abrupt cervical rotation
- Posttraumatic arterial dissection
- Blunt cervical arterial trauma
- Arteriography
- Posttraumatic carotid cavernous fistula
- Coagulation defect with minor trauma
- Amniotic fluid/placental embolism
- Penetrating intracranial trauma

Modified from Roach and Riela. *Pediatric Cerebrovascular Disorders,* New York. Futura Publishing Co., 1995.

## *References*

1. Wiznitzer M, Ruggieri PM, Masaryk TJ, Ross JS, Modic MT, Berman B: Diagnosis of cerebrovascular disease in sickle cell anemia by magnetic resonance angiography. *J Pediatr* 1990; 117:551-555.

2. Ball WS: Cerebrovascular occlusive disease in childhood. *Neuroimaging Clin N Amer* 1994; 4:393-421.

3. Koelfen W, Wentz U, Freund M, Schultze C: Magnetic resonance angiography in 140 neuropediatric patients. *Pediatr Neurol* 1995; 12:31-38.

4. Brower MC, Rollins N, Roach ES: Basal ganglia and thalamic infarction in children (In press). *Arch Neurol* 1996; 53.

5. Schoenberg BS, Mellinger JF, Schoenberg DG: Cerebrovascular disease in infants and children: A study of incidence, clinical features, and survival. *Neurology* 1978; 28:763-768.

6. Broderick J, Talbot T, Prenger E, Leach A, Brott T: Stroke in children within a major metropolitan area: The surprising

importance of intracerebral hemorrhage. *J Child Neurol* 1993;
8:250-255.

7.  Kerr LM, Anderson DM, Thompson JA, Lyver SM, Call GK: Ischemic stroke in the young: Evaluation and age comparison of patients six months to thirty-nine years. *J Child Neurol* 1993; 8:266-270.

8.  Roach ES, Riela AR: Pediatric Cerebrovascular Disorders. 2nd ed. New York: *Futura*, 1995, 359 pp.

9.  Portnoy BA, Herion JC: Neurological manifestations in sickle-cell disease—with a review of the literature and emphasis on the prevalence of hemiplegia. *Ann Intern Med* 1972; 76:643-652.

10. Adeloye A, Odeku EL: The nervous system in sickle cell disease. *Afr J Med* 1970; 1:33-48.

11. Balkaran B, Char G, Morris JS, Thomas PW, Serjeant BE, Serjeant GR: Stroke in a cohort of patients with homozygous sickle cell disease. *J Pediatr* 1992; 120:360-366.

12. deVeber GA, Adams M, Andrew M: Canadian Pediatric Ischemic Stroke Registry (Abstract). *Can J Neurol Sci* 1995; 22:S24.

13. Peters U, Wiener GJ, Gilliam J, Van Nord G, Geisinger KR, Roach ES: Reye's syndrome in adults: A case report and review of the literature. *Arch Intern Med* 1986; 146:2401-2403.

14. Michelson AD, Bovill E, Andrew M: Antithrombotic therapy in children. *Chest* 1995; 108:506S-522S.

15. deVeber G, Andrew M, Adams M, et al: Treatment of pediatric sinovenous thrombosis with low molecular weight heparin (Abstract). *Ann Neurol* 1995; 38:532.

16. Massicotte P, Adams M, Marzinotto V, Brooker L, Andrew M: Low molecular weight heparin in pediatric patients with thrombotic disease: A dose finding study (In press). *J Pediatr* 1996.

17. Kay R, Sing Wong K, Ling Yu Y, et al: Low-molecular weight heparin for the treatment of acute ischemic stroke. *N Engl J Med* 1995; 333:1588-1593.

18. Andrew M, Marzinotto V, Brooker LA, et al: Oral anti-coagulant therapy in pediatric patients: A prospective study. *Thromb Haemostas* 1994; 71:265-269.

19. Leaker M, Massicotte MP, Brooker L, Andrew M: Thrombolytic therapy in pediatric patients: A comprehensive review of the literature (In press). *Thromb Haemostas* 1996.

20. Leaker M, Nitschmann E, Benson L, Mitchell L, Andrew M: Thrombolytic therapy in pediatric *Thromb Haemostas* 1996; 73:948.

21. Higashida RT, Helmer E, Halbach VV, Hieshima GB: Direct thrombolytic therapy for superior sagittal sinus thrombosis. *A J N R* 1989; 10:S4-S6.

22. Wong VK, LeMesurier J, Franceschini R, Heikali M, Hanson R: Cerebral venous thrombosis as a cause of neonatal seizures. *Pediatr Neurol* 1987; 3:235-237.

23. Griesemer DA, Theodorou AA, Berg RA, Soera TD: Local fibrinolysis in cerebral venous thrombosis. *Pediatr Neurol* 1994; 10:78-80.

24. Cohen AR, Martin MB, Silber JH, Kim HC, Ohene-Frempong K, Schwartz E: A modified transfusion program for prevention of stroke in sickle cell disease. *Blood* 1992; 79:1657-1661.

25. Miller ST, Jensen D, Rao SP: Less intensive long-term transfusion therapy for sickle cell anemia and cerebrovascular accident. *J Pediatr* 1992; 120:54-57.

26. Kurokawa T, Tomita S, Ueda K, et al: Prognosis of occlusive disease of the circle of Willis (moyamoya disease) in children. *Pediatr Neurol* 1985; 1:274-277.

27. Taylor BJ, Seibert JJ, Glasier CM, VanDevanter SH, Harrell JE, Fasules JW: Evaluation of the reconstructed carotid artery following extracorporeal membrane oxygenation. *Pediatrics* 1992; 90:568-572.

# Chapter 6

# *Seeking Health Care Following Stroke*

Advances in the diagnosis, management, and acute treatment of stroke present us with the challenge of delivering care to a population that traditionally seeks care hours and even days after the event in a system that does not respond urgently to this disease process. In the past, early treatment interventions for stroke were not available and there was no incentive to seek immediate health care. However, recent evidence indicates that early intervention for stroke increases the chance for recovery and restoration of function.[1] Therefore, it is imperative that persons experiencing signs and symptoms of stroke seek health care immediately to reduce disability and death.

The immediate goal for acute stroke care is to decrease the time it takes from stroke onset to initiation of acute medical intervention. This entire time is described as "delay time." Delay time from first symptoms and signs to the start of treatment has been studied in the cardiac population to determine changes needed to streamline care. These studies are helpful when trying to understand delay time in the stroke population. Knowledge of the factors influencing delay time and the decision-making process of stroke victims and bystanders will help create an effective public education campaign, which is the focus of this chapter.

"Seeking Health Care Following Stroke: Public Education," by Carol A. Barch, M.N., C.R.N.P., C.N.R.N., University of Pittsburgh Medical Center, from the Proceedings of a National Symposium on Rapid Identification and Treatment of Acute Stroke, National Institute of Neurological Disorders and Stroke (NINDS), December 12-13, 1996, reviewed July 1, 2001.

## Delay Time

Delay time—the time between the onset of symptoms and the start of medical intervention—has been well-studied in an effort to understand health-seeking behaviors. The literature on cardiac health-seeking behavior documents the various phases and characteristics of delay time. The six phases adapted by Alonzo[2] from Suchman's stages of illness[3] are outlined:

- *Prodromal period.* The period between the initial awareness of a health deviation (prodromal symptoms) and the onset of acute symptoms.

- *Definition period.* The period of self-evaluation that occurs between the onset of acute symptoms and the seeking of lay advice.

- *Lay consultation period.* The period between the seeking of lay advice and medical consultation. If medical consultation is not sought, the period extends to the initiation of travel to the hospital.

- *Medical consultation period.* The interval between the start of medical consultation and the initiation of travel to the hospital.

- *Travel period.* The time spent traveling to the hospital.

- *Hospital procedural period.* The time spent in the hospital emergency department (ED) or in the admission office until definitive treatment begins. This phase includes patient admission procedures, initial medical evaluation, and diagnostic studies.

The sequence and amount of time spent in each phase described will vary with each individual. To reduce delay time, each period must be understood and specific problems addressed. Once the individual or the bystander has made medical contact, the acute stroke system is considered to be activated. It is then up to the system to decrease the time it takes to start the appropriate medical intervention. Therefore, understanding decision-making in the first three time periods is critical to developing an effective public education program.

## Decision-Making/Delay Time

Typically, in the prodromal period the individual recognizes something is wrong. In the stroke population it is unclear what percent of patients are aware of their symptoms or that their health is impaired. Those with altered cognition following a stroke are at special risk of not recognizing symptoms.

The definition period that leads to attempts to seek help is a multidimensional process. The individual will recognize something is wrong. At that point he or she decides what may be wrong, how serious it is, and what to do about it. Determination of the problem will influence the perceived level of seriousness and the necessity of action. The action may include initiating self-treatment, seeking help from a family member or friend, or contacting a health care professional (family physician, clinic, or 911). Moss et al[4] studied delay time in the cardiac population and concluded that three cognitive factors are required to make a decision to seek medical help: (a) perception of presenting symptoms, (b) appreciation of the meaning and seriousness of the symptoms (recognition), and (c) realization that medical help is indicated for the recognized and appropriately interpreted symptoms. Education programs should focus on these three factors to facilitate specific decision-making behaviors for the stroke population.

The lay consultation period may be even more important in decreasing delay time in the stroke population. If a friend or family member is consulted, the burden of making a decision is shifted to that individual. The lay person must determine if the problem is serious and what should be done. Therefore, understanding stroke and stroke symptoms, as well as the appropriate actions in response to stroke, becomes imperative in the lay population. Anecdotal information indicates that nearly all stroke patients have help from another person when obtaining health care. Therefore, family members or close friends of those at risk for stroke must be a target in a public education campaign.

## Health Belief Model

The Health Belief Model (HBM) is used as the theoretical underpinning for understanding health-seeking behaviors. The HBM evolved from the premise that each individual's perception of the world determines what that individual will do. The concepts of the model include the individual's perceptions of susceptibility to the disease, severity of the disease, and benefits and barriers associated with the choice of action that may prevent the disease process. The theory was developed to explain preventive health behaviors.

The second stage of the model is "illness behavior," described by Kasal and Kobb[5] and by Kirscht[6] as a person's actions when faced with acute symptoms. Illness behaviors include recognizing symptoms and deciding whether to self-treat or seek medical care. The HBM theory represents a universal view of health behaviors. The HBM also relates psychological theories of decision-making, which attempt to explain actions in a situation presenting choices, to an individual's decision about alternative health behaviors.[7] The HBM provides a framework for determining the predictive variables that influence health care choices of stroke survivors or their family members when they are faced with the signs and symptoms of acute stroke.

## Delays in Seeking Health Care for Heart Disease

The problem of delaying health care is not unique to the stroke population. In the late 1960s when a high mortality associated with heart attack was identified, the delay time in seeking medical treatment was recognized as a critical factor.[8] It was evident that if patients sought treatment sooner, lives could be saved by the advanced treatment options available. Over the last 20 years, the literature on delay in seeking health care has been exclusively in the domain of the cardiac population.

Assessments of the characteristics of individuals with heart disease who seek health care have been reported. The studies found no significant difference in hospital arrival time with respect to age, gender, educational level, socioeconomic class, or past history of heart disease.[2, 4, 8-13] A documented medical history of hypertension, diabetes, or angina,[4, 8, 9, 12, 13] self-treatment of symptoms,[2, 9, 12] and the presence of family members who participated in seeking health care [4, 8] all contributed to increased delay time. Chest pain did not shorten delay time unless the patient was unstable.[12] These characteristics specific to the cardiac population have been examined to uncover any similarities or trends in the stroke population.

## Delay Pattern of Stroke Patients

Despite the severity and prevalence of the disease, little is known about how individuals decide to seek medical help when signs and symptoms of stroke appear. We do know that there are barriers that explain the long delay in seeking care in the stroke population.

The first barrier is the inability to recognize the symptoms of stroke. Often the symptoms are not identified as stroke but as another less serious problem. Stroke victims or bystanders may decide to take care of the problem on their own and delay seeking medical care. In a phone survey conducted by the Dupont Company in 1989, the majority of individuals interviewed did not understand what a stroke was or how to recognize the signs and symptoms.[14] In 1996, a Gallup poll conducted by the National Stroke Association revealed that the level of knowledge of stroke symptoms and risk factors has improved since the 1989 poll. However, the improvement was minimal. Face, arm, and leg weakness on one side of the body was the most frequently (58%) reported known symptom of stroke.[15] Stroke recognition remains a significant problem when 42% of the population cannot name the most common and recognizable symptom of stroke.

A stroke can impair cognition and judgment and limit mobility, speech, or vision, preventing one's ability to seek help. Stroke may occur during sleep, in which case the onset time cannot be determined and acute intervention cannot be safely implemented.

A number of studies [16-22] have been published on delay time in the stroke population. These studies varied in methodology and had small sample sizes. Moreover, those studies completed in Europe are difficult to apply to the U.S. population because of differences in the health care delivery system. The Duke/Veterans Administration stroke registry[21] revealed that only 42% of a total of 457 stroke patients presented within 24 hours and 33% presented within 24 to 48 hours following the onset of symptoms. The delay time was greatly reduced after initiating changes in the health care delivery system and increasing awareness among both the public and health care providers. Presently, we do not have sufficient data on the delay time for stroke patients. These data are necessary to measure the impact of education and changes in the health care system on delay time for stroke treatment.

A complete understanding of the causes of delay time for stroke treatment will require studies with a large number of patients. Variables that may need to be examined are:

1.  Actual presenting symptoms of stroke.

2.  Patient and bystander perception of the severity of different symptoms.

3.  Circumstances at the time of stroke (onset during sleep, bystander present, location at home or elsewhere).

4.  Patient and bystander recognition that symptoms are due to stroke, that they represent a serious problem, and that there is a potential treatment of known benefit.

These variables need to be explored further to develop a better model of health-seeking behaviors in acute stroke patients.

## Education Campaigns

Because of the devastating results of delaying immediate medical attention, many experts encourage the development of community educational programs to expedite arrival time at the hospital following stroke or heart attack.[4, 8-11, 13, 18, 20-26] A study by Podell[27] showed that despite educational efforts the number of cardiac patients who did not seek medical attention within 4 hours of the start of symptoms of heart attack in 1976-77 had not changed in comparison to a 1965-66 group.

A community heart disease awareness program was developed, implemented, and measured by Ho et al.[28] The entire educational campaign cost $300,000. Cardiac patients who came to the ED with complaints of pain were examined. This specific group of patients was tested prior to and following the education campaign. Results indicated that delays in arriving at the hospital following onset of symptoms did not change, but the level of education increased. Ho et al concluded that education increased the level of knowledge, but did not change patient behavior. Years of educational efforts and community awareness programs supported by the American Heart Association did not significantly reduce the delay time of individuals with heart disease seeking medical attention.[27] For public education campaigns the most difficult problem is finding ways to effectively change behavior to decrease delay time.

## The Proposed Education Process

The proposed education process is based upon what is known about the stroke population, work previously done with the cardiac population, and the HBM. There are two tiers to the process. The first tier seeks to educate the general public; the goals are to increase awareness of stroke, improve the recognition of stroke symptoms, and reinforce the concept that a stroke is an emergency. This effort should be conducted by all those working in the area of stroke, including professional, governmental, and commercial organizations. The second tier of education would focus on those at risk for stroke and their families. These individuals must understand their susceptibility to stroke, their ability to take preventive measures, their need to recognize the symptoms of stroke, and their need to seek immediate medical attention if they have a stroke. Primary care physicians, specialty physicians, and other health care providers need to provide information to stroke-prone individuals in a one-on-one setting.

Whether this process changes behavior is not known. Data should be collected on patients presenting within 6 hours to determine if public education efforts are beneficial. Based on what is already known, the initial reduction in delay time may be the result of health care system changes and increased awareness of the importance of rapid identification and treatment of stroke within the medical community rather than changes in the behavior of stroke patients and bystanders due to public education campaigns.

## References

1. The National Institute of Neurological Disorders and Stroke rt-PA Stroke Study Group. Tissue plasminogen activator for acute ischemic stroke. *N Engl J Med* 1995;333:1581-1587.

2. Alonzo AA. Acute illness behavior: A conceptual exploration and specification. *Soc Sci Med* 1980;14A:515-526.

3. Suchman EA. Stages of illness and medical care. *J Health Soc Behav* 1965;6:114-123.

4. Moss AJ, Wynar B, and Goldstein S. Delay in hospitalization during the acute coronary period. *Am J Cardiol* 1969;24:651-658.

5. Kasal S, and Kobb S. Health behavior, illness behavior, and sick role behavior. *Arch Environ Health* 1966;12:246-266.

6. Kirscht JP. The health belief model and illness behavior. *Health Education Monographs* 1974;2:387-408.

7. Maiman LA, and Becker MH. The health belief model: Origins and correlates in psychological theory. *Health Education Monographs* 1974;2:336-353.

8. Hackett TP, and Cassem NH. Factors contributing to delay in responding to the signs and symptoms of acute myocardial infarction. *Am J Cardiol* 1969;24:659-665.

9. Simon AB, Feinleib M, and Thompson KH. Components of delay in the prehospital phase of acute myocardial infarction. *Am J Cardiol* 1972;30:476-482.

10.  Tjoe SL, and Luria MH. Delays in reaching the cardiac care unit: An analysis. *Chest* 1972;61:617-621.

11.  Zoltan G, Stone P, Muller J, et al (and the Millis Study Group). Implications for acute intervention related to time of hospital arrival in acute myocardial infarction. *Am J Cardiol* 1986;57:203-208.

12.  Turi ZG, Stone PH, and Muller JE. Implications for acute intervention related to time of hospital arrival in acute myocardial infarction. *Am J Cardiol* 1986;58:203-209.

13.  Schroeder JS, Lamb IH, and Hu M. The prehospital course of patients with chest pain. Analysis of the prodromal, symptomatic, decision-making, transportation and emergency room periods. *Am J Med* 1978;64:742-748.

14.  National Stroke Association Consumer Survey: Are you at risk? DuPont Pharmaceutical Company, unpublished phone survey.

15.  National Stroke Association Gallup Poll, 1996.

16.  Harper GD, Haigh RA, Potter JF, et al. Factors delaying hospital admission after stroke in Leicestershire. *Stroke* 1992;23:835-838.

17.  Davalos A, Castillo J, and Martinez-Vila E. Delay in neurological attention and stroke outcome. Cerebrovascular Study Group of the Spanish Society of Neurology. *Stroke* 1995;26:2233-2237.

18.  Feldmann E, Gordon N, Brooks JM, et al. Factors associated with early presentation of acute stroke. *Stroke* 1993;24:1805-1810.

19.  Fogelholm R, Murros K, Rissanen A, et al. Factors delaying hospital admission after acute stroke. *Stroke* 1996;27:398-400.

20.  Alberts MJ, Perry A, Dawson DV, et al. Effects of public and professional education on reducing the delay time in presentation and referral of stroke patients. *Stroke* 1992; 23:352-356.

21.  Alberts MJ, Bertels C, and Dawson DV. An analysis of time of presentation after stroke. *JAMA* 1990;263:65-68.

22. Barch C. Health seeking behaviors of stroke survivors and/or significant others. 1992; Emory University, Atlanta, GA. Unpublished Master's Thesis.

23. Barsan WG, Brott TG, Broderick JP, et al. Urgent therapy for acute stroke. Effects of a stroke trial on untreated patients. *Stroke* 1994;25:2132-2137.

24. Brott T, Halley C, Levy D, et al. The investigational use of t-PA for stroke. *Ann Emerg Med* 1988;17:1202-1205.

25. Rowley JM, Hill JD, Hampton JR, et al. Early reporting of myocardial infarction: Impact of an experiment in patient education. *Br Med J* 1982;284:1741-1746.

26. Pole D. Delays between onset of acute myocardial infarction and definitive care. *Heart Lung* 1974;3:263-267.

27. Podell RN. Delay in hospitalization for myocardial infarction. *J Med Soc New Jersey* 1980;77:13-16.

28. Ho MT, Eisenberg MS, Litwin PE, et al. Delay between onset of chest pain and seeking medical care: The effect of public education. *Ann Emerg Med* 1989;18:727-731.

# Part Two

# Stroke Triggers and Risks

# Chapter 7

# Stroke Risk Factors and Triggers

## Preventing Stroke: Brain Basics

If you're like most Americans, you plan for your future. When you take a job, you examine its benefit plan. When you buy a home, you consider its location and condition so that your investment is safe. Today, more and more Americans are protecting their most important asset—their health. Are you?

Stroke ranks as the third leading killer in the United States. A stroke can be devastating to individuals and their families, robbing them of their independence. It is the most common cause of adult disability. Each year more than 500,000 Americans have a stroke, with about 145,000 dying from stroke-related causes. Officials at the National Institute of Neurological Disorders and Stroke (NINDS) are committed to reducing that burden through biomedical research.

### What Is a Stroke?

A stroke, or brain attack, occurs when blood circulation to the brain fails. Brain cells can die from decreased blood flow and the resulting

"Preventing Stroke: Brain Basics," National Institute of Neurological Disorders and Stroke (NINDS), NIH Publication No. 94-3440-b, reviewed July 1, 2001; "Study: Jolts May Cause Strokes," February 9, 2002, by Daniel Q. Haney, AP Medical Editor. Reprinted with permission of the Associated Press; and "Weather Conditions May Affect Stroke," published 4/16/2002, reported by Katrina Woznicki. Copyright United Press International, reprinted with permission.

lack of oxygen. There are two broad categories of stroke: those caused by a blockage of blood flow and those caused by bleeding. While not usually fatal, a blockage of a blood vessel in the brain or neck, called an ischemic stroke, is the most frequent cause of stroke and is responsible for about 80 percent of strokes. These blockages stem from three conditions: the formation of a clot within a blood vessel of the brain or neck, called thrombosis; the movement of a clot from another part of the body such as the heart to the neck or brain, called embolism; or a severe narrowing of an artery in or leading to the brain, called stenosis. Bleeding into the brain or the spaces surrounding the brain causes the second type of stroke, called hemorrhagic stroke.

Two key steps you can take will lower your risk of death or disability from stroke: know stroke warning signs and control stroke risk factors. Scientific research conducted by the NINDS has identified warning signs and a large number of risk factors.

### What Are Warning Signs of a Stroke?

Warning signs are clues your body sends that your brain is not receiving enough oxygen. If you observe one or more of these signs of a stroke or brain attack, don't wait, call a doctor or 911 right away!

- Sudden numbness or weakness of face, arm or leg, especially on one side of the body
- Sudden confusion, trouble speaking or understanding
- Sudden trouble seeing in one or both eyes
- Sudden trouble walking, dizziness, loss of balance or coordination
- Sudden severe headache with no known cause

Other danger signs that may occur include double vision, drowsiness, and nausea or vomiting. Sometimes the warning signs may last only a few moments and then disappear. These brief episodes, known as transient ischemic attacks or TIAs, are sometimes called mini-strokes. Although brief, they identify an underlying serious condition that isn't going away without medical help. Unfortunately, since they clear up, many people ignore them. Don't. Heeding them can save your life.

### What Are Risk Factors for a Stroke?

A risk factor is a condition or behavior that occurs more frequently in those who have, or are at greater risk of getting, a disease than in those who don't. Having a risk factor for stroke doesn't mean you'll have a stroke. On the other hand, not having a risk factor doesn't mean you'll avoid a stroke. But your risk of stroke grows as the number and severity of risk factors increases.

Stroke occurs in all age groups, in both sexes, and in all races in every country. It can even occur before birth, when the fetus is still in the womb. In African-Americans, the death rate from stroke is almost twice that of the white population. Scientists have found more and more severe risk factors in some minority groups and continue to look for patterns of stroke in these groups.

### What Are the Treatable Risk Factors?

Some of the most important treatable risk factors for stroke are:

- *High blood pressure*. Also called hypertension, this is by far the most potent risk factor for stroke. If your blood pressure is high, you and your doctor need to work out an individual strategy to bring it down to the normal range. Some ways that work:

    - Maintain proper weight.

    - Avoid drugs known to raise blood pressure.

    - Cut down on salt.

    - Eat fruits and vegetables to increase potassium in your diet.

    - Exercise more.

    Your doctor may prescribe medicines that help lower blood pressure. Controlling blood pressure will also help you avoid heart disease, diabetes, and kidney failure.

- *Cigarette smoking*. Cigarette smoking has been linked to the buildup of fatty substances in the carotid artery, the main neck artery supplying blood to the brain. Blockage of this artery is the leading cause of stroke in Americans. Also, nicotine raises blood pressure; carbon monoxide reduces the amount of oxygen your blood can carry to the brain; and cigarette smoke makes your blood thicker and more likely to clot. Your doctor can recommend programs and medications that may help you quit smoking. By quitting, at any age, you also reduce your risk of lung disease, heart disease, and a number of cancers including lung cancer.

- *Heart disease*. Common heart disorders such as coronary artery disease, valve defects, irregular heart beat, and enlargement of one of the heart's chambers can result in blood clots that may break loose and block vessels in or leading to the brain. The most common blood vessel disease, caused by the buildup of fatty deposits in the arteries, is called atherosclerosis. Your doctor will treat your heart disease and may also prescribe medication, such as aspirin, to help prevent the formation of clots. Your doctor may recommend surgery to clean out a clogged neck artery if you match a particular risk profile. If you are over 50, NINDS scientists believe you and your doctor should make a decision about aspirin therapy. A doctor can evaluate your risk factors and help you decide if you will benefit from aspirin or other blood-thinning therapy.

- *Warning signs or history of stroke.* If you experience a TIA, get help at once. Many communities encourage those with stroke warning signs to dial 911 for emergency medical assistance. If you have had a stroke in the past, it's important to reduce your risk of a second stroke. Your brain helps you recover from a stroke by drawing on body systems that now do double duty. That means a second stroke can be twice as bad.

- *Diabetes.* You may think this disorder affects only the body's ability to use sugar, or glucose. But it also causes destructive changes in the blood vessels throughout the body, including the brain. Also, if blood glucose levels are high at the time of a stroke, then brain damage is usually more severe and extensive than when blood glucose is well-controlled. Treating diabetes can delay the onset of complications that increase the risk of stroke.

## Do You Know Your Stroke Risk?

Some of the most important risk factors for stroke can be determined during a physical exam at your doctor's office. Working with your doctor, you can develop a strategy to lower your risk to average or even below average for your age.

Many risk factors for stroke can be managed, some very successfully. Although risk is never zero at any age, by starting early and controlling your risk factors you can lower your risk of death or disability from stroke. With good control, the risk of stroke in most age groups can be kept below that for accidental injury or death.

Americans have shown that stroke is preventable and treatable. A better understanding of the causes of stroke has helped Americans make lifestyle changes that have cut the stroke death rate nearly in half in the last two decades.

More than a million stroke survivors suffer little or no long-lasting disability from their strokes. Another two million, however, live with the crippling and lifelong disabilities of paralysis, loss of speech, and poor memory. Scientists at the NINDS predict that, with continued attention to reducing the risks of stroke and by using currently available therapies and developing new ones, Americans should be able to prevent 80 percent of all strokes by the end of the decade.

## Jolts May Cause Strokes

Ringing doorbells and other jolts that make people jump appear to be powerful and surprisingly common triggers of strokes, a study concluded. Researchers found that sudden movements, usually ones caused by being startled, increase the risk of stroke by 33 times over the usual level.

Israeli researchers who looked for possible stroke triggers in 150 victims found that 22 percent of them had a sudden movement just before their strokes. Other researchers have identified a variety of triggers for heart attacks—including climbing out of bed in the morning—but the latest study is among the first to search for the events that start strokes.

Dr. Nathan Bornstein noted that many people live with the underlying causes of strokes, such as high blood pressure or diabetes, for years. Then, for no obvious reason, a blood clot lodges in the brain, triggering a stroke. "We are looking for the triggers," he said. "What happened around this moment when the artery is blocked by a clot?" Bornstein presented the results of the study, conducted at Tel Aviv University, at the annual meeting of the American Stroke Association in San Antonio, Texas, February 8, 2002.

The second most common trigger, after sudden movement, was what the researchers called negative emotions. These included feeling distressed, upset, guilty, scared, hostile, irritable, ashamed, nervous, jittery, or afraid. These increased the risk 10-fold and preceded 13 percent of strokes.

Bornstein said that if confirmed, the finding suggests at least some factors that people at high risk of stroke might be warned to control. "We can tell people they have to be careful about exposure to outrageous anger," said Bornstein. "It's easy to say, but it's more difficult to apply."

Dr. Philip Gorelick, director of stroke research at Chicago's Rush-Presbyterian-St. Luke's Medical Center, said that while individual episodes of anger or jumping may trigger strokes, the repeated effects of these kinds of stress on the arteries over the years might be the real hazard. "It's the accumulation of stress that is important," he said, "not simply what happens one day."

## Weather Conditions May Affect Stroke

Stroke appears to occur more frequently when temperatures turn colder, suggesting some weather patterns may play a role in certain types of stroke, according to a new study presented April 16, 2002.

Dr. Dominique Minier of the Service de Neurologie in Dijon, France, and colleagues studied 3,289 first-time stroke patients over a 14-year period. They studied weather conditions including temperature, humidity, air pressure, wind strength, sun, and rain on the day the stroke occurred and five days prior to the attack. They also looked at four types of stroke, including ischemic stroke from large or small cerebral arteries or from a blood clot, transient ischemic attacks that temporarily interrupt blood supply to the brain, and hemorrhages or internal bleeding caused by clot eruption.

During the warmer months, the number of strokes caused by fat blocking the blood vessels in the larger arteries—such as the carotid artery running through the neck—declined significantly compared to the colder months, the researchers reported.

"Cold is associated with higher blood pressure," Minier told United Press International. "Warmer temperature is associated with higher stroke rate in Israel." Minier said it is unclear how weather impacts a person's health or if it can influence an individual's blood flow. And it could vary region to region. "I think that the relationship between weather and stroke is very difficult to understand," she said.

The findings are to help bring about "a better understanding of stroke in the acute phase," Minier said. Whether doctors should be more alert during the colder seasons for patients at a high risk for suffering a stroke is not known.

"Maybe they should," Minier said, "but it is difficult to know what we must do to be more aware. In my practice, I am always aware and I don't look at the sky when I practice." Also, researchers reported there were more overall strokes and strokes caused by a blockage in one of the large arteries in the brain and heart when there had been a temperature drop five days prior to the stroke attack.

The research was presented Tuesday, April 16, 2002 at the American Academy of Neurology annual meeting in Denver. Dr. Larry Goldstein, director of the Duke Center for Cerebrovascular Disease at Duke University in Durham, N.C., who also attended the AAN meeting, said while the research is interesting, it does not appear to have any clinical implications.

"Of stroke risk factors, one of the things that can't be changed is the weather," Goldstein told UPI. "In addition, the relationship is likely a statistical one, and the implications for an individual are likely to be limited." Goldstein added, "Environmental temperature changes can affect cardiac function, but in general I think the link to stroke would be tenuous. I am unaware of any data regarding changes in blood flow related to changes in barometric pressure," he said.

Chapter 8

# Homocysteine, Antibodies, and Inflammation Impact Stroke Risk

## The Functions of Folate

On the back of cereal boxes, where complicated tenets of nutrition have been reduced to their essence, the virtues of many vitamins and minerals are described in simple and familiar terms: vitamin A is good for skin, calcium builds strong bones and teeth, vitamin D is the sunshine vitamin. And folate, for women who are pregnant or trying to conceive, helps to prevent birth defects.

The B vitamin folate, also known as folic acid, has indeed proved effective in reducing the risk of neural-tube defects, particularly spina bifida. In 1992 the U.S. Public Health Service first recommended a daily intake of 400 micrograms of folic acid for women who were pregnant or could become pregnant. To help attain this goal, the Food and Drug Administration (FDA) in 1998 began requiring that cereal grain products (including breakfast cereals) be fortified with 140 micrograms of folic acid per 100 grams of product. But babies and mothers-to-be are not the sole beneficiaries. Several lines of evidence now show

This chapter includes "The Functions of Folate," by Sandra J. Ackerman, *NCRR Reporter*, Fall 1999, National Center for Research Resources; "Study Finds New Risk Factor for Stroke and Heart Attack," by Ellen Beth Levitt, August 2, 2001, University of Maryland Medical News © University of Maryland Medical System, reprinted with permission; and an excerpt from "Biomarkers and Surrogate Endpoints: Advancing Clinical Research and Application: Cardiovascular II," National Institutes of Health and U.S. Food and Drug Administration, 1999 Conference.

that nearly everyone who supplements a healthy diet with folic acid can reduce blood levels of the amino acid homocysteine, thereby controlling a major risk factor for coronary heart disease.

Yet questions remain. Scientists still do not know exactly how folic acid reduces homocysteine levels, how homocysteine may harm the heart and arteries, and what can be done about it. Recent clinical and molecular studies supported in part by NCRR are beginning to provide some much-needed answers.

Among the general public, homocysteine is not a recognized health threat of the caliber of cholesterol. But a recent prospective study shows that homocysteine can indeed be highly hazardous to one's health. At the Oregon Health Sciences University in Portland, a study conducted in part at the NCRR-supported General Clinical Research Center quantified the risk quite clearly. Researchers evaluated more than 350 patients who had a stable baseline level of atherosclerosis and coronary heart disease and tracked their clinical condition over several years. For every increase of just one micromole (135 micrograms) per liter of homocysteine in the blood, the scientists found an individual's risk of death from cardiovascular disease rose by 5.6 percent. This makes homocysteine as important a risk factor in coronary heart disease as any of the usual culprits: smoking, high blood pressure, high cholesterol levels, or advanced age.

"The natural history of atherosclerotic cardiovascular disease as related to homocysteine had only been studied a few times before this study," says Dr. Lloyd M. Taylor, professor of surgery at Oregon Health Sciences University and first author of the study. "We needed to have this baseline information in place before we could begin the treatment phase of our study." In this second phase, now under way, the same study participants will receive either folic acid supplements or a placebo for up to five years. The goal is to determine if reducing homocysteine levels can also lower the risk of death from cardiovascular disease or slow the progression of coronary heart disease. Although it is suspected to be true, no study has yet shown conclusively that homocysteine reduction can improve cardiovascular health.

"In some ways homocysteine is similar to cholesterol: when the level found in blood is within normal range, it poses no significant health risk," says Dr. M. Rene Malinow, professor of medicine at Oregon Health Sciences University and affiliate senior scientist at the NCRR-supported Oregon Regional Primate Research Center in Beaverton. But homocysteine has no apparent redeeming qualities, unlike cholesterol, which is known to play an essential role in embryonic development and cellular activities. The amino acid homocysteine enters the bloodstream as a byproduct "formed when the body metabolizes, or breaks down, the essential amino acid methionine, which we take in from food," Dr. Malinow explains. Homocysteine subsequently can be converted back to methionine or metabolized further to the amino acid cysteine, which is a component of many proteins.

Since homocysteine is known mainly for the apparent damage it causes if it accumulates, Dr. Malinow has focused on reducing its levels in the bloodstream. In a recent NCRR-supported study, he and his colleagues tested the effects of three different levels of folic acid enrichment in breakfast cereals. Seventy-five men and women with coronary artery disease ate preassigned packets of cereal every morning for a total of 15 weeks and had their blood levels of folic acid and homocysteine checked regularly. The study, published last year, demonstrated a clear dose-response effect. At the level of folic acid enrichment recommended by the FDA (the lowest of the three levels in this study), folic acid in the blood increased, but homocysteine did not decrease. But the other two levels of enrichment—roughly four times and five times the level recommended by the FDA—reduced plasma homocysteine levels by 11 percent and 14 percent, respectively. "However," says Dr. Malinow, "these results, which were obtained in well-defined experimental conditions, may not be directly applicable to a large population ingesting folic acid-fortified grain products whose exact folic acid contents are uncertain."

These findings suggest that Americans should consume more folic acid, either through enriched foods or through a daily vitamin pill, to reap the benefits of this compound. Like Dr. Taylor's group, Dr. Malinow's team is now conducting follow-up clinical studies to determine if lowering blood homocysteine levels can reduce the occurrence of heart attack or stroke. Results from Dr. Malinow's group are expected in three to five years.

Although the link between folic acid intake and homocysteine reduction has become well established, the precise mechanisms by which the folic acid lowers homocysteine levels remains more of a mystery. But now biochemists and structural biologists using NCRR-supported instruments and resources are weighing in with a critical piece of the puzzle. By focusing their attention on the structure of an enzyme known as methylenetetrahydrofolate reductase (MTHFR), which furnishes the form of folate that is required to convert homocysteine back to methionine, the researchers have gathered hard evidence that folates stabilize MTHFR, thereby preventing accumulation of homocysteine. These results are based on biochemical studies by Dr. Rowena Matthews and her colleagues and on structural studies by

Dr. Martha Ludwig and her co-workers. In their studies Drs. Matthews and Ludwig, both professors of biological chemistry at the University of Michigan in Ann Arbor, used MTHFR from the bacterium *Escherichia coli*, which is very similar to MTHFR from humans but easier to obtain.

Determining the three-dimensional (3-D) structure of MTHFR at atomic resolution required more than just a good microscope. This was a job for a synchrotron—specifically, the NCRR-supported MacCHESS synchrotron facility at Cornell University in Ithaca, New York. Using a method known as x-ray crystallography, scientists from Dr. Ludwig's group shone a beam of synchrotron light through a crystal of MTHFR, and a detector measured and analyzed how the x-rays were deflected by the molecule's constituent atoms. The intense and tunable x-rays produced by the synchrotron allowed the researchers to use a novel technique called multi-wavelength anomalous diffraction to locate the position of these atoms.

Earlier preliminary studies in Ann Arbor of the molecule's 3-D structure used crystallography equipment purchased through an NCRR Shared Instrumentation Grant. The data from Ann Arbor were combined with measurements from the synchrotron to develop the structure of MTHFR. The picture of the molecule slowly emerged from a dialogue between calculations and model-building, then more calculations and more modeling. "At first we could just see that the structure of MTHFR was a barrel," says Dr. Ludwig. Once they had teased out the detailed structure, though, the researchers could see how folate might stabilize MTHFR. To perform its function, MTHFR must bind tightly to a small molecule called flavin adenine dinucleotide, or FAD. "When folate is added," says Dr. Ludwig, "it sits on top of the flavin, almost pinning it down. The binding of one cofactor [the folate] makes the binding of the other cofactor [FAD] more stable."

In about 12 percent of the population, a mutation in the MTHFR gene causes the enzyme to loosen its binding of FAD, which makes the enzyme unstable and prevents it from functioning properly. These people are at much higher risk both for neural tube defects at birth and for high homocysteine levels later in life. "Our experiments suggested that the mutant form of MTHFR loses its flavin much more easily than the wild type," adds Dr. Matthews.

Drs. Ludwig and Matthews and their co-workers now hope to determine the high-resolution structure for the mutant enzyme, "and for purposes of comparison we want to study the mutant enzyme from both bacteria and humans," Dr. Ludwig says. Resolving these structures will clear up some long-standing biochemical questions, but for

Dr. Matthews the quest has taken on a personal note as well. For two decades, from her appointment as assistant professor to her current post as chair of the biophysics research division, MTHFR has been a focus of her research. To have the full crystal structure revealed, she says, is "like finally seeing your spouse on the day of an arranged marriage, when you've been told how he acts, but you've never before met him in person."

The research described in this article is supported by the Biomedical Technology, Clinical Research, and Comparative Medicine areas of the National Center for Research Resources; the National Institute of General Medical Sciences; the National Heart, Lung, and Blood Institute; and the Medical Research Council of Canada.

## Additional Reading

1. Guenther, B. D., Sheppard, C. A., Tran, P., et al., The structure and properties of methylenetetrahydrofolate reductase from *Escherichia coli* suggest how folate ameliorates human hyperhomocysteinemia. *Nature Structural Biology* 6:359-365, 1999.

2. Taylor, L. M., Moneta, G. L., Sexton, G. J., et al., Prospective blinded study of the relationship between plasma homocysteine and progression of symptomatic peripheral arterial disease. *Journal of Vascular Surgery* 29:8-21, 1999.

3. Malinow, M. R., Duell, P.B., Hess, D. L., et al., Reduction of plasma homocyst(e)ine levels by breakfast cereal fortified with folic acid in patients with coronary heart disease. *New England Journal of Medicine* 338:1009-1015, 1998.

## Study Finds New Risk Factor for Stroke and Heart Attack

Researchers studying the risk factors for stroke and heart attack say they have identified an antibody that seems to double the risk of both health problems in men, independent of other risk factors. Their study, published in the August 2001 issue of the journal *Stroke*, is the first prospective study to show that the risk of ischemic stroke and heart attack is increased among men who have these particular antibodies, known as Beta-2 Dependent Anticardiolipin Antibodies (B2GP1-dependent aCL).

"Our study found that the risk of stroke and heart attack associated with these antibodies was similar to the increased risk from other conditions, such as hypertension and diabetes," says Steven J. Kittner,

M.D., M.P.H., professor of neurology at the University of Maryland School of Medicine and a neurologist at the Baltimore VA Medical Center. Dr. Kittner is the study's senior author.

For the study, the researchers evaluated blood samples from men of Japanese ancestry who were followed over the past 20 years as part of the Honolulu Heart Program. They measured the antibodies in 259 men who went on to have an ischemic stroke (caused by a blockage in a blood vessel) and 374 men who developed a heart attack. They also studied blood from a control group of 1,360 men who remained free of both health problems.

Men with the antibodies had a two-fold increased risk of stroke, and for heart attack the risk was almost twice as high, when adjusted for other risk factors. While it is clear that uncontrolled hypertension, diabetes, high cholesterol, and smoking increase the risk of cardiovascular disease, the researchers say they do not know all of the predisposing risk factors. There are still many people who suffer from these common health problems who do not seem to be at high risk.

Our bodies form antibodies after they are exposed to infection, and the role of inflammation and infection in cardiovascular disease is a major focus of research now, as part of the effort to better prevent, predict, and treat heart disease and stroke. But there are many unanswered questions.

"While we found a striking association between these particular antibodies and heart attack and stroke, we do not know whether they are a cause or merely a precursor for these events," says Dr. Kittner. "We need more research to determine if there is a cause and effect relationship. Or, it could be that something else, such as a particular infection, is causing both the antibodies and the stroke or heart attack," Dr. Kittner adds.

The researchers also want to learn whether people who have these antibodies should be treated differently after they have a heart attack or a stroke. Robin L. Brey, M.D., associate professor of medicine at the University of Texas Health Science Center at San Antonio, says this study will help answer those questions.

"Now that we have proof that these antibodies are markers for increased risk, we can turn our attention to how they are associated with stroke and heart attack. We now need to explore whether these antibodies cause stroke or heart attack, and try to better understand the mechanism, if they are found to be causative," adds Dr. Brey, who was the lead author of the study. "The next step will be to use information about mechanism to develop better strategies to decrease stroke and heart attack risk for people with these antibodies," she adds.

The B2GP1-dependent aCL antibodies were found in about 12 percent of men in the study who did not have cardiovascular disease, but they were prevalent in 17 percent of men who had a stroke and 16 percent of those who had a heart attack. Scientists do not know which type of infection, if there is one, may be responsible for these particular antibodies.

## Biomarkers and Surrogate Endpoints: Advancing Clinical Research and Applications

### Stable Cardiovascular Disease

In patients with stable coronary artery disease (CAD), the atherosclerotic process can induce a host of coronary functional and anatomic abnormalities that eventually affect myocardial performance. A number of factors likely contribute to this process, including procoagulant tendencies, inflammation, metabolic abnormalities, coronary microcalcification, oxygen radicals, and oxidized lipids. The treatment is usually multitargeted, frequently focused on clinical presentation of ischemia. The relevant biomarker might target coronary flow limitations and/or abnormalities, expression of ischemia, such as perfusion, myocardial metabolism or left ventricular function, or factors involved in CAD. Ischemia can be assessed directly by myocardial metabolic assessment (31P or other techniques), indirectly by perfusion techniques, such as nuclear imaging or MRI, or by ECG changes (ambulatory ECG).

### Inflammatory Biomarkers in the Prediction of Future Coronary Events among Apparently Healthy Men and Women by Paul M. Ridker, M.D., M.P.H.

Myocardial infarction and stroke commonly occur among individuals without hyperlipidemia. In an attempt to better predict future coronary events, epidemiologic studies have explored a series of novel risk factors including biomarkers of inflammatory function. Specifically, recent large-scale prospective studies indicate that nonspecific inflammatory markers, such as C-reactive protein and serum amyloid A, as well as direct markers of cellular adhesion (soluble intercellular adhesion molecule 1), and cytokine activation interleukin-6 are all elevated many years in advance among those at high risk for future events. This has been shown for women as well as men and is present in subgroups of patients traditionally considered low risk.

Further, the predictive value of inflammatory markers appears to be additive to that of total and high-density lipoprotein cholesterol. Because these inflammatory changes are present many years in advance and likely reflect the presence of unstable lesions, the use of inflammatory markers in the clinical setting may provide a mechanism for early detection and intervention for those at high risk for future coronary disease.

Chapter 9

# *Atherosclerosis May Lead to Stroke*

## *Atherosclerosis*

Alternative names: Arteriosclerosis; Hardening of the arteries

### *Definition*

The terms can be a little confusing. "Athero"-sclerosis is a disease in which fatty material is deposited on the wall of your arteries, which narrows the arteries and eventually restricts blood flow.

It is one of several types of "Arterio"-sclerosis, a disease characterized by thickening and hardening of artery walls. However, the word "atherosclerosis" is often used to indicate any of the forms of arteriosclerosis.

---

This chapter includes "Atherosclerosis," © 2002, A.D.A.M. Inc. Reprinted with permission; "Enlarged View of Atherosclerosis," (image), © 2002, A.D.A.M., Inc. Reprinted with permission; "Stroke Secondary to Atherosclerosis," © 2002, A.D.A.M. Inc. Reprinted with permission; "Stroke Secondary to Carotid Stenosis," © 2002, A.D.A.M., Inc. Reprinted with permission; and "Carotid Stenosis, X-Ray of the Right Artery," (image), © 2002, A.D.A.M., Inc. Reprinted with permission. Along with an excerpt from "Biomarkers and Surrogate Endpoints: Advancing Clinical Research and Application: Cardiovascular II," National Institutes of Health and U.S. Food and Drug Administration, 1999 Conference; and "Men Are Four Times More Likely Than Women to Suffer a Stroke Due to Large-Vessel Atherosclerosis," *Research Activities*, March 2000, No. 235, Agency for Healthcare Research and Quality (AHRQ).

## Causes and Risks

Atherosclerosis is a common disorder of the arteries. Fat, cholesterol, and other substances accumulate in the walls of arteries and form "atheromas" or plaques. Eventually, the fatty tissue can erode the wall of the artery, diminish the elasticity (stretchiness) of the artery, and interfere with the blood flow.

Clots may form around the plaque deposits, further interfering with blood flow. When blood flow in the arteries to heart muscle becomes severely restricted, it leads to symptoms like chest pain.

Risk factors include smoking, diabetes, obesity, high blood cholesterol, a diet high in fats, and having a personal or family history of heart disease. Cerebrovascular disease, peripheral vascular disease, high blood pressure, and kidney disease involving dialysis are also disorders that may also be associated with atherosclerosis.

## Prevention

Diet recommendations may include low-fat, low-cholesterol, and low-salt diet. Follow the health care provider's recommendations for treatment and control of hypertension, diabetes, and other diseases. Reduce body weight if overweight and stop smoking if a smoker. Get regular exercise to improve the fitness of the heart and circulation.

## Symptoms

Atherosclerosis shows no symptoms until a complication occurs.

## Signs and Tests

Atherosclerosis may not be diagnosed until complications occur. Prior to complications, atherosclerosis may be noted by the presence of a "bruit" (a whooshing or blowing sound heard over the artery with a stethoscope). The affected area may have a decreased pulse.

Tests that indicate atherosclerosis (or complications) include:

- An abnormal difference between the blood pressure of the ankle and arm (ankle/brachial index, or ABI)
- A Doppler study of the affected area
- Ultrasonic Duplex scanning
- A CT scan of the affected area
- Magnetic resonance arteriography (MRA)

- An arteriography of the affected area

- An intravascular ultrasound (IVUS) of the affected vessels

### Treatment

To some extent, the body will protect itself by forming new blood vessels around the affected area.

Medications may be recommended to reduce fats and cholesterol in your blood. These include cholestyramine, colestipol, nicotinic acid, gemfibrozil, probucol, lovastatin, and others. Aspirin, ticlopidine, and clopidogrel (inhibitors of platelet clumping) or anti-coagulants may be used to reduce the risk of clot formation.

Balloon angioplasty uses a balloon-tipped catheter to flatten plaque and increase the blood flow past the deposits. The technique is used to open the arteries of the heart and other arteries in the body. Another widely used technique is stenting, which consists of implanting a small metal device inside the artery (usually following angioplasty) to keep the artery open.

Surgically removing deposits (endarterectomy) may be recommended in some cases. A bypass graft is the most invasive procedure. It uses a normal artery or vein from the patient to create a bridge that bypasses the blocked section of the artery.

### Prognosis

The outcome varies. All people begin to develop atherosclerosis at birth, and in some people, it leads to complications.

### Complications

- Coronary artery disease (atherosclerosis of arteries to the heart) where the blood supply to the heart is insufficient due to obstruction (ischemia). A symptom is angina, or chest pain.

- Heart attack.

- Transient ischemic attack (TIA) or stroke.

- Insufficient blood supply to the limbs (mainly the legs and feet) due to obstruction.

- Damage to organs.

- Atherosclerosis and obstruction of bypass grafts.

Call your health care provider if you are at risk for atherosclerosis, particularly if symptoms of complications occur.

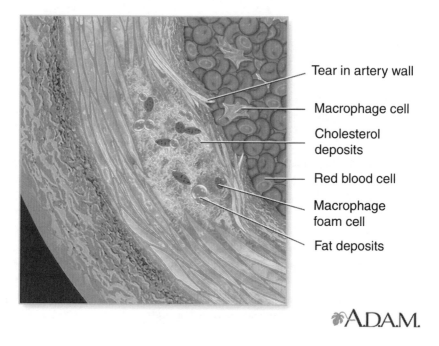

Tear in artery wall

Macrophage cell

Cholesterol deposits

Red blood cell

Macrophage foam cell

Fat deposits

🌿A.D.A.M.

**Figure 9.1.** *Cut-Section of Artery*

## Stroke Secondary to Atherosclerosis

### Definition

A group of brain disorders involving loss of brain functions, caused by complications of atherosclerosis.

### Causes and Risks

Stroke secondary to atherosclerosis affects about 2 out of 1,000 people, or approximately 50% of all those who have strokes. Strokes are the third leading cause of death in most developed countries, including the U.S. Stroke secondary to atherosclerosis is most common in people over 50 years old. The incidence of stroke rises dramatically with age, with the risk doubling with each decade after 35 years old.

About 5% of people over 65 years old have had at least one stroke. The disorder occurs in men more often than women.

Atherosclerosis ("hardening of the arteries") is a condition where fatty deposits occur in the inner lining of the arteries, and atherosclerotic plaque (a mass consisting of fatty deposits and blood platelets) develops. The plaque may obstruct (occlude) the artery by itself, or may trigger a clot (thrombus) at that location, causing cerebral thrombosis (thrombotic stroke). The occlusion of the artery develops slowly.

Atherosclerotic plaque does not necessarily cause stroke. There are many small connections among the various brain arteries. If blood flow gradually decreases, these small connections will increase in size and "by-pass" the obstructed area (collateral circulation). If there is enough collateral circulation, even a totally blocked artery may not cause neurologic deficits. A second safety mechanism within the brain is that the arteries are large enough that 75% of the blood vessel can be occluded, and there will still be adequate blood flow to that area of the brain.

Atherosclerosis occludes the blood vessels, causing ischemia (reduced tissue oxygenation associated with insufficient blood flow) and infarction (tissue death associated with ischemia).

Pieces of atherosclerotic plaque or clot may travel in the bloodstream (embolism); however, strokes caused by embolism are most commonly strokes secondary to cardiogenic embolism (clots that develop because of heart disorders, which then travel to the brain). Whatever the source of the embolism, the clot travels through the bloodstream and becomes stuck in a small artery in the brain. This stroke occurs suddenly with immediate maximum neurologic deficit (loss of brain function).

Risks for stroke secondary to atherosclerosis include: a history of high blood pressure (hypertension is present in about 70% of all victims of stroke); peripheral vascular disease; smoking; transient ischemic attacks or other cerebrovascular disease; atherosclerosis or high blood lipids; diabetes mellitus; obesity; and kidney disease requiring dialysis.

### *Prevention*

The prevention of stroke secondary to atherosclerosis includes control of risk factors. Hypertension, diabetes, heart disease, and other risk factors should be treated as appropriate. Smoking should be minimized or, preferably, stopped.

Treatment of TIA can prevent some strokes.

*Symptoms*

- weakness or total inability to move a body part
- numbness, loss of sensation
- tingling or other abnormal sensations
- decreased or lost vision, may be partial, may be temporary
- language difficulties (aphasia)
- inability to recognize or identify sensory stimuli (agnosia)
- loss of memory
- facial paralysis
- eyelid drooping
- vertigo (abnormal sensation of movement)
- loss of coordination
- swallowing difficulties
- personality changes
- mood and emotion changes
- urinary incontinence (lack of control over bladder)
- lack of control over the bowels
- consciousness changes:
    - sleepy
    - stuporous, somnolent, lethargic
    - comatose, unconscious

*Signs and Tests*

Signs of stroke are present. Testing is the same as for stroke. Serum lipids, especially triglycerides and cholesterol, may be high. Other tests and procedures:

- head CT scan
- head MRI
- ECG (electrocardiogram) may be used to determine underlying heart disorders
- echocardiogram (if the cause is suspected to be cardiac embolus)
- carotid duplex (ultrasound)

## Treatment

Stroke is an acute, serious condition. Immediate treatment is required. Treatment varies depending on the severity of symptoms. For virtually all strokes, there is a need for hospitalization, possibly including intensive care and life support. If a patient with symptoms arrives at the hospital within 3 hours of onset, he or she may be eligible for immediate intervention including thrombolysis (the dissolution of clot) which may immediately open the artery and prevent the stroke from causing permanent deficits. There is risk of serious bleeding with this treatment so patients have to be selected carefully, but the most important factor is arriving at the hospital as early as possible from the onset of symptoms.

For patients not eligible for thrombolysis, treatment will be based on the type of stroke they may have had, however, the focus will be supportive (i.e. blood pressure control, adequate fluids) and prevention of complications such as infections. Rehabilitation is important following stroke to maximize function in affected areas. Treatment is also aimed at prevention of future strokes. Recovery may occur as other areas of the brain take over functioning for the damaged areas. The goal of treatment is to prevent spread (extension) of the stroke and to maximize the ability of the person to function.

Special treatment (in addition to treatment for stroke in general) may include medications to control blood cholesterol levels.

A special diet often follows the American Heart Association recommendations for people with hyperlipidemia (increased fats/lipids in the bloodstream). This may include restriction of fat, especially saturated fat. It may also include restriction of salt/sodium if stroke is accompanied by high blood pressure.

A carotid endarterectomy (removal of plaque from the carotid arteries) may be indicated for some people to prevent new strokes from occurring.

## Prognosis

Stroke is the third leading cause of death in developed countries. About one-fourth of the sufferers die as a result of the stroke or its complications, about one-half have long-term disabilities, and about one-fourth recover most or all function.

## Complications

- pressure sores

- permanent loss of movement or sensation of a part of the body
- orthopedic complications, fractures, contractures, muscle spasticity
- permanent loss of cognitive functions
- disruption of communication, decreased social interaction
- decreased ability to function or care for self
- decreased life span
- multi-infarct dementia
- side effects of medications

## Call Your Health Care Provider If

Go to the emergency room or call the local emergency number (such as 911) if symptoms occur indicating a stroke.

# Stroke Secondary to Carotid Stenosis

## Definition

A group of brain disorders involving loss of brain function caused by obstruction of the carotid arteries. This is usually related to hardening of the arteries (atherosclerosis).

## Causes, Incidence, and Risk Factors

Stroke secondary to carotid stenosis occurs when a major portion of one or both carotid arteries (the arteries in the neck that supply blood to the brain) is narrowed or blocked.

Atherosclerosis (hardening of the arteries) is a condition where fatty deposits occur in the inner lining of the arteries, and atherosclerotic plaque (a mass consisting of fatty deposits and blood platelets) develops. The plaque may obstruct the artery or a clot (thrombus) may occur at the site of the plaque and also cause obstruction. Blockage of the artery usually develops slowly. Sometimes, however, a piece of atherosclerotic plaque (an embolism) may break off and travel to an artery in the brain causing obstruction far from the initial site where the plaque developed.

Atherosclerotic plaque does not always lead to stroke. There are many small blood vessels around the carotid arteries. If blood flow gradually decreases, these small connections will increase in size and by-pass the obstructed area (collateral circulation). If there is enough collateral circulation, even a totally blocked artery may not cause neurologic deficits. A second safety mechanism is that the arteries are large enough that 70 % of the blood vessel can be occluded, and there will still be adequate blood flow to the brain.

Stroke secondary to carotid stenosis is most common in older people, and often, there is underlying atherosclerotic heart disease and/or diabetes mellitus.

Risks are the same as for stroke secondary to atherosclerosis.

### *Signs and Tests*

An examination may include neurologic, motor, and sensory examination to determine the specific neurologic deficits present, because they often correspond closely to the location of the injury to the brain. The examination may show emboli in the retina, changes in reflexes including abnormal reflexes or abnormal extent of "normal" reflexes, muscle weakness, decreased sensation, and other changes. A bruit (an abnormal sound heard with the stethoscope) may be heard over the carotid arteries of the neck.

Additional tests include:

- high serum lipids, especially triglycerides and cholesterol

- carotid artery stenosis or complete occlusion showing on

  - carotid or cerebral angiography
  - carotid Duplex/Doppler ultrasound
  - MRI of the head
  - MRA of the brain vessels and neck vessels (carotid and vertebral arteries)

### *Treatment*

Treatment is the same as for stroke. For additional treatment, antihypertensive medication may be needed to control high blood pressure. Medications to control blood cholesterol levels may be required.

Carotid endarterectomy, surgical removal of plaque from the carotid arteries, may be indicated to prevent new strokes from occurring, especially if there is more than 70% of the carotid artery occluded and there are no contraindications (reasons against the surgery) such as coexisting terminal illness or dementia.

### Expectations (Prognosis)

Stroke is the third leading cause of death in developed countries. About one-fourth of the sufferers die as a result of the stroke or its complications, about one-half have long-term disabilities, and about one-fourth recover most or all function.

### Complications

Complications are the same as for stroke.

### Calling Your Health Care Provider

Go to the emergency room or call the local emergency number (such as 911) if symptoms occur.

### Prevention

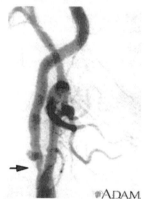

**Figure 9.2.** *Carotid Stenosis, X-ray of the Right Artery*

Prevention includes control of risk factors. Hypertension, diabetes, heart disease, and other risk factors should be treated as appropriate. Smoking should be minimized or, preferably, stopped.

Treatment of TIA (transient ischemic attack, "warning strokes") may prevent some strokes.

## Biomarkers and Surrogate Endpoints: Advancing Clinical Research and Applications

### Stable Cardiovascular Disease

In patients with stable coronary artery disease (CAD), the atherosclerotic process can induce a host of coronary functional and anatomic abnormalities that eventually affect myocardial performance. A number of factors likely contribute to this process, including procoagulant tendencies, inflammation, metabolic abnormalities, coronary microcalcification, oxygen radicals, and oxidized lipids. The treatment is usually multitargeted, frequently focused on clinical presentation of ischemia. The relevant biomarker might target coronary flow limitations and/or abnormalities, expression of ischemia, such as perfusion, myocardial metabolism or left ventricular function, or factors involved in CAD. Ischemia can be assessed directly by myocardial metabolic assessment (31P or other techniques), indirectly by perfusion techniques, such as nuclear imaging or MRI, or by ECG changes (ambulatory ECG).

## *Calcium as a Biomarker for Atherosclerosis Progression and Regression in Coronary Artery Disease by Douglas P. Boyd, Ph.D.*

Atherosclerosis is a silent disease that develops slowly over decades of life until it manifests itself in clinical coronary artery disease with symptoms including angina, heart attack, heart failure, and sudden death. The treatment of atherosclerosis involves lifestyle modifications and medical treatment of lipid disorders. Histologic studies have shown that approximately 20 percent of the volume of plaque in coronary atherosclerosis is marked by detectable levels of calcium (Rumberger et al. 1995). Although soft plaques with no detectable calcium exist, large studies have shown that 96 percent of asymptomatic patients with clinical coronary disease as demonstrated by angiography have detectable coronary calcium (Laudon et al. 1999). Other studies have shown that the prevalence of calcium correlates with increased risk of future coronary events, and the greater the amount of calcium, the higher the risk (Arad et al. 1996). The risk, sometimes expressed as an "odds ratio," can be 20:1 or higher and is independent of the presence or absence or symptoms of cardiac disease. In the past, coronary artery calcification (CAC) could be detected by fluoroscopy. However, the results were variable due to the relative insensitivity of the fluoroscopic technique and the requirement of a skilled operator. Today the "gold-standard" for the detection and quantification of CAC is electron beam CT (EBCT) scanning using a 100 millisecond scan speed. Recent research has focused on the reproducibility of CAC scores and the ability of such quantitation to track the progression and regression of atherosclerotic disease. Callister and colleagues (1998) demonstrated in a retrospective study of 149 patients the ability to track disease progression after 12 to 15 months of treatment with a statin drug. Untreated patients advanced in plaque volume by 52 percent. Those treated who achieved a final low-density lipoprotein (LDL) cholesterol level of less than 120 mg per deciliter had a net regression of about 7 percent. Regression analysis showed an association with the degree of regression and the final LDL level achieved. These kinds of drug studies depend on the accuracy of CAC scoring. With higher accuracy, the longitudinal interval could be shortened and fewer patients would need to be logged into a blind study. Currently, CAC is scored using an Agatston score (Agatston et al. 1990), which approximates the mass of calcium present, and a volume score, which estimates a plaque volume. The major sources of error include motion artifact, electrocardiograph triggering errors, resolution blurring, and variability in background subtraction as determined by a threshold. All of these issues can be addressed by technical improvements, many of which are under way. Some of the improvements will be made in the EBT scanner itself (reduce scan speed to the 35-50 msec range, introduce multiple slices, increase resolution by doubling detector pitch), and others require improvements in the CAC scoring workstation algorithms (interpolation scoring, linearization, and normalization of background using self-calibration). These techniques and others will advance the accuracy of CAC in future years, thus providing an increasingly precise biomarker for early detection, monitoring of treatment, and for interventional research studies in coronary artery disease.

## *Electron Beam-Computed Tomography by Nathaniel Reichek, M.D.*

Electron beam-computed tomography (EBCT) is a highly effective method for detection of calcific coronary atherosclerosis. Thus, the EBCT calcium score is a very useful marker of the extent of coronary atherosclerosis, particularly for studies of clinical epidemiology. Stratification of a population by calcium score correlates well overall with likelihood of coronary stenoses and prevalence of coronary events. In populations with chest pain, those with normal EBCT calcium scores have a much lower likelihood of coronary stenoses than those with high calcium scores. Effective treatment of hyperlipidemia can be associated with a reduction in calcium score. However, the calcium score also has many important limitations that limit use as a biomarker for coronary atherosclerosis at the present time. The variability of calcium score on repeat EBCT is excessively high. Age-dependent increases in score complicate interpretation. The method may not identify patients with early disease and potentially hazardous vulnerable plaques. A high calcium score is sensitive but nonspecific as a marker for coronary stenoses. Although scores may change with lipid-lowering treatment or increase over time as part of the natural history of coronary atherosclerosis, there is no evidence that such changes correlate with changes in the actual extent of atherosclerosis or risk of clinical events.

## Men Are Four Times More Likely Than Women to Suffer a Stroke Due to Large-Vessel Atherosclerosis

Over 400,000 men and women suffer from a first ischemic stroke each year in the United States. Although these strokes may be classified by the several different causes that produce them, scant data exist on the incidence rates and risk factors for different types of ischemic stroke.

A recent study, supported in part by the Agency for Healthcare Research and Quality (Stroke Prevention Patient Outcomes Research Team, PORT, 290-91-0028), examined some of these incidence rates and risk factors. It found that men and women had significantly different rates for strokes due to atherosclerosis with stenosis (narrowing of the blood vessel). After adjustment for age, men had four times the rate of this type of stroke as women (47 vs. 12 per 100,000), a difference in incidence that could explain why U.S. rates of carotid endarterectomy (surgical opening of a blocked carotid artery) are 30 to 60 percent higher in men than in women.

For this study, the researchers used the Rochester Epidemiology Project medical records linkage system to identify all 454 Rochester, MN, residents who suffered a first ischemic stroke between 1985 and 1989. Ninety-six percent of the population of Rochester is white, and 51 percent is female. The age- and sex-adjusted incidence rates of ischemic stroke per 100,000 in this population were 27 were due to large-vessel cervical or intracranial atherosclerosis with over 50 percent stenosis; 40 due to cardioembolic causes (blood clots originating from the heart); 25 due to lacunae (strokes due to blockages in tiny blood vessels deep in the brain); 52 due to uncertain cause; and 4 due to other or uncommon cause. Hypertension occurred with strikingly similar frequency among study patients with stroke due to large-vessel disease, cardioembolic stroke, and lacunae. There was no difference in history of prior transient ischemic attack.

Subtype-specific stroke incidence rates also provide a means of more accurately comparing racial differences and differences between men and women in stroke mechanisms. In comparing this study with a study of blacks in metropolitan Cincinnati, OH, the researchers found that although blacks had a higher overall age- and sex-adjusted ischemic stroke incidence compared with whites (246 vs. 147 per 100,000), the incidence of stroke due to large-vessel atherosclerosis with stenosis was significantly greater among whites than blacks (27 vs. 17 per 100,000). This difference could not be attributed to a disparity in procedure rates since the same proportion (54 percent) of patients in both studies received diagnostic tests to detect carotid stenosis.

Details are in "Ischemic stroke subtypes: A population-based study of incidence and risk factors," by George W. Petty, M.D., Robert D. Brown, Jr., M.D., Jack P. Whisnant, M.D., and others, in the December 1999 *Stroke* 30, pp. 2513-2516.

Chapter 10

# Stroke and Cardiovascular Disease

## Contents

# Section 10.1

# *Stroke Is a Cardiovascular Disease*

Excerpt from "Hearts N' Parks Community Mobilization Guide," National Heart, Lung, and Blood Institute and the National Recreation and Park Association, NIH Publication No. 01-1655, June, 2001.

## *Focused Facts*

- Cardiovascular disease is the leading cause of death for all people in the United States.

- 60.8 million Americans had one or more types of cardiovascular disease in 1998.

- Cardiovascular disease claimed 949,000 lives in the United States in 1998.

- 41 percent of all deaths in 1998 were attributable to cardiovascular disease.

Source: *NHLBI FY 2000 Fact Book*

## *Cardiovascular Disease*

Heart-healthy behavior can prevent the development of cardiovascular disease (CVD) and reduce its severity among those who already have it. CVD includes such diseases as high blood pressure, coronary heart disease (myocardial infarction and angina pectoris), stroke, rheumatic fever/rheumatic heart disease, and congestive heart failure.

The risk factors for cardiovascular disease include high blood cholesterol, high blood pressure, overweight, obesity, diabetes, smoking, and physical inactivity. These factors do not just add up in a simple manner. Instead, each one multiplies the effects of the other risk factors. For example, if you smoke and have high blood pressure and high blood cholesterol, you're eight times more likely to develop coronary heart disease than someone with no risk factors. The good news is that all of these risk factors, except for smoking, can be prevented or controlled by two important behaviors: heart-healthy eating and physical activity.

# Risk Factors for Heart Disease

## *High Blood Cholesterol*

High blood cholesterol plays an important part in deciding a person's chance or risk of getting coronary heart disease. The higher your blood cholesterol, the greater your risk. When you have too much cholesterol in your blood, the excess builds up on the walls of the arteries that carry blood to the heart. This buildup is called atherosclerosis, or hardening of the arteries. It narrows the arteries and can slow down or block blood flow to the heart. With less blood, the heart gets less oxygen. Without enough oxygen to the heart, there may be chest pain (angina or angina pectoris), heart attack (myocardial infarction), or death. Cholesterol buildup is the most common cause of heart disease, but it happens so slowly that people are not aware of it. Blood cholesterol level is influenced by many factors.

These include:

- Diet
- Level of physical activity
- Age
- Weight
- Heredity
- Gender

## *High Blood Pressure*

High blood pressure, also called hypertension, is a risk factor for heart and kidney diseases and stroke. Blood is carried from the heart to all of the body's tissues and organs in vessels called arteries. Blood pressure is the force of the blood pushing against the walls of arteries. Each time the heart beats (about 60-70 times a minute at rest), it pumps blood into the arteries. Some people have blood pressure that stays high all or most of the time. Their blood pushes against the walls of their arteries with higher-than-normal force. If untreated, this can lead to serious medical problems like atherosclerosis, heart attack, enlarged heart, kidney damage, and stroke. High blood pressure is influenced by several factors. These include:

- Diet
- Physical activity
- Family history

- Weight
- Alcohol consumption
- Ethnicity

## Diabetes

Diabetes is a disorder of metabolism—the way our bodies use digested food for growth and energy. Most of the food we eat is broken down into a simple sugar called glucose, which is the main source of fuel for the body. For the glucose to get into the body's cells, insulin must be present. In people with diabetes the body produces little or no insulin, or the cells do not respond to the insulin that is produced. As a result, glucose builds up in the blood, overflows into the urine, and passes out of the body. Thus, the body loses its main source of fuel, even though the blood contains large amounts of glucose.

Diabetes is widely recognized as one of the leading causes of death and disability in the United States. Diabetes is associated with long-term complications that affect almost every major organ of the body. It contributes to blindness, heart disease, strokes, kidney failure, amputations, and nerve damage. Diabetes is not contagious. People cannot catch it from each other. However, certain factors can increase one's risk of developing diabetes. People at risk for diabetes include:

- Those with family members who have diabetes (especially type 2 diabetes)
- Those who are overweight
- Those who are African-American, Hispanic, or Native American

## Overweight and Obesity

Over the past four decades, the number of overweight children, adolescents, and adults has risen. In 1998, a little over one-half of all American adults (about 97 million) and one in five children over the age of 6 were considered overweight or obese, levels unmatched in our nation's history. In 1995, the costs attributed to obesity alone amounted to an estimated $99 billion.

Being overweight or obese puts someone at risk for developing many problems, such as heart disease, stroke, diabetes, cancer, gallbladder disease, arthritis, sleep apnea, and breathing problems. Losing weight helps to prevent and control these diseases and conditions. Obesity is a complex, chronic disease that develops from an interaction

118

of genetics and the environment. Our understanding of how and why obesity develops is incomplete, but involves the integration of social, behavioral, cultural, physiological, metabolic, and genetic factors. Assessment and classification of overweight and obesity uses three key measures:

- Body mass index (BMI)
- Waist circumference
- Risk factors for diseases and conditions associated with obesity.

## Smoking

Smoking is a major risk factor in four of the five leading causes of death, including heart disease, stroke, cancer, and lung diseases like emphysema and bronchitis. For adults 60 and over, smoking is a major risk factor for 6 of the top 14 causes of death. The good news is that stopping smoking reduces these risks and improves outcomes for people who have suffered a heart attack. In some cases, ex-smokers can cut their risk of another heart attack by half or more.

## Physical Inactivity

Physical inactivity increases the risk of heart disease. It contributes directly to heart-related problems and increases the chances of developing other conditions that raise heart disease risk, such as high blood pressure and diabetes. Unfortunately, too few Americans are active enough. Consider:

- About 40 percent of Americans age 18 or older reported no leisure-time physical activity in 1997.

- About 23 percent of U.S. adults engaged in regular vigorous physical activity 3 times a week for at least 20 minutes in 1997.

- Less-active, less-fit persons have a 30-50 percent greater risk of developing high blood pressure.

But the good news is that regular physical activity can help reduce the risk of coronary heart disease. Staying active helps take off extra pounds, helps to control blood pressure, boosts the level of good HDL-cholesterol, helps to prevent diabetes, and helps to prevent heart attacks. For those who have heart disease, regular, moderate physical activity lowers the risk of death from heart-related causes. Physical

119

activity has many other benefits. It strengthens the lungs, tones the muscles, keep the joints in good condition, maintains bone density, improves balance, and helps prevent and treat depression. Many people find that physical activity helps them cope better with stress and anxiety.

To reap benefits from physical activity, you don't need to train for a marathon. You need to engage in only about 30 minutes of moderate-level activity on most—and preferably all—days. A moderate-level activity is one that's about as demanding as brisk walking.

**Table 10.1.** Children and Heart Disease

The evidence shows that the atherosclerotic process begins in childhood and that many American children have risk factors for coronary heart disease. A report card on the state of the cardiovascular health of America's children revealed:

| Health factor | Status |
| --- | --- |
| High Blood Cholesterol | Average blood cholesterol levels in American children and adolescents are too high. Children and adolescents with elevated blood cholesterol levels are more likely to have elevated levels as adults. Research shows that atherosclerosis develops in the late teenage years, and cholesterol levels in young adults predict the risk of coronary disease over the next 40 years. |
| Overweight | Nearly 14 percent of children and 11.5 percent of adolescents are overweight (NHANES III), more than double the percentage of a decade ago. Up to 20 percent of overweight children remain so throughout life. One in five children over the age of 6 is considered overweight, and overweight or obesity acquired during childhood or adolescence may persist into adulthood and increase the risk for some chronic diseases later in life. |
| Physical Activity | Most children accumulate at least 1 hour of activity daily, but a sizable percentage do not get frequent, vigorous, continuous activity. Of high school students, about 70 percent of boys and 55 percent of girls do a vigorous physical activity three or more times per week. Activity levels of girls are below those of boys and tend to decline with age. |

# Section 10.2

# *Heart Disease and Stroke in Women*

"Heart Disease and Stroke in Women," Fact Sheet,
Office on Women's Health, Health and Human
Services (HHS), 1999.

## The Issue

Heart disease and stroke are major health problems for women. Heart disease alone is the leading cause of death among women. One in 10 American women age 45 to 64 years has some degree or type of heart disease; the incidence of heart disease increases to one in five in women older than age 65 years. Stroke is the third leading cause of death in the United States. More than 1 million women in the United States have had a stroke, and each year 90,000 women die of stroke.

## The Facts

Both heart disease and stroke are known as cardiovascular diseases, which are disorders of the heart and blood vessels. Heart disease affects the heart muscle. When an artery (in the heart) becomes blocked, oxygen and nutrients are prevented from getting to the heart, and/or the blood supply is interrupted suddenly or for a long time, muscle cells suffer irreversible injury and die. This is known as a heart attack.

### *Warning Signs of a Heart Attack*

- Uncomfortable pressure, fullness, squeezing, or pain in the center of the chest that lasts for more than a few minutes, numbness or tingling in the left arm.

- Pain that may spread to the shoulders, neck, or arms.

- Indigestion, sweating, nausea, shortness of breath, lightheadedness, fainting, or fatigue.

121

Not all of these symptoms occur before or during a heart attack, especially for women. Likewise, they can be either mild or severe and can subside and then return. Frequently, women mistake pain signaling a heart attack as indigestion.

A stroke occurs when an artery bringing blood to the brain either becomes clogged or ruptures, and a part of the brain is deprived of the oxygen it needs. Without oxygen, nerve cells in the affected area of the brain are unable to function and then die within minutes. This results in loss of function in the part of the body controlled by these cells.

### Symptoms of a Stroke

- Sudden weakness or numbness of parts of one side of the body usually the face, arm, or leg.

- Sudden dimness or loss of vision, particularly in one eye.

- Loss of speech, or trouble talking or understanding speech.

- Sudden, severe headaches with no known cause.

- Unexplained dizziness, unsteadiness, or sudden falls.

Not all of these symptoms occur during a stroke. Symptoms depend on the location and amount of damaged cells.

## Major Risk Factors

Certain risk factors increase the chance of developing heart disease and stroke. As the number of risk factors increases, the more likely the chance of developing cardiovascular disease. They include lifestyle habits, family history, and certain personal characteristics such as:

**Cigarette/Tobacco Smoke:** Women who smoke are twice as likely to have heart disease as nonsmoking women. Women who smoke while using oral contraceptives have an even higher risk of heart attacks.

There is no safe way to smoke. Although low-tar and low-nicotine cigarettes may reduce lung cancer risk somewhat, they do not lessen the risks of heart diseases and other smoking-related diseases. Smoking also increases the risk of stroke.

**High Blood Cholesterol:** Today, about one-fifth of American women have blood cholesterol levels high enough to pose a serious risk for coronary heart disease. Cholesterol levels tend to rise sharply beginning at about age 40 years and continue to increase until about age 60 years. As a woman's blood cholesterol level increases, so does her heart disease risk.

**High Blood Pressure:** High blood pressure, also known as hypertension, is another major risk factor for heart disease and the most important risk factor for stroke. High blood pressure is called the silent killer because most people who have it do not feel sick. It usually has no specific symptoms or early warning signs. When hypertension is present, the heart works harder; over time, the heart enlarges and weakens.

Blood pressure is the result of two forces—one created by the heart as it pumps blood into the arteries. The other is the force of the arteries as they resist the blood flow. A blood pressure reading is in two measurements, given as a fraction such as 120/80. The first, systolic pressure, is the highest pressure in the arteries when your heart beats. The second, diastolic pressure, is the lowest pressure of the blood flow as your heart rests between beats. High blood pressure is defined as readings of 140/90 or greater that stay high over an extended time.

About 24 percent of women age 20 years and older have high blood pressure. Women are at an even greater risk after menopause because older women have a higher risk of developing high blood pressure. More than one-half of all women older than 55 years suffer from this condition. High blood pressure is more prevalent and more severe in black women than in white women.

## Other Risk Factors

**Family History:** If family members have had heart disease, a woman is more likely to develop it. Race is also a factor. African-Americans have a greater risk of heart disease than white Americans—in large part because they have higher average blood pressure levels.

**Physical Inactivity:** Numerous studies have shown that a lack of physical activity is a major risk factor for heart disease. Heart disease is almost twice as likely to develop in inactive people than in those who are more physically active.

**Obesity:** Excess body weight in women is linked with heart disease, stroke, and death from other heart-related causes. As a woman becomes more overweight, her risk for heart disease increases. Individuals who are overweight are more likely to develop heart disease and stroke even if they have no other risk factors. Excess weight contributes not only to cardiovascular disease but also to other conditions, including high blood pressure, high blood cholesterol, and adult-onset diabetes.

Apple-shaped individuals with extra fat at the waistline may have a higher risk than pear-shaped people with heavy hips and thighs. If a woman's waist is nearly as large, or larger, than the size of her hips, she may have a higher risk for heart disease.

Nearly 50 percent of African-American women, more than 48 percent of Mexican-American women, and more than 32 percent of white women are overweight.

**Diabetes:** Diabetes, or high blood sugar, is a serious disorder that raises the risk of heart disease. The risk of death from heart disease is about three times higher in women with diabetes. Diabetes is often called a woman's disease because after age 45 years, about twice as many women as men develop diabetes. Diabetes is present 1.4 to 2.3 times more frequently in blacks than whites, particularly among women. Although there is no cure for this disorder, there are steps a person can take to control it.

**Oral Contraceptives:** Women who use high-dose birth control pills are more likely to have a heart attack or a stroke because blood clots are more likely to form in blood vessels. These risks are lessened once the use of birth control pills is stopped. The risks of using low-dose birth control pills are not fully known.

**Menopause:** Although women of all ages are at risk for heart disease and stroke, the incidence of heart disease is more prevalent among women older than age 55 years. Scientists believe that the loss of estrogen in the body after menopause may contribute to developing heart disease.

## Additional Information

### Office on Women's Health
8550 Arlington Blvd., Suite 300
Fairfax, VA 22301
Toll-Free: 800-994-9662
TTD: 800-220-5446
Website: www.4women.gov

*National Heart, Lung, and Blood Institute*
P.O. Box 30105
Bethesda, MD 20824-0105
Tel: 301-592-8573
Fax: 301-592-8563
Website: www.nhlbi.nih.gov/index.htm
E-mail: NHLBIinfo@rover.nhlbi.nih.gov

## Section 10.3

# *Postmenopausal Hormone Therapy and Stroke Risk*

"Postmenopausal Hormone Therapy: Information for
the Public," National Heart, Lung, and Blood
Institute (NHLBI), 2002.

## What is the purpose of the WHI study on combination hormone therapy?

The long-term studies in the Women's Health Initiative (WHI) were initiated because over the years a number of research studies presented a complicated picture of the risks and benefits of hormone therapy, and its continued use for prevention of cardiovascular diseases was controversial. This situation led the NIH to conduct a large clinical trial of the risks and benefits of hormone therapy. The WHI set out to examine the long-term effect of estrogen plus progestin on the prevention of heart disease and hip fractures, while monitoring for possible increases in risk for breast and colon cancer. The estrogen plus progestin regimen was given to women who have a uterus since progestin is known to protect against endometrial cancer, a known effect of unopposed estrogen. A separate study of estrogen alone in women who had a hysterectomy was also begun.

### Why were the women in the WHI estrogen plus progestin study told to stop study pills at this time?

In its most recent review of the study data, the WHI Data and Safety Monitoring Board saw an increased risk of breast cancer in women taking estrogen plus progestin. The Board also saw that the previously identified risks for heart attacks, strokes, and blood clots to the lungs and legs had persisted. Therefore, in the judgment of the Board, the overall risks outweighed the benefits of taking estrogen plus progestin.

### What were the main findings in the WHI study on estrogen plus progestin?

The main findings show that compared to women taking placebo pills:

- The number of women who developed breast cancer was higher in women taking estrogen plus progestin.

- The numbers of women who developed heart attacks, strokes, or blood clots in the lungs and legs were higher in women taking estrogen plus progestin.

- The numbers of women who had hip and other fractures or colorectal cancer were lower in women taking estrogen plus progestin.

- There were no differences in the number of women who had endometrial cancer (cancer of the lining of the uterus) or in the number of deaths.

### What are the increased risks for women taking estrogen plus progestin?

For every 10,000 women taking estrogen plus progestin pills:

- 38 developed breast cancer each year compared to 30 breast cancers for every 10,000 women taking placebo pills each year.

- 37 had a heart attack compared to 30 out of every 10,000 women taking placebo pills.

- 29 had a stroke each year, compared to 21 out of every 10,000 women taking placebo pills.

- 34 had blood clots in the lungs or legs, compared to 16 women out of every 10,000 women taking placebo pills.

## *What are the reduced risks for women taking estrogen plus progestin?*

For every 10,000 women taking estrogen plus progestin pills:

- 10 had a hip fracture each year, compared to 15 out of every 10,000 women taking placebo pills each year.

- 10 developed colon cancer each year, compared to 16 out of every 10,000 women taking placebo pills.

## *What are the conclusions from these findings?*

The main conclusions are:

- The estrogen plus progestin combination studied in WHI does not prevent heart disease.

- For women taking this estrogen plus progestin combination, the risks (increased breast cancer, heart attacks, strokes, and blood clots in the lungs and legs) outweigh the benefits (fewer hip fractures and colon cancers).

## *What were the actual hormones that women in the estrogen plus progestin study were taking?*

Women who were randomized to receive active hormones were taking conjugated equine estrogens 0.625 mg each day and medroxyprogesterone acetate 2.5 mg each day. This is the most commonly prescribed postmenopausal hormone therapy in the United States for women who have a uterus (used each day by more than six million women).

## *How does this new information affect women in the WHI study of estrogen alone?*

The Data and Safety Monitoring Board of the WHI will be reviewing the information about the risks for ovarian cancer and provide their input to the NIH. The NIH will also send letters to the study investigators updating them with information which they can discuss with study participants.

### Do you have recommendations about other hormone alternatives (lower-dose estrogens, micronized progesterone, natural hormones)?

We cannot make specific recommendations about other hormone medications, such as different estrogens or progestins. We also cannot make recommendations about hormones women take in lower dosages or in different ways, such as patches instead of pills. Further, without scientific clinical trial data, one cannot assume that alternative estrogen plus progestin treatments are any safer than those studied in WHI.

### I am taking prescription hormones, what should I do?

We recommend that you talk with your health care provider about your individual health risk profile and the hormones you are currently taking.

### Does this new information apply to selective estrogen receptor modulators (SERMS) or phytoestrogens?

These preparations were not studied in the WHI Hormone Program, and therefore, we cannot make any conclusions about the risks or benefits of SERMs, such as raloxifene (Evista®), tamoxifen (Nolvadex®), or phytoestrogens.

### How does all of this new information affect my decision to use HRT for relief from hot flashes, sleep problems, and mood swings?

The WHI and the observational studies on the risk of ovarian cancer were long-term studies which were not meant to address the shorter-term use of HRT. Thus, the information from these studies should be used by women considering use of HRT for longer than 3 or 4 years.

Chapter 11

# Stroke May Be Caused by Diabetes

## Diabetes Mellitus: A Major Risk Factor for Cardiovascular Disease

Diabetes mellitus has long been recognized as an independent risk factor for several forms of cardiovascular disease in both men and women (e.g., coronary heart disease (CHD), stroke, peripheral arterial disease, cardiomyopathy, and congestive heart failure). Indeed, cardiovascular complications are now the leading causes of illness and death in the diabetic patient.

Type 2 diabetes, the most common form of the disease, affects approximately 90 percent of the 10.3 million Americans diagnosed with diabetes. An additional 5.4 million persons also are estimated to have type 2 diabetes but remain undiagnosed. Rates of diabetes and milder forms of glucose abnormalities are increasing in the U.S. Above age

This chapter includes "Diabetes Mellitus: A Major Risk Factor for Cardiovascular Disease," Statement from Dr. Claude Lenfant, Director, National Heart, Lung, and Blood Institute, and Dr. Phillip Gorden, Director, National Institute of Diabetes and Digestive and Kidney Diseases, *Word on Health*, Press Release, October 1999, National Heart, Lung, and Blood Institute (NHLBI); "Diabetes—A Growing Public Health Concern," by Carol Lewis, *FDA Consumer*, January-February 2002; "A 'Touch' of Diabetes?" by Christopher D. Saudek, M.D., The Last Word (Opinion), January-February 2002, *FDA Consumer*, U.S. Food and Drug Administration; and "Another Reason to Avoid a Sugar High: Study Links High Blood Sugar to Mortality after Stroke," Friday, August 23, 2002, by Tania Zeigler, National Institute of Neurological Disease and Stroke (NINDS).

65 years, almost half of Americans have abnormal glucose levels. Type 2 diabetes most often occurs in overweight or obese adults after the age of 30 and typically is preceded by insulin resistance, which also is related to coronary heart disease. Factors that contribute to insulin resistance and type 2 diabetes are genetics, obesity, physical inactivity, and advancing age, all of which are also the major predisposing risk factors for cardiovascular disease.

The increasing prevalence of type 2 diabetes is related to a variety of factors, many of which also are associated with an increased risk of CVD. These factors include: the rising prevalence of obesity in the United States (an estimated 97 million American adults are overweight or obese); the relatively low levels of physical activity among American adults (approximately 25 percent of adult Americans engage in regular physical activity of any intensity); increasing age of the population; the rapid growth in the United States of populations that are particularly susceptible to type 2 diabetes—African-Americans, Hispanics, Native Americans, Pacific Islanders, and Asians; and improved medical care which prolongs life, thus increasing the risk for development of type 2 diabetes and its CVD complications.

NHLBI and NIDDK emphasize that both CVD and type 2 diabetes may be prevented or at least postponed by lifestyle changes that maintain normal weight and physical activity. Thus, modification of life habits is at the heart of the public health strategy for reducing rates of type 2 diabetes and its cardiovascular complications.

Drug therapy may be required to control diabetes and CVD risk factors, especially when diet and exercise are not sufficient. Highly effective medications are now available to control high levels of blood sugar, blood pressure, and cholesterol. In recent years, several new drugs have been introduced that can lead to greatly improved control of diabetes and CVD risk factors. Unfortunately, many patients with type 2 diabetes still have high levels of these risk factors and efforts are necessary to get health providers and patients to improve risk factor control.

Much of what we know about the cardiovascular complications of diabetes—and how they can be prevented or treated—has come from studies supported by NHLBI and NIDDK. In fact, in recent years these NIH institutes have substantially increased research in this area.

Surveys show that physicians often are not emphasizing approaches to reduce the risk of cardiovascular disease in their patients with diabetes.

# Diabetes: A Growing Public Health Concern

## *Either You Have It or You Don't*

That's the message that the American Diabetes Association (ADA) is driving home to millions of people who believe they may be "borderline diabetic," or that their "sugar is just a bit high." Convenient phrases and stereotypes such as these don't adequately describe one of the nation's leading causes of death and disability. In fact, they tend to only minimize problems associated with the disease. The bottom line? An accurate diagnosis is essential, because while a person can live a long and healthy life with diabetes, ignoring it or not taking it seriously can be deadly.

"It's crucial to know when you have diabetes, to hear the diagnosis, and to pay attention to it," says ADA president Christopher D. Saudek, M.D. Saudek, who also heads up the diabetes center at Johns Hopkins University School of Medicine in Baltimore, says he's seen people deny their diabetes "almost to the point of death."

Diabetes mellitus is a chronic disease in which the pancreas produces too little or no insulin, impairing the body's ability to turn sugar into usable energy. Doctors often use the full name diabetes mellitus, rather than diabetes alone, to distinguish this disorder from diabetes insipidus—a different disease altogether that is characterized by excess urination, but is unrelated to blood sugar.

The number of people diagnosed with diabetes has increased more than six-fold from 1.6 million in 1958 to 10 million in 1997, according to the Centers for Disease Control and Prevention (CDC) in Atlanta. Today, some 16 million people have the disease—making it a leading cause of death in the United States—yet 5 million don't know they have it. And nearly 800,000 new cases of diabetes are diagnosed each year.

There is no cure for the disease, and the resulting health complications from poorly controlled diabetes are what make it so frightening. Consistently high blood sugar levels can, over time, lead to blindness, kidney failure, heart disease, limb amputations, and nerve damage. In fact, diabetes is the leading cause of new cases of blindness in adults between the ages of 20 and 74, and it accounts for 40 percent of people who have kidney failure. Cardiovascular disease is 2 to 4 times more common among people with diabetes, and is the leading cause of diabetes-related deaths. The risk of stroke is also 2 to 4 times higher in people with diabetes, and 60 percent to 65 percent have high blood pressure.

Despite these numbers, Saudek says diabetes can be very well-managed and that people can expect to live full and productive lives. Much of the treatment, however, depends largely on self-care practices. It's important, Saudek says, not only to target good behaviors, but also to consistently follow through with them.

Monitoring blood sugar levels is a key component in treatment and management of the disease. Research has indicated that people who keep their blood sugar levels within individual target ranges set by their doctor stand a good chance of reducing the risk of complications from diabetes. Moreover, in many cases intensive lifestyle changes in diet and exercise actually can prevent, reduce, or delay the risk of developing one type of the disease.

## Understanding Diabetes

Blood sugar, or blood glucose, refers to the amount of sugar in the blood. The brain's only food is glucose; therefore, blood sugar must be maintained at a certain level for the brain to function normally. After eating any meal that contains carbohydrate or protein, a person's blood sugar normally rises, often to between 120 and 130 milligrams per deciliter (mg/dL), but generally not above 140 mg/dL. Every day, every hour, blood sugar levels vary, even in people who don't have diabetes.

If the blood sugar level drops too low (hypoglycemia), a person's ability to reason can become impaired. When the blood sugar levels are too high (hyperglycemia), diabetes is diagnosed. Often the diagnosis is obvious to doctors because symptoms such as thirst, fatigue, weight loss, frequent urination, and persistent vaginal infections in women are evident. In the presence of these symptoms, diabetes can be confirmed by a random test of blood sugar, meaning that the blood is drawn at any time during the day, rather than specifically before eating breakfast. If the person is thirsty and urinating large amounts, the blood sugar usually will be well over 200 mg/dL, sometimes up in the 300s and 400s, or higher.

But when the classic symptoms are not present, the criteria for diagnosing diabetes include a fasting blood glucose test. This means that the blood glucose is drawn at least 10 hours following a meal early in the morning, when it is usually at its lowest point in the day. A random blood glucose higher than 200 mg/dL and a fasting glucose of 125 mg/dL or more confirms a diagnosis of diabetes.

To understand diabetes it's important to know something about insulin. Insulin is a hormone made in the pancreas, a large, elongated gland located behind the stomach. Its purpose is to unlock the cells of the body so that glucose carried by the blood can be used for energy. When you eat carbohydrates, your blood sugar rises. This increase triggers a release of insulin from cells in the pancreas called beta cells. The insulin opens the doors of the cells throughout the body to glucose. As glucose enters the cells, the blood sugar level falls back to normal—and the release of insulin ebbs until the next time protein or carbohydrates are eaten. The basic problem in type 1 diabetes is that the pancreas quits making insulin. In type 2, it either doesn't make enough or something interferes with the action of the insulin that is made. Someone with type 1 diabetes must inject replacement insulin to stay alive. Blood sugar levels in type 2 diabetes usually are controlled by drugs that lower blood sugar as well as diet and exercise. Sometimes, injections of replacement insulin are needed to maintain normal blood sugars. The increasing emphasis on the importance of reducing weight and other lifestyle changes, combined with the latest advances in medical therapies, all have had dramatic effects on diabetes control.

While it is fairly easy to diagnose, determining what type of diabetes a person has can be both challenging and critical. An accurate diagnosis matters because there are different ways to treat the different types of diabetes in order to stave off potential long-term complications.

## *Type 1 Diabetes*

People with type 1 diabetes, such as 56-year-old Paul Keister of Arlington, Va., must inject replacement insulin to control the levels of glucose in their blood. Frequent tests (several times a day) using blood obtained from finger pricks are required to maintain good blood sugar control.

In type 1 diabetes, the beta cells of the pancreas are destroyed by the body's immune system, which is responsible for recognizing and destroying outside invaders such as viruses or bacteria.

In a process that is not well-understood, the body begins to think that its own pancreatic beta cells are foreign and sets off an autoimmune response that ends up destroying the cells. As a result, no insulin can be produced.

Type 1 diabetes accounts for 5 percent to 10 percent of all people with the disease. This type is sometimes called juvenile diabetes because it most commonly appears initially in children or adolescents. However, people older than 30 also may develop the condition.

133

Scientists believe that some environmental factor—possibly a viral infection or something related to nutrition—causes the immune system to destroy the insulin-producing cells. At 30 years old, Keister was diagnosed with type 1 diabetes following a stomach illness and after a stubborn tooth infection refused to go away.

The resulting insulin deficiency is usually severe. Without injections of enough insulin to control increases in the blood sugar, diabetic ketoacidosis (coma and potentially death) can result. Today, type 1 diabetes is treatable, and ketoacidosis preventable by taking sufficient amounts of insulin and by following dietary guidelines set by doctors and the ADA.

## Type 2 Diabetes

Type 2 diabetes accounts for more than 90 percent of cases in the United States. In this type, the pancreas continues to produce insulin; however, the body develops resistance to its effects, resulting in a different kind of insulin deficiency than in type 1. Although the blood sugar rises in type 2 diabetes for different reasons than in type 1, the symptoms and potential complications are similar.

Certain racial and ethnic groups, including African-Americans, American Indians, Mexican-Americans, and other Hispanics, are at increased risk for getting the disease. And obesity is a risk factor for type 2 diabetes. Although doctors don't know exactly why, they say it's clear that the muscle cells (where most of the sugar breakdown occurs) of obese people are far less responsive to insulin than are muscle cells of thinner people. An obese person's pancreas has to put out large amounts of insulin to keep blood sugars normal. The likelihood of developing type 2 diabetes in people who are at risk increases with age and weight gain.

The typical person with type 2 diabetes is older, overweight, and often has a family history of diabetes. Dale Driscoll of Frederick, MD, was diagnosed with type 2 diabetes at about the same age that Paul Keister was diagnosed with type 1—an indication that age alone is not a reliable diagnostic criterion. And there is little evidence to suggest that diabetes runs in Driscoll's family.

It's important, says Saudek, to know that some people don't fit neatly into either of these diagnostic boxes. Like Driscoll, none of Keister's relatives on either parent's side has ever had diabetes, even though type 1 occurs in people with a genetic susceptibility. There are exceptions to the general rule that diabetes occurring in the young is type 1, and that diabetes occurring in older people is type 2. Likewise, taking insulin does not mean you have type 1 diabetes, just as obesity is not a sure diagnostic sign of type 2.

Type 2 diabetes is nearing epidemic proportions in the United States, according to diabetes experts, due to an increased number of older Americans and a greater prevalence of obesity and sedentary lifestyles.

### *Gestational Diabetes*

Between 3 percent and 5 percent of pregnant women in the United States develop gestational diabetes—elevated blood sugar due to certain hormones that occurs only during pregnancy. It is important to diagnose and treat gestational diabetes properly because it increases the risk of a baby growing larger than he or she would have been, and a large baby may have difficulty during delivery, or may be born by cesarean section.

Keeping blood sugar within a normal range during the pregnancy reduces these risks. Women who experience gestational diabetes have a greater risk of developing diabetes later in life. One large study found that more than half of women who had gestational diabetes eventually developed type 2 diabetes.

### *Controlling Diabetes—Treatment Goals*

Daily monitoring and careful control of blood sugar levels are the most important steps that people with diabetes can take, says David G. Orloff, M.D., director of the FDA's division of metabolic and endocrine drugs. Over the past decade, tight control of blood sugar with a goal of achieving and maintaining near-normal levels has become the standard of care for both type 1 and type 2 diabetes. Maintaining normal levels is difficult, Orloff says, "but good glycemic control is key to preventing long-term complications." Another reason for good blood sugar control, Orloff adds, "is that it does make a difference in how people feel."

Joanna K. Zawadzki, M.D., of the FDA's metabolic and endocrine drugs division, cautions that "just having a blood glucose monitor is not adequate follow-up to your diabetic treatment." People need better blood sugar control than just enough to avoid symptoms, she says. Keeping blood sugars always between 150 mg/dL and 200 mg/dL, for instance, may help a person avoid obvious symptoms, but may not be good enough to avoid the long-term complications. "Diabetes treatment is a complex approach that comprises a team of professionals, the patient, his or her family, and treatment and goals agreed upon by the team." Zawadzki adds, "Work with your doctor to come up with reasonable expectations for your individual treatment plan."

People with type 1 diabetes need insulin from the time they are initially diagnosed, throughout life. Type 2 diabetes may often mean a prescribed regimen of diet and exercise in the initial phases of the disease. Frequently, however, and certainly over time, changes in diet and exercise aren't enough to keep blood sugar at near-normal levels. The next step for these people is taking a medicine that lowers the blood sugar. There are two basic kinds: insulin therapy and oral medications.

### Insulin Replacement Therapy

Before the availability of insulin, treatments for people with type 1 diabetes were unpleasant and often ineffective. A low-carbohydrate, semi-starvation diet and exercise were all doctors had to offer. People lost more and more weight, and many of them died within the first year of diagnosis. Like many scientific advances, the discovery of replacement insulin in the 1920s was nothing short of a miracle.

Insulin lowers blood sugar by both increasing the removal of glucose from the blood and reducing the production of glucose by the liver. In type 1 diabetes, since there is virtually no insulin produced by the pancreas, people need insulin all the time—more at mealtimes to cover the carbohydrates and protein eaten, and less during other times to maintain as even a level as possible. In people with type 2 diabetes, insulin injections sometimes are needed to supplement the amount produced by the pancreas.

Insulin injections are given under the skin (subcutaneously) into the fat layer, usually in the arm, thigh, or abdomen. Insulin cannot be given by mouth because it is destroyed by digestive enzymes in the stomach. Small syringes with very thin needles make the injections nearly painless. In recent years, several external insulin pumps, which deliver insulin continuously through a thin, flexible tube placed under the skin, have been developed.

There are more than 20 types of insulin available in four basic forms, each with a different time of onset and duration of action. The decision as to which insulin to choose is based on an individual's lifestyle, a physician's preference and experience, and the person's blood sugar levels. Among the criteria considered in choosing insulin are: how soon it starts working (onset), when it works the hardest (peak time), and how long it lasts in the body (duration).

## *Oral Medications*

Pills to treat diabetes—antidiabetic agents—are used only in type 2 treatment. Four general classes of drugs work in different ways to lower blood sugar. There are some risks associated with the use of these drugs. For example, sulfonylureas, which stimulate the beta cells in the pancreas to release more insulin, can be associated with severe low blood sugar levels, particularly when the person has other medical problems or is taking other medications. And in order for them to work, a person's pancreas must be making at least some insulin. That is why oral medications will not work for the treatment of type 1 diabetes.

For best results, oral medications must be taken regularly every day, not irregularly or started and stopped according to blood sugar. Since many dosages are available, a physician can change the dosage if blood sugars are running too high or too low. Many of these drugs can be used in combination with one another, but any change in their use should be done only at the direction of a health care professional.

Driscoll's doctor found that oral medications were not effective in controlling his blood sugar, and he replaced them with insulin injections. In retrospect, Driscoll says, "while the pills were easier to deal with, insulin has made the greatest difference in my life." In addition, Driscoll has shed 40 of the 100 pounds recommended by his doctor as part of his treatment plan.

## *Organ Transplants*

Pancreas transplants and kidney transplants are options for people with type 1 diabetes, if they have kidney failure (about one-third of type 1 patients). Since the 1970s, doctors have performed pancreas transplants along with kidney transplants in hopes of halting or reversing the complications of diabetes. The procedure has met with some success. Kidneys alone are transplanted to replace kidneys that have totally failed. Pancreas transplants may be done simultaneously or after kidney transplants, to try to cure diabetes. But pancreases are often not transplanted unless a kidney is also needed, says Saudek, "because the surgery is so major and the need for continuous immune suppression is more dangerous than taking insulin." Saudek adds that unavailability of transplantable kidneys and pancreases is also a factor.

A kidney transplant for people with type 1 and type 2 diabetes can restore the body's ability to perform a number of crucial functions, including filtering wastes from the blood and controlling the body's fluid and chemical balance. Receiving a new pancreas at the same time may actually improve kidney survival. In addition, a new pancreas can improve blood sugar levels to normal, or close to it.

Organ transplants aren't always successful. Besides the risk inherent in any major surgery, the body can reject the new organ days or even years after the transplant. Because of this, transplant recipients will likely need to take immunosuppressive drugs the rest of their lives. The drugs themselves carry significant health risks, such as cancer, but they work to prevent the immune system from rejecting the new organ.

Another noteworthy therapeutic intervention, and one that Keister hopes to be considered for, is a procedure called islet cell transplantation. Researchers have known for some time that transplanting these insulin-producing cells may provide a possible cure for type 1 diabetes. The process to date is still not perfected, but there is some evidence that researchers may be getting closer to their goal.

"From the biologics perspective," says Philip Noguchi, M.D., director of the FDA's division of cellular and gene therapy, "emphasis on products for diabetes is clearly experimental at this time, but potentially very promising." In islet cell transplantation, doctors extract islet cells from the pancreas of a person who has recently died and then infuse them via a catheter into the liver of the person with diabetes. The liver instead of the pancreas is the location for the transplant because it is easier and less invasive to access the large vein in the liver than a pancreatic vein, and islet cells that grow in the liver closely mimic normal insulin secretion.

Because the cells are very fragile, the procedure is fraught with problems. One of the biggest obstacles is the availability of fresh islet cells. There is a shortage of organ donors in the United States, and the supply of islet cells, like kidneys and pancreases, is limited. Another challenge is the ability to isolate the cells. It takes several donor pancreases to isolate enough islet cells for a single transplant.

Still, "when it comes to trying new treatments," says Keister, "I'm going to push the envelope." Since his diabetes was detected prior to glucose meters, Keister says the greatest contribution he can give back to society is his "participation in new trials using the latest technology to learn more about the effects of treatment on the disease."

While additional studies are underway to learn more about the long-term effects of islet cell transplantation, Noguchi says, "at the moment there are a number of well-established procedures for type 1 and type 2 diabetes that let people live normal lives."

## Prognosis

Saudek says it's a scientific fact that the outlook for people with diabetes can be excellent if the disease is well taken care of. Several major studies, including the Diabetes Control and Complications Trial Research Group, in which people with type 1 diabetes have been followed for years, compared the effects of standard and more intensive diabetes treatments on the development and progression of long-term complications. The more intensive treatments prevented or slowed diabetes complications.

So, says Saudek, "It's doable. Taking advantage of what's available puts people in the best possible position to be strong and healthy when diabetes is ultimately cured."

## Characteristics of Type 1 Diabetes

- Age of onset under 40 years old, most common in children; some older people develop this type

- Thin to normal body weight

- Quick onset with thirst, frequent urination, and weight loss symptoms developing and worsening over days to weeks

- Usually no known family history, but in rare cases there may be

- No major risk factors; risk is increased if strong family history exists

- Usually more than one shot daily of insulin treatment always needed to control diabetes

- Difficult to keep fluctuating blood sugar in ideal range

- Blood sugar is sensitive to small changes in diet, exercise, and insulin dose

- Can be caused by a combination of heredity and exposure to some factor during life that triggers autoimmune destruction of the insulin-producing beta cells in the pancreas

## Characteristics of Type 2 Diabetes

- Age of onset over 40 years old, most common in adults; some younger people develop this type

- Overweight; occasionally occurs in people of normal weight

- Usually slow onset with thirst, frequent urination, and weight loss symptoms developing over weeks to months, or even years

- Can be silent disease

- Usually runs in families

- Treatment usually begins with diet and exercise, progressing to pills, and later to insulin

- Easier to control without fluctuating blood sugar range

- Blood sugar may respond to weight loss, and/or change in diet and exercise; blood sugar may be less responsive to small changes in insulin dose

- Can be caused by combination of heredity, insulin resistance, and deficiency of the insulin-producing beta cells of the pancreas

### *Advances at a Glance*

- **GlucoWatch:** Glucose monitoring device worn like a watch; detects blood glucose levels through the skin; must be calibrated to a glucose meter; approved March 2001. Cygnus Inc., Redwood City, Calif.

- **Sof-Tact:** Semi-automated home blood glucose monitor that uses light suction vacuum to hold skin in place while integrated apparatus lances skin. Device automatically transfers small amount of blood to a biosensor strip, and blood glucose test result is delivered in 20 seconds. Eliminates need for traditional finger-stick method; can be used on forearm or upper arm; approved November 2000. Abbott Laboratories, Abbott Park, IL.

- **Continuous Glucose Monitoring System:** Continuous measure of tissue glucose levels in adults with diabetes. Records levels at five-minute intervals for up to three days; information is then downloaded on computer for review by health care practitioner; must be used in conjunction with finger-stick tests; approved June 1999. MiniMed Inc., Sylmar, CA.

- **Lasette:** Portable, battery-operated laser; means for drawing blood without using traditional lancets (small, razor-sharp devices for puncturing skin); for adults and children; approved December 1998. Cell Robotics International Inc., Albuquerque, NM.

- **Q-103 Needle Management System:** Used to remove certain hypodermic needles from insulin syringes and store them safely for later disposal; device holds up to 5000 removed needles; approved December 2000. QCare International LLC, Marietta, GA.

- **Apligraf:** Wound dressing that helps heal diabetic foot ulcers, open foot sores that can lead to amputation; approved June 2000. Organogenesis Inc., Canton, MA.

- **Dermagraft:** Skin substitute used to help in the wound closure of diabetic foot ulcers; helps replace and rebuild damaged tissue in diabetic foot ulcers; approved September 2001. Advanced Tissue Sciences, La Jolla, CA.

- **Other devices:** Over 100 glucose meters and several external insulin pumps approved in the last several years.

## A Touch of Diabetes? By Christopher D. Saudek

Christopher D. Saudek, M.D., is president of the American Diabetes Association and director of the diabetes center at the Johns Hopkins School of Medicine in Baltimore.

Sometimes, inside the health care professions and health care regulatory agencies, we hear the opinion that type 2 diabetes isn't that big a deal. It isn't cancer and it isn't AIDS. It's just a lifestyle disease. People shouldn't have let themselves get overweight. There are lots of pills available, and then there's always insulin. It is amazing how often physicians don't even bother to tell people that they have diabetes; they soften the message with euphemisms like, "We'll have to watch your sugar," or the oldest of all, "You only have a touch of diabetes."

Statistics do not support this casual attitude. Available through the American Diabetes Association's website, www.diabetes.org, the numbers are sobering: 15.7 million people have diabetes in the United States, and about 5.4 million don't even know it. Over 200,000 people will die of diabetes this year. About 15 percent of diagnosed people already have long-term complications when they are first told they have diabetes, and the mean time between onset and diagnosis is estimated to be seven years. Type 2 diabetes is the leading cause of end-stage renal disease, preventable amputations, working-age blindness, and a major cause of heart disease and stroke. It cost over $98 billion in the United States in 1997. The stats go on, and paint an ugly picture of inadequate treatment with devastating results.

But isn't diabetes easily treated? Isn't it a disease people can easily take care of, if they would only pay attention? Easily is a huge misconception. It may be easy to say, "Diet and exercise, give up on the sweets, check your numbers, know your blood pressure and cholesterol, and stop smoking, have your eyes checked, your feet, your lipids, and your A1c. Oh yes, and keep losing the weight." But have you, the reader, ever tried to take such good care of your health? Probably only if you have diabetes.

Adding things up, people with diabetes are expected to think about their disease perhaps 20 to 30 times a day, between worrying every time they eat, exercise, check their blood sugar, or take a medication.

As new medications and new technologies are developed, it is worth thinking about what they mean for the person with diabetes. The new is too often dismissed by a summary comment: "Too expensive;" "a convenience item;" "too complicated for the average patient;" "not proven to be better." These put-downs were probably used when disposable syringes replaced boiling glass syringes, when ultrafine needles replaced thick needles. (I talked with a person the other day who had found the pan her deceased mother used to boil her glass syringe). Better drugs, better meters, insulin pens and pumps translate into better self-care and fewer complications. And too complicated almost never applies: very little is too complicated for the average patient, and they need all the help they can get.

What about too complicated for the health care professional? Those of us specializing in diabetes may be able to keep the medication options and the monitoring guidelines reasonably straight in our minds. But when diabetes is only a small part of a person's professional practice, it does present a huge challenge. In my opinion, the best thing to come along in the treatment of diabetes is the Certified Diabetes Educator, or CDE. It is a whole profession of people trained and certified in helping people with diabetes take care of themselves. People with diabetes and physicians who care for them should take advantage of the CDE.

So if diabetes is so complicated, so difficult to manage for the patient and health care professional alike, is there any point trying? The evidence all points to a resounding "Yes." Large, definitive clinical trials such as the Diabetes Control and Complications Trial and the United Kingdom Prospective Diabetes Study have proven conclusively that not only do blood glucose control and control of other risk factors matter, but they are achievable.

I believe, therefore, that it is up to us in the health care professions and the health segment of the government to keep pushing the medications and the technologies forward. A safe, reliable pill to help people lose weight, regardless of whether it independently affects blood glucose, would have an enormous effect in controlling diabetes, since obesity-related insulin resistance is the major underlying cause of type 2 diabetes. Thousands of people with diabetes will benefit from any new medication that some people will respond well to, that has fewer side effects, or that will keep some people off insulin for a while longer. Dramatic advances like continuous or non-invasive blood glucose monitoring will come gradually and incrementally.

It must always be remembered that the cost of diabetes is in the complications and in the personal toll it takes. The incremental expense of new drugs and new technologies makes up a relatively small part of the total cost of diabetes. We therefore have to continue the progress in making safe, effective drugs and devices available until treatment is as easy as taking an aspirin a day.

## Another Reason to Avoid a Sugar High: Study Links High Blood Sugar to Mortality after Stroke

Stroke has long been regarded as an untreatable condition with potentially devastating consequences. But in recent years, new treatments have markedly improved patients' ability to recover from stroke, and researchers now have a new clue about how to further improve stroke treatment.

A study published in the July 9, 2002, issue of the journal *Neurology* shows that stroke victims who have high blood sugar have a higher risk of dying than stroke patients with normal blood sugar levels. The researchers reviewed 5 years of medical records from 656 adults who were hospitalized because of a stroke. More than 40 percent of those patients had abnormally high blood sugar levels when they were admitted to the hospital.

Patients were studied from 1 to 5 years after their strokes, depending on availability of hospital records. Those with high blood sugar (glucose) when they were admitted to the hospital were at higher risk of dying within 30 days, 1 year, or 5 years after their stroke. They also had longer hospital stays and higher hospital costs than patients with normal blood sugar levels.

Although most of the patients had a previous history of diabetes, their blood sugar levels were not under control and often were not managed during hospitalization. Study author Askiel Bruno, M.D., associate professor of neurology at Indiana University (IU) School of Medicine, says finding high glucose levels, or hyperglycemia, in stroke patients was not surprising. "Glucose levels tend to rise during acute stress, especially in people with diabetes," says Bruno.

What was surprising, says co-author Linda Williams, M.D., assistant professor of neurology at IU, was that blood sugar levels remained high in about 90 percent of the patients. When blood glucose levels rise, a substance called lactic acid begins to build up in various tissues, including the brain. When there is insufficient blood flow, as in stroke, this acid build-up accelerates a series of reactions that cause cell death following a stroke. With the incidence of diabetes on the rise, this link between high blood sugar and death after stroke suggests that glucose management with insulin needs to be an important part of inpatient care after stroke.

It's possible that patients with one poorly controlled risk factor may also have other poorly controlled risk factors for stroke, says Dr. Williams. Hyperglycemia occurring with stroke also could indicate something unique about a patient's response to stress in general, she adds.

Bruno, Williams, and their colleagues have teamed up again to study the effectiveness and safety of intravenous insulin treatments for hyperglycemia beginning within 12 hours after stroke. Their goal is to see if strict control of blood sugar in the first 3 days after stroke will result in better outcomes than standard treatments. The pilot clinical trial, which is funded by the National Institute of Neurological Disorders and Stroke (NINDS), will begin in 2002 and is expected to last 3 years.

"We're very interested in reducing functional deficits after stroke, since the overwhelming majority of stroke patients become disabled in some way," says Dr. Bruno. "We hope there will be a significant difference in cognitive and motor function between the aggressive and the standard treatment groups."

If the trial is successful, managing blood sugar would likely add to the existing ammunition against stroke, such as the clot-busting drug tissue plasminogen activator (tPA), which is used to treat strokes caused by blood clots. "You can think of insulin treatment as complementary to current stroke treatments," says Dr. Bruno. However, stroke patients would still need emergency care, he adds.

While tPA, or thrombolysis, takes care of treating the clot, insulin would deal with the negative effects of high blood sugar. "If it works, it would be easier to use than some new drug, because most physicians are familiar with insulin," says Dr. Bruno. One possible risk associated with insulin treatment is hypoglycemia, or low blood sugar, but the researchers say intensive monitoring during treatments will allow them to detect rapidly dropping blood sugar levels.

## Reference

Williams LS, Rotich J, Qi R, Fineberg N, Espay A, Bruno A, Fineberg SE, and Tierney WR. "Effects of Admission Hyperglycemia on Mortality and Costs in Acute Ischemic Stroke." *Neurology*, Vol. 59, No. 1, July 9, 2002, pp. 67-71.

## Additional Information

### American Diabetes Association
Attn: Customer Service
1701 N. Beauregard St.
Alexandria, VA 22311
Toll-Free: 800-DIABETES (1-800-342-2383)
To contact your local affiliate, call toll-free: 888-DIABETES (1-888-342-2383)
Website: www.diabetes.org; E-mail: askda@diabetes.org

### National Center for Chronic Disease Prevention and Health Promotion
Centers for Disease Control and Prevention (CDC)
Division of Diabetes Translation
P.O. Box 8728
Silver Spring, MD 20910
Toll-Free: 877-CDC-DIAB (877-232-3422)
Fax: 301-562-1050
Website: www.cdc.gov/diabetes; E-mail: diabetes@cdc.gov

### Juvenile Diabetes Foundation International
120 Wall Street
New York, NY 10005
Toll-Free: 800-533-CURE (800-533-2873)
Tel: 212-785-9500; Fax: 212-785-9595
Website: www.jdfcure.org; E-mail: info@jdrf.org

### National Institute of Diabetes and Digestive and Kidney Diseases
National Diabetes Information Clearinghouse
1 Information Way
Bethesda, MD 20892
Toll-Free: 800-860-8747
Website: www.niddk.nih.gov/health/diabetes/diabetes.htm

Chapter 12

# High Blood Pressure Increases Stroke Risk

## Hypertension in the U.S.

- Percent of Americans ages 20-74 with hypertension: 23% (1988-1994).

- Hypertension is most prevalent in the black population.

- Over three-quarters of women aged 75 and over have hypertension.

- Sixty-four percent of men aged 75 and over have hypertension.

- Deaths annually: 14,308 (1998).

- Death Rate: 5 deaths per 100,000 (1998).

- In 1999, there were 32 million office visits for hypertension.

This chapter includes "Hypertension," National Center for Health Statistics (NCHS), reviewed January 28, 2002; "Your Guide to Lowering High Blood Pressure," National Heart, Lung, and Blood Institute (NHLBI); "NHLBI Study Finds High-Normal Blood Pressure Increases Cardiovascular Risk," NIH News Release October 31, 2001, National Heart, Lung, and Blood Institute; "NHLBI Study Shows Vast Majority of Middle-Aged Americans at Risk of Developing Hypertension," NIH News Release February 26, 2002, National Heart, Lung, and Blood Institute (NHLBI); "Blood Pressure Drugs Relax Heart, Reduce Heart Failure Risk," reprinted with permission from the American Heart Association World Wide Web Site, www.americanheart.org. © 2002, Copyright American Heart Association; and "Moderate Rise in Blood Pressure Linked to Drop in Thinking Skills," reprinted with permission from the American Heart Association World Wide Web Site, www.americanheart.org. © 2002, Copyright American Heart Association.

## Your Guide to Lowering High Blood Pressure

### What Is Blood Pressure?

Blood pressure is the force of blood against the walls of arteries. Blood pressure is recorded as two numbers—the systolic pressure (as the heart beats) over the diastolic pressure (as the heart relaxes between beats). The measurement is written one above or before the other, with the systolic number on top and the diastolic number on the bottom. For example, a blood pressure measurement of 120/80 mm Hg (millimeters of mercury) is expressed verbally as "120 over 80."

Normal blood pressure is less than 130 mm Hg systolic and less than 85 mm Hg diastolic. Optimal blood pressure is less than 120 mm Hg systolic and less than 80 mm Hg diastolic.

### Understanding High Blood Pressure

High blood pressure increases your chance (or risk) for getting heart disease and/or kidney disease, and for having a stroke. It is especially dangerous because it often has no warning signs or symptoms. Regardless of race, age, or gender, anyone can develop high blood pressure. It is estimated that one in every four American adults has high blood pressure. Once high blood pressure develops, it usually lasts a lifetime. You can prevent and control high blood pressure by taking action.

### What Is High Blood Pressure?

Blood pressure is the force of blood against the walls of arteries. Blood pressure rises and falls during the day. When blood pressure stays elevated over time, it is called high blood pressure or hypertension.

Blood pressure is typically recorded as two numbers—the systolic pressure (as the heart beats) over the diastolic pressure (as the heart relaxes between beats). A consistent blood pressure reading of 140/90 mm Hg or higher is considered high blood pressure, another term for hypertension.

### What Is Systolic Blood Pressure?

Systolic pressure is the force of blood in the arteries as the heart beats. It is shown as the top number in a blood pressure reading. High blood pressure is 140 and higher for systolic pressure. Diastolic pressure does not need to be high for you to have high blood pressure. When that happens, the condition is called "isolated systolic hypertension," or ISH.

*Is isolated systolic high blood pressure common?*

Yes. It is the most common form of high blood pressure for older Americans. For most Americans, systolic blood pressure increases with age, while diastolic increases until about age 55 and then declines. About 65 percent of hypertensives over age 60 have ISH. You may have ISH and feel fine. As with other types of high blood pressure, ISH often causes no symptoms. To find out if you have ISH—or any type of high blood pressure—see your doctor and have a blood pressure test. The test is quick and painless.

*Is isolated systolic high blood pressure dangerous?*

Any form of high blood pressure is dangerous if not properly treated. Both numbers in a blood pressure test are important, but, for some, the systolic is especially meaningful. That's because, for those persons middle-aged and older, systolic pressure gives a better diagnosis of high blood pressure.

If left uncontrolled, high systolic pressure can lead to stroke, heart attack, congestive heart failure, kidney damage, blindness, or other conditions. While it cannot be cured once it has developed, ISH can be controlled.

Clinical studies have proven that treating a high systolic pressure saves lives, greatly reduces illness, and improves the quality of life. Yet, most Americans do not have their high systolic pressure under control.

*Does it require special treatment?*

Treatment options for ISH are the same as for other types of high blood pressure, in which both systolic and diastolic pressures are high. ISH is treated with lifestyle changes and/or medications. The key for any high blood pressure treatment is to bring the condition under proper control. Blood pressure should be controlled to less than 140/90 mm Hg. If yours is not, then ask your doctor why. You may just need a lifestyle or drug change, such as reducing salt in your diet or adding a second medication.

## What Is Diastolic Blood Pressure?

Diastolic pressure is the force of blood in the arteries as the heart relaxes between beats. It's shown as the bottom number in a blood pressure reading.

The diastolic blood pressure has been and remains, especially for younger people, an important hypertension number. The higher the diastolic blood pressure the greater the risk for heart attacks, strokes, and kidney failure. As people become older, the diastolic pressure will begin to decrease and the systolic blood pressure begins to rise and becomes more important. A rise in systolic blood pressure will also increase the chance for heart attacks, strokes, and kidney failure. Your physician will use both the systolic and the diastolic blood pressure to determine your blood pressure category and appropriate prevention and treatment activities.

## Why Is High Blood Pressure Important?

High blood pressure is dangerous because it makes the heart work too hard. It also makes the walls of the arteries hard. High blood pressure increases the risk for heart disease and stroke, the first- and third-leading causes of death for Americans. High blood pressure can also cause other problems, such as heart failure, kidney disease, and blindness.

## Effect of High Blood Pressure on Your Body

### Impaired Vision

High blood pressure can eventually cause blood vessels in the eye to burst or bleed. Vision may become blurred or otherwise impaired and can result in blindness.

### Stroke

High blood pressure is the most important risk factor for stroke. Very high pressure can cause a break in a weakened blood vessel, which then bleeds in the brain. This can cause a stroke. If a blood clot blocks one of the narrowed arteries, it can also cause a stroke.

### Heart Attack

High blood pressure is a major risk factor for heart attack. The arteries bring oxygen-carrying blood to the heart muscle. If the heart cannot get enough oxygen, chest pain, also known as angina, can occur. If the flow of blood is blocked, a heart attack results.

### Congestive Heart Failure

High blood pressure is the number one risk factor for congestive heart failure (CHF). CHF is a serious condition in which the heart is unable to pump enough blood to supply the body's needs.

*Kidney Damage*

The kidneys act as filters to rid the body of wastes. Over time, high blood pressure can narrow and thicken the blood vessels of the kidneys. The kidneys filter less fluid, and waste builds up in the blood. The kidneys may fail altogether. When this happens, medical treatment (dialysis) or a kidney transplant may be needed.

*Arteries*

As people get older, arteries throughout the body harden, especially those in the heart, brain, and kidneys. High blood pressure is associated with these stiffer arteries. This, in turn, causes the heart and kidneys to work harder.

## What Causes High Blood Pressure?

The causes of high blood pressure vary. Causes may include narrowing of the arteries, a greater than normal volume of blood, or the heart beating faster or more forcefully than it should. Any of these conditions will cause increased pressure against the artery walls. High blood pressure might also be caused by another medical problem. Most of the time, the cause is not known. Although high blood pressure usually cannot be cured, in most cases it can be prevented and controlled.

## Who Can Develop High Blood Pressure?

High blood pressure is common. More than 50 million American adults—1 in 4—have high blood pressure. It is very common in African-Americans, who may get it earlier in life and more often than whites. Many Americans tend to develop high blood pressure as they get older, but this is not a part of healthy aging. About 60% of all Americans age 60 and older have high blood pressure. Others at-risk for developing high blood pressure are the overweight, those with a family history of high blood pressure, and those with high-normal blood pressure (130-139/85-89 mm Hg).

## African-Americans

High blood pressure occurs more often among African-Americans than whites. It begins at an earlier age and is usually more severe. Further, African-Americans have a higher death rate from stroke and kidney disease than whites. The good news is treatment can control high blood pressure. In addition, lifestyle changes can prevent and control high blood pressure. These include losing weight if overweight (losing 10 lbs. can help); increasing physical activity (walking 30 minutes per day can help); following a healthy eating plan that emphasizes fruits, vegetables, and low-fat dairy foods; choosing and preparing foods with less salt and sodium; and if you drink alcoholic beverages, drinking in moderation. If lifestyle changes alone are not effective in keeping your blood pressure controlled, there are many blood pressure medications to help you.

### High Blood Pressure Detection

You can find out if you have high blood pressure by having your blood pressure checked regularly. Most doctors will diagnose a person with high blood pressure on the basis of two or more readings, taken on several occasions. A consistent blood pressure reading of 140/90 mm Hg or higher is considered high blood pressure, another term for hypertension.

Some people experience high blood pressure only when they visit the doctor's office. This condition is called white-coat hypertension. If your doctor suspects this, you may be asked to monitor your blood pressure at home or asked to wear a device called an ambulatory blood pressure monitor. This device is usually worn for 24 hours and can take blood pressure every 30 minutes. In this section you will learn more about diagnosing high blood pressure.

### How Do I Know if I Have High Blood Pressure?

High blood pressure often has no signs or symptoms. The only way to find out if you have high blood pressure is to be tested for it. Using the familiar blood pressure cuff, your doctor or nurse can easily tell if your blood pressure is high.

## How Is Blood Pressure Tested?

Having your blood pressure tested is quick and easy. Blood pressure is measured in millimeters of mercury (mm Hg) and recorded as two numbers systolic pressure over diastolic pressure. For example, the doctor or nurse might say "130 over 80" as a blood pressure reading.

Both numbers in a blood pressure reading are important. As we grow older, systolic blood pressure is especially important.

To test your blood pressure, your doctor will use a familiar device with a long name. It is called a sphygmomanometer (pronounced sfig'-mo-ma-nom-e-ter). Some blood pressure testing devices use electronic instruments or digital readouts. In these cases, the blood pressure reading appears on a small screen or is signaled in beeps, and no stethoscope is used.

### *Tips for Having Your Blood Pressure Taken*

• Don't drink coffee or smoke cigarettes 30 minutes before having your blood pressure measured.

• Before the test, sit for five minutes with your back supported and your feet flat on the ground. Rest your arm on a table at the level of your heart.

**Table 12.1.** Categories for Blood Pressure Levels in Adults*
(Ages 18 Years and Older)

| Category | Blood Pressure Level (mm Hg) | |
| --- | --- | --- |
| | Systolic | Diastolic |
| Optimal** | < 120 | < 80 |
| Normal | < 130 | < 85 |
| High Normal | 130-139 | 85-89 |
| | | |
| High Blood Pressure | | |
| Stage 1 | 140-159 | 90-99 |
| Stage 2 | 160-179 | 100-109 |
| Stage 3 | ≥180 | ≥110 |

*For those not taking medicine for high blood pressure and not having a short-term serious illness. These categories are from the National High Blood Pressure Education Program.

**Optimal blood pressure with respect to heart disease risk is below 120/80 mm Hg. However, unusually low readings should be evaluated for clinical significance.

Legend
< means *less than*
≥ means *greater than or equal to*

- Wear short sleeves so your arm is exposed.

- Go to the bathroom prior to the reading. A full bladder can change your blood pressure reading.

- Get two readings, taken at least two minutes apart, and average the results.

- Ask the doctor or nurse to tell you the blood pressure reading in numbers.

When systolic and diastolic blood pressures fall into different categories, the higher category should be used to classify blood pressure level. For example, 160/80 mm Hg would be stage 2 hypertension (high blood pressure).

## What Device Can I Use to Take My Own Blood Pressure?

Tests at home can be done with the familiar blood pressure cuff and a stethoscope, or with an electronic monitor, such as a digital readout monitor. Also, be sure that the person who will use the device reads the instructions before taking blood pressure readings. Your doctor, nurse, or pharmacist can help you check the device and teach you how to use it. You also may ask for their help in choosing the right one for you. Blood pressure devices can be bought at various places, such as discount chain stores and pharmacies.

## Treatment of High Blood Pressure

It is important to take steps to keep your blood pressure under control. The treatment goal is blood pressure below 140/90 and lower for people with other conditions, such as diabetes and kidney disease. Adopting healthy lifestyle habits is an effective first step in both preventing and controlling high blood pressure. If lifestyle changes alone are not effective in keeping your pressure controlled, it may be necessary to add blood pressure medications.

# High Blood Pressure Study Results

## NHLBI Study Finds High-Normal Blood Pressure Increases Cardiovascular Risk

High-normal blood pressure significantly increases the risk of heart attack, stroke, and heart failure, according to a new study supported by the National Heart, Lung, and Blood Institute (NHLBI). The adverse effects of high-normal blood pressure held for both men and women and at all ages, although it was especially high for those age 65 and older.

The study found that those with high-normal blood pressure had a 1.5 to 2.5 times greater risk of suffering a heart attack, a stroke, or heart failure in 10 years than those with optimal blood pressure.

While earlier research had shown that high-normal blood pressure increases the risk of cardiovascular death, this study looked at the risk not only of that but also of nonfatal cardiovascular events. The findings support current clinical practice guidelines calling for lowering of high-normal blood pressure.

High-normal blood pressure is a systolic pressure of 130-139 mm Hg and/or a diastolic pressure of 85-89 mm Hg. About 13 percent of Americans have high-normal blood pressure. By contrast, about 23 percent have hypertension, which is a systolic pressure of 140 mm Hg or higher, or a diastolic pressure of 90 mm Hg or higher.

The study used data from the NHLBI-supported Framingham Heart Study, a landmark epidemiological study that began in 1948. Results appeared in the November 1, 2001, issue of the *New England Journal of Medicine.*

"This study underscores that, when it comes to blood pressure, any elevation over normal puts people at a significant cardiovascular risk," said NHLBI Director Dr. Claude Lenfant. "While more research is needed on this topic, it's advisable that high-normal blood pressure be treated." He added that, for most, treatment would consist of such lifestyle changes as following a healthy eating plan lower in saturated fat and cholesterol, choosing foods low in salt and other forms of sodium, losing extra weight, becoming physically active, and limiting alcoholic beverages.

Dr. Ramachandran Vasan, Associate Professor of Medicine at Boston University School of Medicine and a co-author of the study, agreed: "This finding is important in order to help Americans add healthy years to their life. Anyone with a high-normal blood pressure should undertake lifestyle changes to lower it to a healthier level.

"Older Americans in particular should do this," Vasan continued, "since they are especially likely to have other cardiovascular disease risk factors, such as high cholesterol and diabetes, which multiply their risk even more."

The research involved 6,859 men and women of the original Framingham Heart Study and its Offspring Study. When their initial blood pressure measurements were taken, none of the participants had cardiovascular disease or hypertension. At the outset, about a quarter of the participants had high-normal blood pressure, about a third had normal blood pressure (systolic pressure of less than 130 and diastolic pressure of less than 85 mm Hg), and about two-fifths had optimal blood pressure (systolic pressure of less than 120 mm Hg and diastolic pressure of less than 80 mm Hg).

Participants were followed for about 12 years. During that time, 397 participants had a cardiovascular event, including 72 who died from cardiovascular disease, 190 who had a heart attack, 85 who had strokes, and 50 who had congestive heart failure.

Cardiovascular events were analyzed separately for men and women for three blood pressure categories (optimal, normal, and high-normal), and for two age groups (35-64 years, and 65 years and older).

Results showed a stepwise increase in cardiovascular events across the three blood pressure categories. In women, the 10-year rates of cardiovascular events when adjusted for age differences were 1.9 percent for those with optimal blood pressure, 2.8 percent for those with normal blood pressure, and 4.4 percent for those with high-normal blood pressure. In men, the 10-year rates of cardiovascular events when adjusted for age differences were 5.8 percent for those with optimal blood pressure, 7.6 percent for those with normal blood pressure, and 10.1 percent for those with high-normal blood pressure.

The incidence of cardiovascular events also increased continuously with age. After 10 years of follow-up, the overall risk of cardiovascular disease in those age 35-64 who had high-normal blood pressure was 4 percent for women and 8 percent for men; in those age 65 or older, the overall risk was 18 percent for women and 25 percent for men.

## NHLBI Study Shows Vast Majority of Middle-Aged Americans at Risk of Developing Hypertension

Middle-aged Americans face a 90 percent chance of developing high blood pressure at some time during the rest of their lives, according to a new study supported by the National Heart, Lung, and Blood Institute (NHLBI). However, the study also had some good news for Americans: The risk of developing severe degrees of high blood pressure has decreased in the past 25 years, due partly to improved treatment.

The study, based on data from NHLBI's landmark Framingham Heart Study (FHS), appeared in the February 27, 2002, issue of the *Journal of the American Medical Association*. The National Institute of Neurological Disorders and Stroke also contributed support to the research.

"Ninety percent is a staggering statistic and cause for concern," said Health and Human Services Secretary Tommy G. Thompson. "This finding should energize Americans to take steps to protect themselves against high blood pressure. By adopting some simple healthy behaviors, most people can reduce their risk of high blood pressure. Prevention gives people the power to protect their health."

"Americans have to better understand their risk of developing high blood pressure," agreed NHLBI Director Dr. Claude Lenfant. "They cannot adopt a wait and see approach. If they do, chances are they will find themselves with high blood pressure and that puts them at increased risk for heart disease and stroke."

"Fortunately," Lenfant continued, "high blood pressure is easily diagnosed and can be prevented by adopting certain lifestyle measures—don't smoke, follow a healthy eating plan that includes foods lower in salt and sodium, maintain a healthy weight, be physically active, and if you drink alcoholic beverages, do so in moderation. For those who already have high blood pressure, it's important that they properly control it with these lifestyle measures and medication."

High blood pressure, or hypertension, is a measure of the force of blood within blood vessels. It is recorded as two numbers—the systolic (the force of the blood as the heart beats) over the diastolic (the force of the blood as the heart relaxes between beats). If either or both are high—140/90 mm Hg or above—then that is hypertension.

Lifetime risk estimates the chance that someone at a given age will develop a particular disease during his or her remaining years of life.

FHS began in 1948 with 5,209 participants who were aged 28 to 62 and without cardiovascular disease. Participants underwent medical examinations every 2 years. The current study includes 1,298 of the original participants—those who had not developed hypertension by 1975. Researchers calculated lifetime risk for two ages—55 and 65.

Additionally, the researchers compared lifetime risk from two time periods—1952-75 and 1976-98. They examined the results to see if any trends emerged in participants' risk for developing hypertension.

Calculations were based on the current U.S. life expectancies for 55- and 65-year-olds, which are 80 and 85 years, respectively. "We chose to calculate estimates for ages 55 and 65 because that's when the risk of developing hypertension dramatically increases," said Dr. Ramachandran Vasan, Associate Professor of Medicine at Boston University School of Medicine and a co-author of the study.

The investigators found that the lifetime risk of developing hypertension was about 90 percent for men and women at both ages. Further, more than half of the participants aged 55 and about two-thirds of those aged 65 went on to develop hypertension within 10 years. Both men and women had a nearly 60 percent chance of being prescribed blood pressure-lowering drugs.

Other study results include:

- Nearly 85 percent of the participants developed Stage I or greater hypertension over 20-25 years. Thirty-five to 44 percent of them went on to develop Stage II or greater hypertension.

- For women, there were no differences in lifetime risk between the earlier and later time periods. By contrast, men had a higher lifetime risk of developing hypertension during the later time period.

- Both men and women had a greater lifetime risk of receiving a hypertension medication in the more recent time period.

- The risk of developing Stage II or greater hypertension (160/100 mm Hg or higher) decreased for both men and women in the more recent time period.

"The trends over time may be due in part to an increase in obesity among the men in the study," said Vasan. "Their average body mass index rose between the two periods. Women in the study did not have such a rise in body mass index." He added that, "The decrease in the lifetime risk of developing Stage II or greater hypertension for both men and women probably resulted from an increased use of hypertension lowering drugs through the years."

Vasan cautions that the study was not ethnically diverse. He stresses that the lifetime risk of developing hypertension varies among individuals and depends on the presence of risk factors. "Americans should see their doctor and have their blood pressure checked," Vasan said. "They can talk about their risk factors and the steps they can take to reduce their risk of hypertension. Americans don't necessarily have to develop high blood pressure as they get older. What they have to do is take preventive action."

### American Heart Association Journal Reports Blood Pressure Drugs Relax Heart, Reduce Heart Failure Risk

People who take medications to lower blood pressure may also be improving their heart's pumping action, thus reducing their risk of congestive heart failure, according to research in the February 11, 2002 rapid access issue of *Circulation: Journal of the American Heart Association.*

"The new findings suggest that a year or more of treatment with antihypertensive drugs can improve the way the heart's pumping chamber fills with blood, and that improvement may prevent the development of congestive heart failure," says Kristian Wachtell, M.D., Ph.D., lead author of the study and an assistant professor of medicine at Copenhagen County University Hospital, Glostrup, Denmark.

This study marks the first time that researchers can link changes in the geometry of the left ventricle, the heart's main pumping chamber, to improved diastolic function. "That's important, because diastolic dysfunction is the cause of congestive heart failure in about 40 percent of older people," says Wachtell.

Diastolic ventricular dysfunction means that the left ventricle fails to properly fill during the relaxed or "diastolic" phase of the heart's pumping action. The thickened left ventricle is stiff, making it unable to fully relax. The result is that the left side of the heart pumps too little blood while the right side pumps normally, filling the lungs with blood, which ultimately can result in pulmonary edema and death.

High blood pressure, or hypertension, is a recognized risk factor for diastolic ventricular dysfunction. High blood pressure is defined in an adult as a systolic pressure (top number in a blood pressure reading) of 140 millimeters of mercury (mmHg) or higher and/or a diastolic pressure (bottom number) of 90 mmHg or higher.

Wachtell's group used echocardiograms to measure heart wall thickness and ventricular filling in 728 hypertensive patients with enlarged hearts. They were participating in the Losartan Intervention for Endpoint Reduction in Hypertension (LIFE) Study. Participants were randomized to receive blood pressure reducing drugs: either losartan, which is an angiotensin II receptor blocker, or atenolol, a beta-blocker. After a year, participants were examined again with an echocardiogram.

Blood pressure reductions averaged 23 mmHg systolic and 11 mmHg diastolic after a year of treatment. Heart mass was reduced by about 10 percent on average, which led to improved blood flow into the left ventricle. At baseline, 15 percent of patients had normal left ventricular filling. After one year of treatment, the prevalence of normal filling was about 26 percent.

In addition, there was improvement in the heart's ability to relax and a reduction in stiffness, which was significant among patients who had a reduction or regression in left ventricular mass, notes Wachtell.

For the patients who showed a reduction in left ventricular mass, relaxation time decreased from 116 milliseconds (ms) at baseline to 104 ms after one year of treatment.

The LIFE study is ongoing, and the investigators don't know yet which of the two antihypertensive drugs each patient is taking. For that reason, they are unable to predict if one drug is more effective than the other.

The American Heart Association estimates that 4.8 million Americans have congestive heart failure, while as many as 50 million Americans have high blood pressure.

AHA Journal Report 02/11/02, Co-authors are Jonathan N. Bella, M.D.; Jens Rokkedal, M.D.; Vittorio Palmieri, M.D.; Vasilios Papademetriou, M.D.; Björn Dahlöf, M.D., Ph.D.; Tapio Aalto, M.D.; Eva Gerdts, M.D., Ph.D.; and Richard B. Devereux, M.D.

## *American Heart Association Study Indicates Moderate Rise in Blood Pressure Linked to Drop in Thinking Skills*

Mild to moderate high blood pressure seems to slow thinking skills in older people, researchers reported December 14, 2000 in *Hypertension: Journal of the American Heart Association.*

This study indicates that people should view moderately high blood pressure more seriously, says Gary A. Ford, M.D., professor of pharmacology at the Institute for the Health of the Elderly at the University of Newcastle Upon Tyne, United Kingdom. "Our work suggests that the effects of mild to moderate high blood pressure on cognitive function should be explored."

"A lot of older people are not well treated for this condition and the effects appear to be more serious than previously thought. In nearly every aspect of cognitive function we studied, the people with high blood pressure performed worse than those with normal blood pressure," Ford says. "This suggests that treating high blood pressure may prevent dementia, but we need further studies to establish that." Participants were tested for memory, word and picture recognition, and spatial memory.

Although the changes in thinking skills are too mild to interfere with a person's day-to-day functioning, they might increase the risk of developing dementia, or impaired mental abilities, later on, he says.

The prevalence of dementia doubles with every 5-year age increase, from 2.8 percent at 70 to 74 years of age to 38.6 percent at 90 to 95 years, and the U.K. population—like that of the United States—is aging, says Ford. As a result, the number of people with cognitive impairment in the U.K. is expected to double in the next 50 years.

"Currently, there are no treatments proven to slow or prevent the development of dementia. It's important that we identify interventions that will reduce the incidence of dementia in older people," Ford says.

Blood pressure also tends to rise with age. Studies indicate that by age 75, an estimated 41 percent of men and 54 percent of women have high blood pressure, which is defined as systolic pressure (the top number) above 140 millimeters of mercury (mm/Hg), and diastolic pressure (the lower number) above 90 mm/Hg. Systolic pressure is when the heart beats, whereas diastolic pressure measures the pressure between heartbeats.

Researchers have speculated that high blood pressure and dementia are related. Long-term studies have found that high blood pressure in mid-life results in reduced thinking skills four to 20 years later. However, other long-term studies have shown conflicting results, perhaps because of certain variables, Ford says.

For instance, blood pressure tends to drop with the onset of dementia or any other condition that causes weight loss, he says. In addition, stroke is associated with dementia and earlier studies did not attempt to control for stroke. In fact, only one small study of 25 patients with severe high blood pressure tried to exclude the effects of stroke. In addition, drugs to reduce blood pressure might affect the results.

This study attempted to control for variables by matching individuals in the normal and high blood pressure groups. It is the largest study to attempt to exclude the effects of cerebrovascular disease—such as stroke—and the only one to do so when examining moderately high blood pressure. Although none of the subjects with high blood pressure were taking medication for the condition during the study, all of them subsequently started treatment.

Ford and his colleagues compared 107 men and women with moderately high blood pressure (averaging 164/89 mm Hg) to a control group of 116 subjects with normal blood pressure (131/74 mm Hg). The average age in both groups was 76.

They gave participants several tests to determine reaction time, and various kinds of short- and long-term memory such as the ability to remember a list of words, numbers, or the details of pictures they had seen.

The people with high blood pressure had slower reaction times and had more trouble remembering things. For instance, the subjects with high blood pressure were on average 10 percent slower in simple reaction time than those with normal blood pressure. While this is significant, it is still less than the reaction times seen in individuals with mild dementia. The reaction times of individuals with high blood pressure are one-third to one-half of that seen in people with mild dementia, say researchers.

"These differences are likely a direct effect of hypertension," Ford says. The groups were well matched for other factors known to influence cognitive function: age, education level, depressive disorder, and psychotropic medication.

Co-authors: Frances Harrington, M.D.; Brian K. Saxby, B.Sc.; Ian G. McKeith, M.D.; and Keith Wesnes, Ph.D. April 17, 2002.

# Chapter 13

# *Obesity and Stroke*

## *Abdominal Obesity Identified as Independent Risk Factor for Stroke*

Abdominal obesity has been found to be an independent factor for ischemic stroke, according to a population-based study. "The effect of abdominal obesity on stroke risk may be greatest among persons younger than 65," said Seung-Han Suk, MD, Northern Manhattan Stroke Study investigator and research fellow in the department of neurology at Columbia-Presbyterian Medical Center in New York, reported on Feb. 8, 2002 at the International Stroke Conference.

Although obesity is a well-established risk factor for coronary heart disease and mortality, its association with ischemic stroke is unclear. Therefore, a four-year, population-based, case-control study was conducted to assess the relationship between abdominal obesity and ischemic stroke in a multi-ethnic community in the northern part of Manhattan, in New York City.

The researchers calculated the waist/hip ratio, an indicator of abdominal obesity, of 576 subjects and 1,142 control subjects. The average age was 69.1 (±12.4) years. Fifty-six percent were women, 56 percent were Hispanic, 26 percent were African-American, and 17 percent were Caucasian. The median waist/hip ratio was 0.95 for men and 0.88 for women.

Reprinted with permission, "ISC: Abdominal Obesity Identified as Independent Risk Factor for Stroke" by Bruce Sylvester, San Antonio, TX, February 14, 2002, Copyright © 2002 Doctor's Guide Publishing Limited (www.docguide.com).

Subjects with greater than the average waist/hip ratio had almost triple the risk for ischemic stroke compared to subjects with below average waist/hip ratio.

The median waist/hip ratio was greater in men than in women (0.95 vs. 0.88), therefore, gender-specific quartiles (GQ) were used for waist/hip ratio. Compared to the first quartile, each waist/hip ratio quartile had an increased adjusted risk of ischemic stroke (GQ2 or 1.43, GQ3 or 2.79, GQ4 or 3.39). WHR-GQ4 had a greater effect among women (or 4.13) than among men (or 2.4).

The correlation of stroke to higher waist/hip ratio was greater among younger participants. Those under 65 with an above average waist/hip ratio had an odds ratio of 5.81 for increased risk of stroke compared to persons with an above average waist/hip ratio who were 65 and older, who had an odds ratio of 2.55 for increased risk.

The effect of waist/hip ratio was greater for atherosclerotic compared to nonatherosclerotic stroke (odds ratio 4.29 vs. 2.77, respectively).

Waist/hip ratio was associated with increased stroke risk in all three ethnic groups in the trial.

Abdominal obesity is independently associated with increased risk of ischemic stroke overall, in men and women, and among all three race-ethnic groups, Dr. Suk noted. The impact of waist/hip ratio may be greater for women, those aged less than 65 years, and for the atherosclerotic stroke subtype, he said.

"The effects of abdominal obesity as an independent and modifiable risk factor for ischemic stroke are not adequately emphasized in stroke prevention and weight reduction programs," Dr. Suk said. "The danger is real, and the information needs to become part of the preventative health mainstream."

# Chapter 14

# Sleep Disorders and Stroke

## International Stroke Conference (ISC): Risk of Death from Stroke Predicted by Oversleeping/ Daytime Napping

Daytime nappers and people who routinely sleep more than eight hours a night have a greater chance of dying from stroke than those with more standard sleep habits, a study by stroke researchers at the University at Buffalo (UB) has shown.

And while the relationship between unusual sleep patterns and mortality was strongest for cerebrovascular diseases, a link also was found between such sleep habits and death from any cause, said Adnan Qureshi, MD, UB assistant professor of neurosurgery and lead author of the study. The research, conducted at UB's Toshiba Stroke Research Center in the School of Medicine and Biomedicine Sciences, was presented by Dr. Qureshi at the 27th International Stroke Conference (ISC) in San Antonio, Texas, in February 2002.

The findings do not suggest that people who regularly sleep more than normal could cut their risk by spending less time under the covers, however. What they indicate, Dr. Qureshi said, is the possible existence of an underlying sleep disorder that is hazardous to health.

---

"ISC: Risk of Death from Stroke Predicted by Oversleeping/Daytime Napping," Source: University of Buffalo, © 2002 Doctor's Guide Publishing Limited (www.docguide.com), reprinted with permission; and "Heart Memo: National Center on Sleep Disorders Research," National Heart, Lung, and Blood Institute (NHLBI), 2000.

"The mechanism behind this association between sleep patterns and mortality is not clear," he stated, "but we hypothesize it may signal there are other conditions that need to be addressed, such as sleep apnea."

People with sleep apnea stop breathing briefly and repeatedly during the night. They wake frequently gasping for breath, which robs them of restful sleep and can lead to drowsiness during the day. The condition is recognized as a contributor to heart disease and stroke.

Earlier research conducted by Dr. Qureshi with 1,348 adults who participated in a stroke-screening program in Buffalo showed that those who regularly slept more than eight hours a night had 9 percent more strokes than those who slept less. Persons who were regularly sleepy during the day showed a 10 percent increase in stroke.

The current study involved a national cohort of 7,844 adults who participated in the first National Health and Nutritional Examination Survey and its 10-year follow-up.

Participants in the initial survey, conducted in a random sample of the U.S. population, provided extensive information on health status and lifestyle habits, including sleep patterns. The follow-up study assessed changes in health since the initial survey.

After adjusting for several conditions that could influence a participant's risk of death from most chronic diseases, results showed that both those who slept more than eight hours a day and those who were regularly sleepy during the day had a 50 percent increased risk of dying compared to participants without those habits. More telling, those persons were nearly three times as likely to have died from stroke than persons with normal sleep patterns, results showed.

"The message here is that a person's unusual sleep habits should raise a red flag," Dr. Qureshi said. "Something is happening in the lives of these people that is increasing their risk of death, especially from stroke."

"It could be related to an underlying sleep disorder. There is a higher prevalence of hypertension and other risk factors in patients with sleep disorders such as sleep apnea. Or their unusual sleep patterns may be a result of underlying social or psychological factors, such as stress or depression. It's something both patients and their doctors should pay attention to," Dr. Qureshi said.

## Sleep Apnea and Snoring Linked to Hypertension

Editor's Note: Hypertension is a risk factor for stroke.

Reports from three studies provide new evidence that persons who experience sleep apnea are at an increased risk for hypertension.

Although further evidence is needed to fully establish how much the risk of hypertension varies with sleep apnea severity, the results point to a strong association. One of the studies also found a relationship between snoring and hypertension.

Researchers in the large Sleep Heart Health Study (SHHS), which is ongoing, provided preliminary results in the April 12, 2000 issue of the *Journal of the American Medical Association* (2000;283[14]: 1829-36). They found that middle-aged and older adults with sleep apnea had a 45 percent greater risk of hypertension than persons who did not experience sleep apnea. The study involved more than 6,000 adults, ages 40 and over, during 1995-98, who were participating in a number of National Heart, Lung, and Blood Institute (NHLBI) cohort studies of cardiovascular and respiratory diseases. The risk of hypertension was found to increase with the severity of the sleep apnea in all participants, regardless of age, sex, race, or weight. Even moderate levels of sleep apnea were associated with increased risk.

NHLBI Director Dr. Claude Lenfant said about the SHHS results, "This is the first study large enough to examine the relationship between sleep apnea and hypertension, independent of other cardiovascular risk factors. Although these results must be verified, they offer hope that we may be able to reduce cardiovascular mortality in hypertensives by more aggressively diagnosing the apnea."

About 12 million Americans experience sleep apnea, a condition characterized by brief interruptions in breathing during sleep. The breathing pauses last at least 10 seconds, and there may be 20 to 30 or more pauses per hour.

The Wisconsin Sleep Cohort Study (WSCS) further established the association between sleep apnea and hypertension. Researchers from the University of Wisconsin Medical School measured the presence of sleep apnea in 700 participants, then assessed their health, including blood pressure, 4 or 8 years later. They considered the range of 5 to 15 breathing pauses per hour to represent mild-to-moderate sleep apnea. They reported in the May 11, 2000 *New England Journal of Medicine* (2000;342[19]:1378-84) that sleep apnea played a significant and independent role in risk for hypertension. Even persons with minimal sleep apnea had an increased risk of becoming hypertensive compared with those without apnea. Persons with moderate-to-severe sleep apnea were three times as likely to become hypertensive.

"This study dramatically enhances our understanding of the role of sleep apnea in hypertension and provides additional evidence that it may be an independent risk factor for hypertension," said Dr.

Lenfant. "Once we have additional follow-up data from the large NHLBI Sleep Heart Health Study, we should be able to make a more reliable determination of the precise role of sleep apnea as a risk factor for cardiovascular disease."

In a third study, researchers at Penn State's College of Medicine showed that patients with moderate-to-severe sleep apnea are 7 times more likely to develop hypertension compared with patients with no sleep problems, and that hypertension risk increases with the severity of the sleep problem. The study also showed that people, especially the young, who snore with no other sleep disorder problems have an increased risk of hypertension.

People who snore and have mild sleep apnea were 2½ times as likely to be affected by hypertension as those with no sleep disordered breathing. Those who snore without evidence of sleep apnea were 1½ times more likely to have hypertension. The 5-year study, involving 1,741 people ages 20 to 100, was the largest sleep laboratory study of its kind. This study was reported in the August 14, 2000 issue of the journal *Archives of Internal Medicine* (2000;160[15]:2289-95). "This study extends earlier findings with evidence that even minimal sleep disordered breathing may be a risk factor for hypertension," said Dr. Lenfant.

Unlike earlier studies, all three studies weeded out other factors that might play a role in developing hypertension, including age, gender, and weight. All three studies were funded by the NHLBI.

## Additional Information

### National Heart, Lung, and Blood Institute
Health Information Center
P.O. Box 30105
Bethesda, MD 20824-0105
Tel: 301-592-8573
Fax: 301-592-8563
TTY: 240-629-3255
Website: www.nhlbi.nih.gov
E-mail: NHLBIinfo@rover.nhlbi.nih.gov

The NHLBI Health Information Center offers these publications on sleep apnea.

- *Facts About Sleep Apnea.* This 4-page brochure discusses sleep apnea, its causes and effects, and how it is diagnosed and treated. Copies can be ordered from the NHLBI Health Information Center.

- *Sleep Apnea: Is Your Patient At Risk?* This 10-page booklet gives health care providers an overview of sleep apnea, including its consequences and comorbidity, how to identify at-risk patients, diagnosis, treatment options, and management considerations.

# Chapter 15

# *Stroke and Young Women*

## *Genes Linked to Hemorrhagic Strokes in Young White Women*

Two genetic variants affecting a clotting factor have been linked to hemorrhagic strokes in young white women, researchers report in the November 2001 issue of *Stroke: Journal of the American Heart Association*.

Hemorrhagic strokes are caused by bleeding in the brain. The genetic variations appeared to increase the risk three to four times in women with hemorrhagic strokes compared with women who did not have brain hemorrhages.

"At this point it would be difficult to predict what kind of impact the findings will have, but eventually we hope to identify some of the genetic determinants that underlie cerebrovascular disease, including hemorrhagic stroke," says Alexander P. Reiner, M.D., research professor of epidemiology at the University of Washington in Seattle. "That would allow us to screen families or other groups of people who have demonstrated a predisposition for hemorrhagic stroke."

"Genes Linked to Hemorrhagic Strokes in Young White Women," *Stroke News* 11/01/2001. Reprinted with permission from the American Heart Association World Wide Web Site, www.american heart.org. © 2002, Copyright American Heart Association; and "University of Maryland Study Links Vitamin B Deficiency to Risk of Stroke in Younger Women," 1999 releases, © University of Maryland Medical System, reprinted with permission.

If the genetic variants in the clotting factor can be confirmed as factors in bleeding strokes, strategies focusing on the clotting factor might be developed to treat or prevent the strokes, he adds.

Hemorrhagic stroke occurs when a blood vessel in the brain or an aneurysm ruptures. An aneurysm is a weak vessel that balloons out. Among young adults, brain hemorrhage is the most common type of stroke and is frequently fatal. Although studies of stroke-prone families have suggested that genetics play a role, little information has emerged to implicate specific genetic variants.

Bleeding strokes that result from ruptured aneurysms have been linked to genetic disorders affecting connective tissues that form the structural framework of blood vessels. Thus, most studies of the genetics of brain hemorrhage have focused on proteins that affect the structural integrity of these blood vessels.

This investigation focused on genetic variations in factor XIII, a protein involved in clotting, blood vessel architecture and tissue repair. The researchers looked at three types of genetic variants, called polymorphisms, affecting factor XIII and a variation involving plasminogen activator inhibitor 1 (PAI-1), which helps regulate the body's natural clot-dissolving capabilities.

The study involved women between the ages of 18 and 44. Forty-two had survived brain hemorrhages and 345 had no history of hemorrhagic stroke. About two-thirds of the strokes involved aneurysms. Blood samples were taken from both groups and researchers analyzed genetic material related to factor XIII subunit A, which is required to produce the activated form of factor XIII, as well as genetic material involved in the regulation of blood levels of PAI-1.

The analysis showed that the women who had hemorrhagic strokes were significantly more likely than the control group to have abnormal variations in two amino acids, which are the building blocks of the genetic material DNA. One variation involved an amino acid called Phe204 and had occurred almost three times as often in the stroke group. A variant of the amino acid called Leu564 was more than four times as common in the stroke patients as in the control group.

The findings do not prove that the genetic variations predispose people to brain hemorrhages, Reiner emphasizes, noting that the findings came from a small group of patients. Until this work is confirmed in a larger group, Reiner discourages genetic testing to determine who might carry the gene variants.

"More research also is needed to further elucidate the importance of these particular mutations with respect to the biology of stroke, particularly hemorrhagic stroke," he says.

## University of Maryland Study Links Vitamin B Deficiency to Risk of Stroke in Younger Women

In the first large population study of its kind, researchers at the University of Maryland School of Medicine have found that higher levels of the naturally occurring substance called homocysteine increase the risk of stroke among younger women.

Deficiency in B vitamins or a genetic predisposition can cause higher levels of homocysteine, which is an amino acid. Results of the study were published in the August 1999 issue of the journal *Stroke*.

"We found that younger women who had the highest levels of homocystine had double the risk of stroke compared to women with lower levels," says Steven J. Kittner, M.D., M.P.H., professor of neurology, epidemiology, and preventive medicine at the University of Maryland School of Medicine.

Dr. Kittner adds that it is possible to lower homocysteine levels by increasing the amount of folic acid and vitamins $B_6$ and $B_{12}$ in the diet. "We may have the potential to significantly improve the public health and reduce the risk of stroke and other forms of cardiovascular disease with nutritional intervention," Dr. Kittner says.

Stroke is the third leading cause of death in the U.S. and is a major cause of disability. Among women under age 45, stroke is more common than Multiple Sclerosis.

The study included 167 white and African-American women age 15 to 44 who had suffered an ischemic stroke in Maryland, Washington, DC, southern Pennsylvania, or Delaware. They were compared to 328 randomly selected women who had not had a stroke, but were matched with the participants for similar characteristics, such as age and location of residence. The researchers also looked at factors such as smoking, socioeconomic status, and vitamin use, in addition to homocysteine levels.

The women in the study whose homocysteine levels were within the top 40 percent of the whole group had a 2.3 percent higher risk of stroke. When cigarette consumption, socioeconomic status, and regular vitamin use were taken into account, the risk was still 1.6 percent higher.

"The magnitude of the increase in stroke risk was similar to that of smoking a pack of cigarettes per day. Even moderately higher homocysteine levels—those that would be considered normal among older people—conferred a greater risk of stroke among the women in our study," says Dr. Kittner.

He adds that the increased stroke risk from elevated homocystine levels was the same for both African-American and white women.

The next step is to find out whether it is possible to prevent stroke by lowering homocysteine levels. The University of Maryland School of Medicine is participating in a study to see if treating high homocysteine levels with B vitamins can reduce the risk of stroke or heart disease. In this new study, men and women of all ages who have had a recent stroke are randomly assigned to take multivitamins with or without a high dose of B vitamins.

Until the answers are in, Dr. Kittner recommends that people get their folic acid and B vitamins from eating a balanced, healthy diet that includes seven servings of vegetables and fruit each day, along with moderate consumption of meat and dairy products.

Chapter 16

# Elderly Patients Have High Stroke Risk within Six Months of Heart Attack

Twenty percent of older patients who have had a heart attack have a one in 25 chance of being hospitalized for a stroke within six months of discharge from the hospital, according to research at Yale University. The study, published in the March 2002 issue of *Circulation*, provides what is believed to be the most accurate estimates of stroke after heart attack among elderly patients. This is because it includes the largest and most geographically diverse sample of older heart attack patients who have not been excluded from the study based on other illnesses or older age.

"The importance of stroke after myocardial infarction (MI) has been under-appreciated, especially among older persons," said Judith Lichtman, PhD, assistant professor in the Department of Epidemiology and Public Health at Yale School of Medicine. "Our results demonstrate that stroke after MI is much more common than previously reported." Dr. Lichtman said the rate of stroke following a heart attack has frequently been based on clinical studies that often exclude older patients and those with more significant medical problems. Yet, among patients hospitalized with a stroke, 77 percent are 65 years of age or older and half are older than 75 years of age. "With improved survival after MI and an increasing number of elderly people in the population, stroke after MI will be increasingly common problem in the coming decades," she said.

"Elderly Patients Have High Stroke Risk within Six Months of Heart Attack," April 3, 2002, Source: Yale University, © Doctor's Guide Publishing Limited, reprinted with permission.

*Stroke Sourcebook, First Edition*

Dr. Lichtman and her co-authors analyzed the data from more than 111,000 elderly patients included in the Cooperative Cardiovascular Project, which is a large, geographically diverse population-based group of patients hospitalized with acute myocardial infarction (AMI). "Overall, 2.5 percent were admitted with an ischemic stroke within six months of discharge," Dr. Lichtman said. She said older patients, African-American patients, and patients with any frailty are at increased risk for a stroke after a heart attack.

Conditions associated with higher stroke admission rates included prior stroke, hypertension, diabetes, atrial fibrillation, heart failure, and peripheral vascular disease. History of hypertension, diabetes, and peripheral vascular disease, are generally accepted as risk factors for stroke, but have not been previously identified as predictors of stroke after a heart attack.

Dr. Lichtman also noted that Aspirin (acetylsalicylic acid) at discharge was associated with reduced stroke admission rates. The risk of stroke among the 20 percent of patients who had at least four of the eight identified factors was four times higher than patients with none of these factors. Patients in this group had a one in 25 chance of being hospitalized for a stroke in the six months after discharge.

This data, Dr. Lichtman said, can be used to target high-risk patients for more aggressive therapies and counseling, including information about the signs and symptoms of a stroke and the appropriate action if these signs are present. Studies have shown that most patients do not recognize the signs and symptoms of a stroke, which results in delays that limit the ability to use time-dependent acute therapies.

Source: Yale University

# Chapter 17

# *Multi-Infarct Dementia Is Caused by Stroke*

## *Multi-Infarct Dementia*

Serious forgetfulness, mood swings, and other behavioral changes are not a normal part of aging. They may be caused by poor diet, lack of sleep, or too many medicines. Feelings of loneliness, boredom, or depression also can cause forgetfulness. These problems are serious and should be treated. Often they can be reversed.

Sometimes, however, mental changes are caused by diseases that permanently damage brain cells. The term dementia describes a medical condition that is caused by changes in the normal activity of very sensitive brain cells. These changes in the way the brain works can affect memory, speech, and the ability to carry out daily activities.

Alzheimer's disease (AD) is the most common cause of dementia in older people. The second most common cause of dementia in older adults is vascular dementia, which affects the blood vessels in the brain.

Multi-infarct dementia is the most common form of vascular dementia, and accounts for 10-20% of all cases of progressive, or gradually worsening, dementia. It usually affects people between the ages of 60-75, and is more likely to occur in men than women.

"Dementia, Before or After Stroke, Increases Risk of Death," August 2002. Reprinted with permission from the American Heart Association World Wide Web Site, www.americanheart.org. © 2002, Copyright American Heart Association; and "Multi-Infarct Dementia Fact Sheet," National Institute on Aging/ Alzheimer's Disease Education and Referral, NIH Publication No. 02-3433, May 2002.

Multi-infarct dementia is caused by a series of strokes that disrupt blood flow and damage or destroy brain tissue. A stroke occurs when blood cannot get to part of the brain. Strokes can be caused when a blood clot or fatty deposit (called plaque) blocks the vessels that supply blood to the brain. A stroke also can happen when a blood vessel in the brain bursts.

Some of the main causes of strokes are:

- untreated high blood pressure (hypertension)
- diabetes
- high cholesterol
- heart disease

Of these, the most important risk factor for multi-infarct dementia is high blood pressure.

Because strokes occur suddenly, loss of thinking and remembering skills—the symptoms of dementia—also occur quickly and often in a step-wise pattern. People with multi-infarct dementia may even appear to improve for short periods of time, then decline again after having more strokes.

## Symptoms

Sudden onset of any of the following symptoms may be a sign of multi-infarct dementia:

- confusion and problems with recent memory
- wandering or getting lost in familiar places
- moving with rapid, shuffling steps
- loss of bladder or bowel control
- laughing or crying inappropriately
- difficulty following instructions
- problems handling money

Multi-infarct dementia is often the result of a series of small strokes. Some of these small strokes produce no obvious symptoms and are noticed only on brain imaging studies, so they are sometimes called silent strokes. A person may have several small strokes before noticing serious changes in memory or other signs of multi-infarct dementia.

Transient ischemic attacks, or TIAs, are caused by a temporary blockage of blood flow. Symptoms of TIAs are similar to symptoms of stroke and include mild weakness in an arm or leg, slurred speech, and dizziness. Symptoms generally do not last for more than 20 minutes. A recent history of TIAs greatly increases a person's chance of suffering permanent brain damage from a stroke. Prompt medical attention is required to determine what may be causing the blockage in blood flow and to start proper treatment (such as aspirin or warfarin).

If you believe someone is having a stroke—if a person experiences sudden weakness or numbness on one or both sides of the body, or difficulty speaking, seeing, or walking—call 911 immediately. If the physician believes the symptoms are caused by a blocked blood vessel, treatment with a clot buster, such as tPA (tissue plasminogen activator), within 3 hours can reopen the vessel and may reduce the severity of the stroke.

## Diagnosis

People who show signs of dementia and who have a history of strokes should be evaluated for possible multi-infarct dementia. The doctor usually will ask the patient and the family about the person's diet, medications, sleep patterns, personal habits, past strokes, and other risk factors (such as high blood pressure, diabetes, high cholesterol, and heart disease). The doctor also may ask about recent illnesses or stressful events, like the death of someone close or problems at home or work, which may account for the symptoms. To look for signs of stroke, the doctor will check for weakness or numbness in the arms and legs, difficulty with speech, or dizziness. To check for other health problems that could cause symptoms of dementia, the doctor may order office or laboratory tests. These tests may include a blood pressure reading, an electroencephalogram (EEG), a test of thyroid function, or blood tests.

The doctor also may ask for x-rays or special tests such as a computerized tomography (CT) scan or a magnetic resonance imaging (MRI) scan. Both CT scans and MRI scans take pictures of sections of the brain. The pictures are displayed on a computer screen to allow the doctor to see inside the brain and check for signs of stroke, tumors, or other sources of brain injury. Specialists called radiologists and neurologists interpret these scans. In addition, the doctor may send the patient to a psychologist or psychiatrist to assess reasoning, learning ability, memory, and attention span.

Sometimes multi-infarct dementia is difficult to distinguish from AD because their symptoms can be very similar. It is possible for a person to have both diseases, making it hard for the doctor to diagnose either.

## Treatment

While no treatment can reverse brain damage that has already been caused by a stroke, treatment to prevent further strokes is very important. For example, high blood pressure, the primary risk factor for multi-infarct dementia, and diabetes are treatable. To prevent more strokes, doctors may prescribe medicines to control high blood pressure, high cholesterol, heart disease, and diabetes. They will counsel patients about good health habits such as exercising, avoiding smoking and drinking alcohol, and eating a low-fat diet.

To reduce symptoms of dementia, doctors may change or stop medications that can cause confusion, such as sedatives, antihistamines, strong painkillers, and other medications. Some patients also may have to be treated for additional medical conditions that can increase confusion, such as heart failure, thyroid disorders, anemia, or infections.

Doctors sometimes prescribe aspirin, warfarin, or other drugs to prevent clots from forming in small blood vessels. Medications also can be prescribed to relieve restlessness or depression or to help patients sleep better.

To improve blood flow or remove blockages in blood vessels, doctors may recommend surgical procedures, such as carotid endarterectomy, angioplasty, or stenting. Studies are underway to see how well these treatments work for patients with multi-infarct dementia. Scientists are also studying drugs that can improve blood flow to the brain, such as anti-platelet and anti-coagulant medications; drugs to treat symptoms of dementia, including Alzheimer's disease medications; as well as drugs to reduce the risk of TIAs and stroke, such as cholesterol-lowering statins and blood pressure medications.

## Helping Someone with Multi-Infarct Dementia

Family members and friends can help someone with multi-infarct dementia cope with mental and physical problems. They can encourage individuals to maintain their daily routines and regular social and physical activities. By talking with them about events and daily experiences, family members can help their loved ones use their mental abilities as much as possible. Some families find it helpful to use reminders such as lists, alarm clocks, and calendars to help the patient remember important times and dates.

A person with multi-infarct dementia should see their primary care doctor regularly. Health problems such as high blood pressure, diabetes, high cholesterol, and heart disease should be carefully monitored. If a person has additional medical conditions, such as depression, mental health experts may be consulted as well.

Help for home caregivers is available from a variety of sources, including nurses, family doctors, social workers, and physical and occupational therapists. Home health care and respite or neighborhood day care services can provide much-needed relief to caregivers. Support groups offer emotional support for family members caring for a person with dementia. A State or local health department, a local hospital, or the patient's doctor may be able to provide telephone numbers for such services.

## The American Heart Association Reports Dementia, Before or After Stroke, Increases Risk of Death

Stroke survivors who have symptoms of dementia before or after a stroke have a significantly greater risk for stroke-related death, according to new research reported in the August 2002 issue of *Stroke*: *Journal of the American Heart Association*.

An analysis of data from a stroke registry compiled in Spain indicates that patients who have post-stroke dementia have a more than eight-fold increase in risk of death within two years of stroke than patients who have no signs of dementia after stroke. When dementia was diagnosed before the stroke, the risk for death was twice as high as the death risk for patients who had no dementia before or after stroke. When dementia is related to stroke, the risk for death within two years increased more than six-fold.

Researchers found that dementia—declines in memory, cognitive function, and capacity to perform daily living activities—is an independent risk factor for death after stroke and one of the most important determinants of death in stroke patients, explains the study's lead author Raquel Barba, M.D., Ph.D., a clinical investigator in the department of medicine at Fundación Hospital Alcorcón, Madrid, Spain.

A possible explanation for the poor survival rate among stroke survivors with dementia is that these patients may not receive the same treatment as stroke survivors who have no cognitive impairment, says Barba. For example, the study found that a patient with

181

dementia was less likely to be treated with oral anticoagulants than one without dementia, even if atrial fibrillation was diagnosed. Atrial fibrillation is an abnormal heart rhythm associated with increased risk for blood clots. It's often treated with anticoagulants to prevent stroke. But these drugs require careful compliance with dosing guidelines and patients with dementia are less likely to comply with medication regimens.

Patients with dementia did receive the same antihypertensive medications and antiaggregant treatments as stroke patients without dementia. But, after discharge from the hospital, dementia patients were less likely to have their blood sugar levels closely monitored, which is recommended to prevent complications associated with diabetes.

Currently, stroke prevention focuses on patients without dementia, but based on the study, Barba believes antiplatelet therapy, blood sugar control, and blood pressure control are important keys even in patients with dementia. For patients who have pre-existing dementia, stroke likely worsens the dementia resulting in poor functional, neurologic, and vital prognosis so preventing stroke is also important in these patients, she says.

The stroke registry included data from 324 patients admitted to a Madrid hospital for stroke treatment between May 1, 1994, and September 30, 1995. When the patients were admitted a close relative or caregiver completed a detailed questionnaire on cognitive decline called the Informant Questionnaire on Cognitive Decline in the Elderly (IQCODE). Information from that questionnaire, as well as medical history and neurological evaluation, identified pre-stroke dementia in 49 patients.

Three months after the stroke neurological evaluation, another IQCODE and a mental status questionnaire identified 75 cases of post-stroke dementia, including 50 cases in which the dementia was stroke-related.

After adjusting for other known risk factors for stroke-related mortality—age, gender, high blood pressure, diabetes, history of previous stroke, heart disease, and severity of stroke—dementia remained a predictor of stroke mortality, says Barba.

After correcting for the other risk factors, the relative risk of mortality for patients with pre-stroke dementia was 2.1. It was 6.4 for those with stroke-related dementia and 8.5 for those who with post-stroke dementia.

After nearly two years of follow-up, 58.3 percent of patients with stroke-related dementia survived compared to 95.4 percent of patients without it.

Dementia is commonly associated with Alzheimer's disease, but another type of dementia is caused by narrowing of the blood vessels inside the brain. This narrowing reduces the supply of blood that carries oxygen and nutrients to keep brain cells alive and functioning. This type of dementia is called vascular dementia and has been associated with stroke. In this study, 63 of the 75 patients with post-stroke dementia had vascular dementia, while 12 had "degenerative dementia plus stroke," says Barba.

Also in the August 2002 issue of *Stroke*, a team of Canadian researchers report that administering a battery of neuropsychological tests can help physicians predict which patients who have slight cognitive impairment caused by vascular disease will lead to dementia. A third study, by researchers from Texas, also suggests that mild cognitive impairment may predict vascular dementia in much the same way that neurologists consider it to be a precursor for Alzheimer's disease.

Barba's co-authors are Maria-del-Mar Morin, M.D.; Carlos Cemillán, M.D.; Carlos Delgado, Ph.D.; Julio Domingo, M.D.; and Teodoro Del Ser, M.D., Ph.D. The research was partly funded by Bayer S.A.

## Additional Information

### *Alzheimer's Association*
919 N. Michigan Ave., Suite 1100
Chicago, IL 60611-1676
Toll-Free: 800-272-3900
Tel: 312-335-8700
Fax: 312-335-1110
Website: www.alz.org
E-mail: info@alz.org

The Alzheimer's Association has a free information packet about multi-infarct dementia and information about support groups for families.

### *Alzheimer's Disease Education and Referral (ADEAR) Center*
P.O. Box 8250
Silver Spring, MD 20907-8250
Toll-Free: 800-438-4380
Website: www.alzheimers.org
E-mail: adear@alzheimers.org

The ADEAR Center is a service of the National Institute on Aging, funded by the Federal Government. It offers information and publications on diagnosis, treatment, patient care, caregiver needs, long-term care, education, and training, and research related to AD and dementia. Staff answer telephone and written requests and make referrals to local and national resources.

### American Stroke Association (a division of the American Heart Association)
7272 Greenville Avenue
Dallas, TX 75231
Toll-Free: 888-4-STROKE (478-7653)
Website: www.strokeassociation.org
E-mail: strokeconnection@heart.org

Information about stroke and recovery, as well as related research, programs, and events is available.

### National Institute of Neurological Disorders and Stroke
P.O. Box 5801
Bethesda, MD 20824
Toll-Free: 800-352-9424
Tel: 301-496-5751
TTY: 301-468-5981
Website: www.ninds.nih.gov

Information about stroke and current research on stroke-related conditions is available.

### National Stroke Association
9707 E. Easter Lane
Englewood, CO 80112
Toll-Free: 800-STROKES (787-6537)
Tel: 303-649-9299
Fax: 303-649-1328
Website: www.stroke.org

Information about stroke and support for stroke survivors and their families is available.

## National Heart, Lung, and Blood Institute
Health Information Center
P.O. Box 30105
Bethesda, MD 20824-0105
Tel: 301-592-8573
Fax: 301-592-8563
TTY: 240-629-3255
Website: www.nhlbi.nih.gov
E-mail: NHLBIinfo@rover.nhlbi.nih.gov

Information about preventing stroke, including information about risk factors such as high blood pressure, high cholesterol, heart disease, and smoking.

## National Diabetes Information Clearinghouse
1 Information Way
Bethesda, MD 20892-3560 (please use full, 9-digit zip code)
Toll-Free: 800-860-8747
Website: www.niddk.nih.gov/health/diabetes/ndic.htm
E-mail: ndic@info.niddk.nih.gov

Information about controlling diabetes.

## Eldercare Locator
National Association of Area Agencies on Aging
927 15th Street N.W., 6th Floor
Washington, DC 20005
Toll-Free: 800-677-1116
Website: www.eldercare.gov
E-mail: eldercare_locator@aoa.gov

Information about services and resources in your area, such as adult day care programs, transportation, and meal services.

# Chapter 18

# *Recurrent Stroke Risks*

## *Patients with Recurrent Stroke Have Poorer Outcomes and Higher Care Costs Than Those with a First Stroke*

Typically, patients who suffer a second or third stroke have poorer outcomes and greater costs than those who suffer a first stroke. Fewer of these patients survive, and those who do are more disabled. These are the findings of a study by the Stroke Prevention Patient Outcomes Research Team (PORT), which is supported by the Agency for Health Care Policy and Research (PORT contract 290-91-0028) and led by David B. Matchar, M.D., of Duke University.

The researchers found that 57 percent of first stroke survivors were alive 24 months after the stroke compared with only 48 percent of those who suffered a recurrent stroke. Costs were similar for the initial hospital stay and in the first 1 to 3 months after stroke. However, for months 4 to 24 after stroke, total costs were higher among those with recurrent stroke by about $375 per patient per month.

The difference was greatest for younger patients and least for patients aged 80 years and older. Most of the difference in total monthly

This chapter includes "Outcomes/Effectiveness Research: Patients with Recurrent Stroke Have Poorer Outcomes and Higher Care Costs Than Those with a First Stroke," Agency for Healthcare Research and Quality (AHRQ), May 1999. Also, reprinted with permission "Recurrent Cerebrovascular Events Associated with Patent Foramen Ovale, Atrial Septal Aneurysm, or Both," Abstracts: Mas et al. 345 (24): 1740, *The New England Journal of Medicine*, Copyright 2001 Massachusetts Medical Society. All rights reserved.

cost was attributable to nursing home use (averaging about $150 per patient per month) and acute hospitalization (averaging about $120 per patient per month). Decision and cost-effectiveness models should use different estimates of survival and cost outcomes depending on whether the patient has a first or recurrent stroke, according to Dr. Matchar.

The researchers used administrative claims files from a random 20 percent sample of nearly 50,000 Medicare patients admitted to U.S. hospitals with a primary diagnosis of cerebral infarction during 1991. Data from hospitalizations during the previous 4 years were used to classify patients as having either first or recurrent stroke. Patients' survival and direct medical costs were followed for 24 months after stroke.

## Abstract: Recurrent Cerebrovascular Events Associated with Patent Foramen Ovale, Atrial Septal Aneurysm, or Both

By Jean-Louis Mas, M.D., Caroline Arquizan, M.D., Catherine Lamy, M.D., Mathieu Zuber, M.D., Laure Cabanes, Ph.D., Geneviève Derumeaux, M.D., Joël Coste, Ph.D., for the Patent Foramen Ovale and Atrial Septal Aneurysm Study Group.

### Background

Patent foramen ovale and atrial septal aneurysm have been identified as potential risk factors for stroke, but information about their effect on the risk of recurrent stroke is limited. We studied the risks of recurrent cerebrovascular events associated with these cardiac abnormalities.

### Methods

A total of 581 patients (age, 18 to 55 years) who had had an ischemic stroke of unknown origin within the preceding three months were consecutively enrolled at 30 neurology departments. All patients received aspirin (300 mg per day) for secondary prevention.

### Results

After four years, the risk of recurrent stroke was 2.3 percent (95 percent confidence interval, 0.3 to 4.3 percent) among the patients with patent foramen ovale alone, 15.2 percent (95 percent confidence interval, 1.8 to 28.6 percent) among the patients with both patent foramen ovale and atrial septal aneurysm, and 4.2 percent (95 percent confidence interval, 1.8 to 6.6 percent) among the patients with neither of these cardiac abnormalities. There were no recurrences among the patients with an atrial septal aneurysm alone. The presence of both cardiac abnormalities was a significant predictor of an increased risk of recurrent stroke (hazard ratio for the comparison with the absence of these abnormalities, 4.17; 95 percent confidence interval, 1.47 to 11.84), whereas isolated patent foramen ovale, whether small or large, was not.

## Conclusions

Patients with both patent foramen ovale and atrial septal aneurysm who have had a stroke constitute a subgroup at substantial risk for recurrent stroke, and preventive strategies other than aspirin should be considered.

## Source Information

From the Department of Neurology, Sainte-Anne Hospital, Paris V University, Paris (J.-L.M., C.A., C.L., M.Z.); the Departments of Cardiology (L.C.) and Biostatistics (J.C.), Cochin Hospital, Paris V University, Paris; and the Department of Cardiology, Charles Nicolle Hospital, Rouen University, Rouen, France (G.D.).

## Additional Reading

"Epidemiology of recurrent cerebral infarction: A Medicare claims-based comparison of first and recurrent strokes on 2-year survival and cost," by Gregory P. Samsa, Ph.D., John Bian, M.S., Joseph Lipscomb, Ph.D., and Dr. Matchar, in *Stroke* 30, pp. 338-349, 1999.

# Chapter 19

# *Tests Help Predict Stroke Risk*

## *Ultrasonography Predicts Heart Attack/Stroke Risk*

National Heart, Lung, and Blood Institute (NHLBI)-supported scientists report that ultrasonography, a non-invasive test, predicts the risk of heart attack and stroke in older persons with no cardiovascular disease symptoms. The test was used to measure the thickness of the walls of two arteries in the neck. The result gave vital information beyond that available from an assessment of the standard cardiovascular disease risk factors, such as high blood pressure and high blood cholesterol.

The NHLBI is part of the National Institutes of Health. The finding appeared in the January 7, 1999 issue of *The New England Journal of Medicine*. "This study shows that ultrasonography has great

---

This chapter includes, "Ultrasonography Predicts Heart Attack/Stroke Risk," National Heart, Lung, and Blood Institute (NHLBI), 01/06/1999; "Carotid Duplex," © 2002 A.D.A.M., Inc. Reprinted with permission; and "Scanning Carotid Artery with MRI May Help Predict Stroke Risk" Reprinted with permission from the American Heart Association World Wide Web Site, www.americanheart.org. © 2002, Copyright American Heart Association. The following abstracts are also included: "Stroke Is Associated with Coronary Calcification as Detected by Electron-Beam CT" (Abstract), Vliegenthart et al. 33 (2): 462; (*Stroke*. 2002;33:462); © 2002 Lippincott, Williams, and Wilkins, reprinted with permission; and "Twenty-Four Hour Blood Pressure and MRI as Predictive Factors for Different Outcomes in Patients with Lacunar Infarct" (Abstract), Yamamoto (*Stroke*. 2002;33:297); © Lippincott, Williams, and Wilkins, reprinted with permission.

potential in the prevention of heart attack and stroke," said NHLBI Director Dr. Claude Lenfant. "By identifying high risk patients, ultrasonography would allow doctors to provide aggressive treatment early." Such treatment includes control of high blood pressure and high blood cholesterol, weight loss, increased physical activity, and aspirin and other drug therapies, he added.

Heart disease and stroke are the first and third leading causes of death among Americans. Each year, about 500,000 Americans die of coronary heart disease and about 160,000 of stroke. One in five Americans has some form of cardiovascular disease.

Ultrasonography is a relatively inexpensive, painless test in which sound waves above the range of human hearing are sent into the neck. Echoes bounce off the moving blood and the tissue in the artery and are then formed into an image. The test is currently used in stroke prevention to diagnose advanced disease in the carotid arteries. The new study found that the test detects disease much earlier and identifies those at risk of heart attack as well as stroke.

The study involved 4,476 men and women, aged 65 and older, drawn from the NHLBI-supported Cardiovascular Health Study (CHS), a multi-center investigation of older Americans. CHS centers are in California, Maryland, North Carolina, and Pennsylvania. About 40 percent of the ultrasound study's participants were men and 60 percent women. Blacks comprised about 15 percent of the participants; the rest were white. Participants were followed for an average of 6.2 years.

Scientists used ultrasound to measure the thickness of walls in the common and internal carotid arteries. The measures assessed patients' degree of atherosclerosis, a condition in which fat and cholesterol are deposited in artery walls. The walls thicken and become less flexible, and the narrowed opening impedes blood flow. If an artery becomes blocked, a heart attack or stroke can occur.

Atherosclerotic buildup is not uniform. By combining the measures from both arteries, scientists gained a more complete picture of the patients' conditions than either measure alone could yield.

Results showed that patients' risk of heart attack and stroke increased in direct proportion with the thickness of their artery walls. Those with the thickest arteries had an almost fivefold greater risk of heart attack or stroke than those with the thinnest measures. Even after accounting for standard cardiovascular disease risk factors— such as cigarette smoking, high blood pressure, high blood cholesterol, and diabetes—patients with the thickest artery walls still had more than double the risk of a heart attack or stroke than those with the thinnest walls.

# Carotid Duplex

Alternative names: Scan—carotid duplex

## Definition

This procedure uses ultrasound (high-frequency sound waves that echo off the body). The echo is registered with devices that project a 2-dimensional image showing the carotid artery walls and their lumen (interior).

This test also looks at the rate the blood flows through the carotid artery (in the neck), which supplies blood to the brain. The test can detect atherosclerotic plaque and blood clots.

## How the Test Is Performed

The test is done in the peripheral vascular lab or radiology department of the hospital. You are placed on your back and your head will be supported to prevent movement.

A water-soluble gel is placed on the skin where the transducer probe (a hand-held device that directs the high-frequency sound waves to the arteries being tested) is to be placed to help transmit the sound to the skin surface. The ultrasound is turned on and images of the carotid artery and pulse wave forms are obtained.

## How to Prepare for the Test

**Adults:** No special preparation is necessary.

**Infants and children:** The physical and psychological preparation you can provide for this or any test or procedure depends on your child's age, interests, previous experience, and level of trust.

## How It Feels

The test is noninvasive and painless.

## Risks

There are no risks.

## Why the Test Is Performed

The test assesses blood flow and is used to detect stenotic ("hardening"), thrombotic ("clots"), and occlusive diseases (in which the arteries are closed).

### Normal Values

The artery is free of any obstructions, stenosis, or thrombosis, and there is no flow abnormality. There is no turbulence or disruption in the arterial blood flow.

### What Abnormal Results Mean

There is a disturbance of the blood flow in the artery related to stenotic, obstructive, or thrombotic diseases.

### Special Considerations

Not applicable.

## American Heart Association Journal Report: Scanning Carotid Artery with MRI May Help Predict Stroke Risk

Co-authors were Shao-xiong Zhang, M.D.; Nayak L. Polissar, Ph.D.; Denise Echelard, B.S.; Geraldo Ortiz, B.S.; Joseph W. Davis, B.S.; Elizabeth Ellington, B.S.; Marina S. Ferguson, B.S.; and Thomas S. Hatsukami, M.D.

A simple imaging test identified people with dangerous clogging in their carotid (neck) arteries according to researchers who say the test may someday help identify individuals who need immediate surgery to prevent stroke. Their findings were reported in the January 15, 2002, *Circulation: Journal of the American Heart Association.*

The researchers caution that because the study was small the results need to be confirmed in a large prospective study. For that reason, they say it is too soon to recommend using MRI to guide clinical decisions.

"However, these early, promising results suggest that in the future it may be possible to use MRI to track the progress of atherosclerosis and to better select patients for surgical intervention," says Chun Yuan, Ph.D., a professor of radiology at the University of Washington, Seattle.

Yuan says the new technique, which uses high resolution magnetic resonance imaging (MRI), helps identify unstable plaque in patients with atherosclerosis—a disease that narrows arteries and increases the risk for stroke.

Plaque is a hard fatty substance that accumulates in the blood vessels of people with atherosclerosis. This build-up can become unstable and break off. When the plaque breaks or ruptures, a blood clot can form around the broken tissue and block blood flow. In the heart this process causes a heart attack. When it happens in the carotid arteries, which supply blood to the brain, it can cause a stroke.

Yuan explains that the core of plaque in the carotid arteries has an outside covering of fibrous tissue. This fibrous cap can be thick, thin, or ruptured. By studying the tissue, researchers discovered that the plaque becomes unstable and prone to rupture when the cap thins.

The researchers used high-resolution MRI to study the condition of fibrous caps in the carotid arteries of 53 patients (49 men, average age 71) who were scheduled for carotid endarterectomy, the surgical procedure in which plaque is removed from the carotid artery. They found subtle differences in the images of the fibrous cap that allowed researchers to identify "intact thick cap, intact thin cap, and ruptured cap."

People with atherosclerosis who had unstable plaque, as detected by MRI, were 23 times more likely to have a stroke than people with the same amount of artery narrowing, but no unstable plaque.

In addition to MRI scans, participants underwent a thorough neurological evaluation to determine if they had a history of stroke or "mini strokes," which are called transient ischemic attacks, or TIAs, within the previous 90 days. Patients with a positive history were classified as symptomatic. He then compared the MRI results to the patient's neurological symptoms.

"There was a clear and consistent association between the condition of the fibrous cap as seen by MRI, and the patient's clinical status," Yuan says. There was an association between history of recent stroke or TIA and cap status. Only 9 percent of those with intact caps had a positive stroke/TIA history, compared to 70 percent of those with ruptured caps. For those with intact, but thin caps, 50 percent had a history of recent stroke or TIA. He adds that MRI is uniquely suited for serial, repeated examinations of plaque because it is non-invasive.

Stroke is the third leading cause of death in the United States, ranking behind disease of the heart and cancer. Each year about 600,000 people suffer a stroke, and every 3.1 minutes someone dies of stroke.

This research was funded in part by the National Institutes of Health.

## Stroke Is Associated with Coronary Calcification as Detected by Electron-Beam CT

Source: Vliegenthart et al. 33 (2): 462; (*Stroke*. 2002;33:462.); © 2002 Lippincott, Williams, and Wilkins, reprinted with permission.

## The Rotterdam Coronary Calcification Study

Co-authors: Rozemarijn Vliegenthart, MSc; Monika Hollander, MD; Monique M.B. Breteler, MD, PhD; Deirdre A.M. van der Kuip, MD, PhD; Albert Hofman, MD, PhD; Matthijs Oudkerk, MD, PhD; Jacqueline C.M. Witteman, PhD

### Background and Purpose

Coronary calcification as detected by electron-beam CT measures the atherosclerotic plaque burden and has been reported to predict coronary events. Because atherosclerosis is a generalized process, coronary calcification may also be associated with manifest atherosclerotic disease at other sites of the vascular tree. We examined whether coronary calcification as detected by electron-beam CT is related to the presence of stroke.

### Methods

From 1997 onward, subjects were invited to participate in the prospective Rotterdam Coronary Calcification Study and undergo electron-beam CT to detect coronary calcification. The study was embedded in the population-based Rotterdam Study. Calcifications were quantified in a calcium score according to Agatston's method. Calcium scores were available for 2013 subjects (mean age [SD], 71 [5.7] years). Fifty subjects had experienced stroke before scanning.

### Results

Subjects were 2 times more likely to have experienced stroke when their calcium score was between 101 and 500 (odds ratio [or], 2.1; 95% CI, 0.9 to 4.7) and 3 times more likely when their calcium score was above 500 (or, 3.3; 95% CI, 1.5 to 7.2), compared with subjects in the lowest calcium score category (0 to 100). Additional adjustment for cardiovascular risk factors did not materially alter the risk estimates.

### Conclusions

In this population-based study, a markedly graded association was found between coronary calcification and stroke. The results suggest that coronary calcification as detected by electron-beam CT may be useful to identify subjects at high risk of stroke.

Key Words:

- atherosclerosis
- calcium
- epidemiology
- stroke
- tomography

# Twenty-Four–Hour Blood Pressure and MRI as Predictive Factors for Different Outcomes in Patients with Lacunar Infarct

Source: Co-authors Y. Yamamoto, PhD; I. Akiguchi, PhD; K. Oiwa, PhD; M. Hayashi, MD; T. Kasai, MD; K. Ozasa, PhD. Yamamoto (*Stroke.* 2002;33:297.); © Lippincott, Williams, and Wilkins, reprinted with permission.

## Background and Purpose

A long-term follow-up study was conducted in patients with lacunar infarct to assess how 24-hour blood pressure monitoring values and MRI findings, in particular lacunar infarcts and diffuse white matter lesions, can predict subsequent development of dementia and vascular events, which include cerebrovascular and cardiovascular events.

## Methods

One hundred seventy-seven patients were tracked for a mean of 8.9 years of follow-up. Documented events comprise the development of dementia and the occurrence of vascular events. The predictors for developing dementia and vascular events were separately evaluated by Cox proportional hazards analysis.

## Results

Twenty-six patients developed dementia (0.17/100 patient-years). Male sex (relative risk [RR], 4.2; 95% CI, 1.2 to 14.7), cognitive impairment (RR, 3.0; 95% CI, 1.0 to 8.5), confluent DWML (moderate: RR, 7.1; 95% CI, 1.6 to 31.5; severe: RR, 35.8; 95% CI, 7.2 to 177.3), and nondipping status (RR, 7.1; 95% CI, 2.2 to 22.0) were independent predictors for dementia. Forty-six patients suffered from vascular events (3.11/100 patient-years). Diabetes mellitus (RR, 5.7; 95% CI, 2.7 to 11.9), multiple lacunae (moderate: RR, 6.4; 95% CI, 2.5 to 15.8; severe: RR, 8.5; 95% CI, 3.1 to 23.3), and high 24-hour systolic blood pressure (>145 mm Hg versus <130 mm Hg) (RR, 10.3; 95% CI, 1.3 to 81.3) were independent predictors for vascular events.

## *Conclusions*

Predictors for developing dementia and vascular events appear to differ. Male sex, confluent diffuse white matter lesions, and nondipping status were independent predictors for subsequent development of dementia, while diabetes mellitus, multiple lacunae, and high 24-hour systolic blood pressure were independent predictors for vascular events.

Key Words:

- blood pressure monitoring, ambulatory
- dementia, vascular
- lacunar infarction
- white matter

# Part Three

# Diagnosis and Treatments for Stroke

Chapter 20

# Tests and Procedures Used for Stroke Diagnosis

## Lab Tests and Procedures Used for Stroke Diagnosis

If you have had a stroke or stroke warning signs, your doctor may need additional information to fully understand your problem or plan the best treatment. In addition to blood tests, you may need to schedule special tests or procedures to examine your brain, heart, or blood vessels. Here are the tests doctors use most often in stroke diagnosis.

### *Tests That View the Brain, Skull, or Spinal Cord*

- **CT scan (CAT Scan, Computed axial tomography):** CT scan uses x-rays to produce a 3-dimensional image of your head. A CT scan can be used to diagnose ischemic stroke, hemorrhagic stroke, and other problems of the brain and brainstem.

---

This chapter includes the following documents reprinted with permission of the Internet Stroke Center © 1997-2002 Internet Stroke Center at Washington University, www.strokecenter.org: "Lab Tests and Procedures Used for Stroke Diagnosis," "Blood Tests and Procedures Used for Stroke Diagnosis," "Electrocardiogram," "Echocardiogram," "Carotid Ultrasound," "Cerebral Angiography," "CAT Scan," and "MRI." Also included are "Backpack-Sized Ultrasound Device Detects Neck Artery Blockages," and "Spiral Scan Sees Stroke Blockage More Clearly," both reprinted with permission from the American Heart Association World Wide Web Site, www.americanheart.org. © 2002, Copyright American Heart Association.

- **MRI scan (Magnetic resonance imaging, MR):** MR uses magnetic fields to produce a 3-dimensional image of your head. The MR scan shows the brain and spinal cord in more detail than CT. MR can be used to diagnose ischemic stroke, hemorrhagic stroke, and other problems involving the brain, brainstem, and spinal cord.

## Tests That View the Blood Vessels That Supply the Brain

- **Carotid doppler (Carotid duplex, Carotid ultrasound):** Painless ultrasound waves are used to take a picture of the carotid arteries in your neck, and to show the blood flowing to your brain. This test can show if your carotid artery is narrowed by arteriosclerosis (cholesterol deposition).

- **Transcranial doppler (TCD):** Ultrasound waves are used to measure blood flow in some of the arteries in your brain.

- **MRA (Magnetic resonance angiogram):** This is a special type of MRI scan (see above) which can be used to see the blood vessels in your neck or brain.

- **Cerebral arteriogram (Cerebral angiogram, Digital subtraction angiography, [DSA]):** A catheter is inserted in an artery in your arm or leg, and a special dye is injected into the blood vessels leading to your brain. X-ray images show any abnormalities of the blood vessels, including narrowing, blockage, or malformations (such as aneurysms or arteriovenous malformations). Cerebral arteriogram is a more difficult test than carotid doppler or MRA, but the results are the most accurate.

## Tests That View the Heart or Check Its Function

- **Electrocardiogram (EKG, ECG):** This is a standard test to show the pattern of electrical activity in your heart. 3-10 electrical leads are attached to your chest, arms, and legs. Sometimes the EKG is recorded continuously over days, with the signals sent to a portable recorder (Holter monitor) or by radio to a hospital monitoring station (telemetry).

- **Echocardiogram (2-d echo, Cardiac echo, TTE, TEE):** Painless ultrasound waves are used to take a picture of your heart and the circulating blood. The ultrasound probe may be placed on your chest (trans-thoracic echocardiogram, TTE) or deep in your throat (trans-esophageal echocardiogram, TEE).

## Routine Screening Tests

- **Chest X-ray (CXR):** An x-ray of the heart and lungs is a standard test for patients with acute medical problems. Abnormalities may alert your doctor to important problems such as pneumonia or heart failure.

- **Urinalysis (UA):** A urine sample is often obtained to screen for bladder infection or kidney problems. If infection is suggested, a urine culture test may be required.

- **Pulse oximetry (Blood oxygen):** This painless test is sometimes done in the emergency room or hospital to determine if your blood is receiving enough oxygen from the lungs. A small probe with a red light is usually attached to one finger.

## Other Neurologic Tests

- **Electroencephalogram (EEG):** The EEG measures your brain waves through several electrical leads painlessly attached to your head. EEG is not routinely used for stroke diagnosis, but would be ordered if your doctor thinks that you may have had a seizure.

- **Lumbar puncture (LP, spinal tap):** A needle is inserted in your lower back to obtain a sample of the fluid (cerebrospinal fluid, CSF) which surrounds your brain and spinal cord. LP is not routinely used for diagnosis of ischemic stroke. However, LP is often required if subarachnoid hemorrhage (bleeding from a cerebral aneurysm) is suspected. LP may also be needed if your doctor suspects a nervous system infection (such as meningitis) or inflammation.

- **Electromyogram/Nerve conduction test (EMG / NCV):** This test records the electrical activity of the nerves and muscles. EMG is not used for stroke diagnosis, but might be needed if your doctor suspects a problem with the nerves in your arms or legs.

- **Brain biopsy:** This is a surgical procedure in which a small piece of the brain is removed for microscopic examination. Biopsy is used to diagnose lesions (such as tumors) which cannot be identified by CT or MRI scan. It is very rarely used for stroke diagnosis, when cerebral vasculitis is suspected.

## Blood Tests and Procedures Used for Stroke Diagnosis

If you are being evaluated for stroke, it is likely that your doctor will order some blood tests. Stroke cannot be diagnosed by a blood test alone. However, these tests can provide information about stroke risk factors and other medical problems which may be important. Please note that the first set of tests are commonly used for routine or emergency evaluation of stroke, while the others are used only in very specific situations. Unless otherwise noted, each of these tests require just one tube of blood (a few teaspoons) drawn from a vein.

### Commonly Used Blood Tests

- **CBC (Complete blood count):** This is a routine test to determine the number of red blood cells, white blood cells, and platelets in your blood. Hematocrit and hemoglobin are measures of the number of red blood cells. A complete blood count might be used to diagnose anemia (too little blood) or infection (shown by too many white blood cells).

- **Coagulation tests:**
  - PT (Prothrombin time)
  - PTT (Partial thromboplastin time)
  - INR (International normalized ratio)
    These tests measure how quickly your blood clots. An abnormality could result in excessive bleeding or excessive clotting (which is difficult to measure). If you have been prescribed a blood-thinning medicine such as warfarin (Coumadin or similar drugs), the INR is used to be sure that you receive the correct dose. It is very important that you obtain regular checks. If you are taking heparin, the PTT (or aPTT) test is used to determine the correct dose.

- **Blood chemistry tests:** These tests measure the levels of normal chemical substances in your blood. The most important test in emergency stroke evaluation is glucose (or blood sugar), because levels of blood glucose which are too high or too low can cause symptoms which may be mistaken for stroke. A fasting blood glucose is used to help in the diagnosis of diabetes, which is a risk factor for stroke. Other blood chemistry tests measure serum electrolytes, the normal ions in your blood (sodium, potassium, calcium), or check the function of your liver or kidneys.

- **Blood lipid tests (Cholesterol, total lipids, HDL, and LDL):** Elevated cholesterol (particularly bad cholesterol, or LDL) is a risk factor for heart disease and stroke.

### Blood Tests for Specific Situations

This is a partial list of less common blood tests sometimes ordered for specific stroke situations, or where the cause of stroke is unclear (for example, in a young person without known stroke risk factors). Abnormal results may suggest a cause for the stroke.

- Antinuclear antibodies (ANA)
- Antiphospholipid antibodies (APL), Anticardiolipin antibodies (ACL), Lupus anticoagulant (LA)
- Blood culture
- Cardiac enzymes: Troponin, Creatine kinase (CPK, CK), LDH isoenzymes
- Coagulation factors: Antithrombin III, Protein C, Protein S; Factor VIII; activated Protein C resistance (Factor V Leiden)
- Erythrocyte sedimentation rate (ESR)
- Hemoglobin electrophoresis
- Homocysteine
- Syphilis serology (VDRL, FTA, others)
- Toxicology screen (serum or urine)

Please note that this listing applies only to the use of these tests for stroke diagnosis. Be sure to discuss any questions or concerns with your doctor or health care provider.

## Electrocardiogram (EKG, ECG)

ECG is done so often and routinely that most people do not even consider it a special test. However, a lot can be learned from an ECG about the regularity (or irregularity) of the heartbeat. The fact that irregularities in the rhythm of the heartbeat can lead to stroke makes it an important tool in stroke evaluation.

## What Is an Electrocardiogram?

An ECG is a painless test that is used to get information about the electrical activity of the heart, such as the rate and regularity of the heartbeat. The size and position of the heart chambers as well as any damage to the heart can also be obtained through an ECG. If you use an implanted device, like a pacemaker, its effect on the heart can also be studied through the results of this test.

## Why Do Doctors Use ECG's?

ECG is sometimes the only method of detecting irregularities in heart rhythm—such as atrial fibrillation—that can lead to the forming of blood clots that can later get flow to the brain. These blood clots can cause stroke by forming in the heart, coming loose and then getting lodged in a small artery of the brain. ECG is performed on every stroke patient as part of the routine evaluation. However, the test shows only a "snapshot" of the electrical activity of the heart (about 5 minutes), and other devices may be used to find irregularities that occur less frequently.

## What Happens during an ECG?

You will be asked to lie down while the sites where the sticky electrodes will be attached are cleaned and shaven, if necessary. About 12 electrodes are attached to various parts of your body, six of which will be attached to the chest. The other six (called limb leads) will be attached accordingly: one on each arm, one on each leg, and two on the abdomen.

You must usually lie still during the test, while holding your breath for short periods at a time. The test requires ten to 15 minutes to complete.

## What Are the Risks of ECG?

Since ECG is done without entering the body and does not use dyes or x-rays, there is no pain or risk associated with having an ECG.

## How Does an ECG Work?

The electrodes contain wires that can detect the electrical signals of the heart through the skin. These wires are connected to a machine that traces the heart rhythm on graph paper. Because the results are immediately known, your doctor will instantly know the basic vital signs of your heart.

## Echocardiogram

An echocardiogram can be used to find out if there is an abnormality of the heart that could lead to stroke. There are two types of echocardiograms: one that examines the heart through the chest (called transthoracic echocardiogram, or TTE), and one that examines the heart through the throat (called transesophageal echocardiogram, or TEE). The information that follows applies only to the use of these procedures in a stroke evaluation.

**Transthoracic echocardiogram** is most commonly performed, and it is a test that gives information about the size of the heart chamber, the motion of the heart walls, the movements of the heart valves, and changes in structure in and around the heart. Ultrasound waves (the same ones used in imaging the fetus in a pregnant woman) are used to make an image of the heart's walls and valves.

**Transesophageal echocardiogram** provides images of the internal structures of the heart and its blood vessels using the same ultrasound technology.

### Why Do Doctors Use Echocardiogram?

Doctors often use TTE on patients in whom they suspect blood clotting (called cardiac embolus), since clots that form in the heart can be detected using this procedure. Blood clots are a leading cause of stroke, as 80% of all clots in the heart eventually come loose and travel to the brain. An echocardiogram can help determine how to treat or prevent a stroke (if a blood clot is found in the heart, a blood-thinner such as Warfarin may be prescribed). TTE is performed routinely after heart attack and as part of a stroke evaluation.

Transesophageal echocardiogram (TEE) is usually prescribed after an abnormality is found in the results of a TTE. The images from TEE can provide more information about the condition of the heart because they have better resolution and are taken from the inside of the body rather than the outside.

### What Happens during Echocardiogram?

In TTE, a clear gel is placed on the area of the chest where the heart is located. This lubricating gel allows a device that both puts out and detects ultrasound signals (called an ultrasound transducer) to slide around easily on the skin. When the transducer is placed against the skin, a picture of the area is shown on a video screen. Depending on how the transducer is positioned, the heart can be viewed from several different angles. Due to blood flowing through the heart, a sound similar to your heartbeat will be heard.

A dye, called agitated saline, may be injected to find any leaking between the chambers of the heart. The images, stored as a 15-minute recording, will be viewed later by the physician. TTE requires about 45 minutes to complete.

TEE, unlike TTE, requires preparation before the test can be done. You will be asked not eat or drink anything except water during the eight hours before the test. You should also not smoke for six hours before the test is done. Be sure to ask your doctor how you should adjust your daily medications, such as insulin if you are diabetic.

During the actual procedure, you will be sedated intravenously to make it less uncomfortable. The doctor will then ask you to swallow a thin, flexible tube with a special tip (called a probe). You may be asked to gargle an anesthetic that will numb your throat and tongue so that you can swallow the probe more easily. The test takes 60-90 minutes to complete, but you may have to stay for one or two hours so that the sedative can wear off.

### What Are the Risks of Echocardiogram?

Since TTE is done without entering the body and does not use dyes, there is no risk or pain in having a TTE. In TEE, the swallowing of the probe may cause some discomfort or pain. However, anesthetics are usually given to make the procedure less uncomfortable.

### How Does Echocardiogram Work?

The transducer, or probe, emits high-frequency ultrasound waves that pass into the body and bounce off the valves of the heart and the muscles of the heart walls. The sound waves are reflected differently by different parts of the body. The transducer detects the different reflections of the sound waves, which are then measured and converted into live pictures of the heart by a computer. These images are recorded on videotape and later viewed by your doctor.

## Carotid Ultrasound (Carotid Doppler, Carotid Duplex)

Carotid ultrasound is a test that shows the carotid arteries (vessels in the neck that provide blood flow to the brain), as well as how much blood flows and how fast it travels through them. Ultrasound waves—the same ones used in imaging the fetus in a pregnant woman—are used to make an image of the arteries. This image can be used to find out if there is an abnormality or blockage of the carotid arteries that could lead to stroke. This test can be used to investigate the carotid arteries for several reasons, but the information here applies only to stroke evaluation.

### Why Do Doctors Use Carotid Ultrasound?

Doctors often use carotid ultrasound on patients who have had a stroke or who might be at high risk for a stroke. Narrowing of the carotid arteries—often caused by cholesterol deposits—and blood clots can be detected using this procedure. These conditions can cause problems with the blood flow to the brain and lead to a stroke. The actual blood flow through the carotid arteries can also be imaged by this test.

### What Happens during Carotid Ultrasound?

You will be asked to lie down on an examination table. The technician (or physician) will place a clear gel on the area of the neck where the carotid artery is located. The gel is simply a lubricant that allows the transducer (a device that both puts out and detects ultrasound signals) to slide around easily on your skin.

When the transducer is placed against the skin, an image of the artery is shown on a video screen. To view the arteries from many different angles, your doctor will re-position the transducer several times. Because blood is flowing through the artery, a sound similar to your heartbeat will be heard.

The procedure is repeated for the carotid artery on the other side of the neck. A carotid ultrasound usually only takes 15 to 30 minutes to complete and the results are immediately known by your doctor.

### What Are the Risks of Carotid Ultrasound?

Since the procedure is done without entering the body and does not use dyes or x-rays, there is no risk or pain involved in having a carotid ultrasound.

### How Does Carotid Ultrasound Work?

The transducer emits high-frequency, ultrasound waves that pass into the body and bounce off the carotid arteries and the red blood cells moving through them. The sound waves are reflected differently by different parts of the body. The transducer detects the different reflections of the sound waves, which are then measured and converted by a computer into live pictures of the arteries and the blood flow.

## Cerebral Angiography (Cerebral Angiogram, Cerebral Arteriogram, Digital Subtraction Angiography [DSA])

Cerebral angiography is used to image the blood vessels of the brain and the blood flowing through them. Angiography involves entering a catheter into the body to inject a dye (a contrast medium) into the carotid arteries, the vessels of the neck that lead to the brain. Then regular x-ray is used to image the dye that is flowing through the blood vessels. Although cerebral angiography can be used to investigate many abnormalities, only its relevance to stroke is discussed here.

### Why Do Doctors Use Cerebral Angiography?

Cerebral angiography shows the brain's blood vessels. Doctors use cerebral angiography to detect abnormalities in the brain's blood vessels, such as narrowing or blockage. It is usually done after another test (such as a CT scan) has already detected an abnormality. Angiography is useful in detecting and diagnosing acute stroke and is especially beneficial since the images taken through cerebral angiography cannot be taken through other techniques.

### What Happens during a Cerebral Angiography?

You will be asked to remove all clothing and jewelry and wear a patient gown before undergoing the procedure. While you are lying on an x-ray table, a local anesthetic is given, usually in the thigh, where an incision is made. The catheter (a long, narrow flexible tube) is put into your body through the incision navigated to the carotid arteries, where the dye is injected.

After you are properly placed on the exam table, your head is positioned in the desired field of view, and regular x-ray is used to take pictures of the blood vessels in the brain. While the procedure is being done, both the technologist and radiologist remain by your side. Although you are awake during the procedure, a medication may be given to help you relax. The entire procedure can take from one to two hours to complete.

## What Are the Risks of Cerebral Angiography?

The use of a catheter in cerebral angiography may cause you some discomfort or pain, although an anesthetic is usually given to help alleviate most discomfort.

There is also a risk of stroke caused by the catheter. While being navigated through the carotid arteries the catheter could break off a plaque that could block a smaller blood vessel in the brain and lead to stroke.

## How Does Cerebral Angiography Work?

The basic principle behind cerebral angiography is the same as that of regular x-ray imaging. As the x-rays pass through the body, they are absorbed at different levels. The absorption of the x-rays by the injected dye allows the blood vessels in the brain to be imaged. The differences in absorption become one of many images detected by a camera, which finally become a movie of the blood flow (and the flow of the intravenous dye) through the vessels.

## Computed Axial Tomography (CAT Scan, CT Scan)

The CAT scan (also called CT scan) is well-known by name, but do you really know what it is and understand how it works? A CT scan is usually one of the first tests done in a stroke evaluation, particularly during an acute stroke in the emergency room. This test can show areas of abnormalities in the brain, and can help to determine if these areas are caused by insufficient blood flow (ischemic stroke), a ruptured blood vessel (hemorrhage), or a different kind of a problem. CT scans can be obtained on any part of the body, but the information here applies only to CT scans of the head.

## What Is a CT Scan?

A CT scan uses x-rays to take pictures of your skull and brain. The patient lies in a tunnel-like machine. The inside of the machine rotates and takes x-rays of the head from different angles, which are later used by computers to make an image of a slice (or cross-section) of the brain.

## Why Do Doctors Use CT Scans?

CT scans use computers and rotating x-ray machines to create images of slices, or cross-sections, of the brain. Unlike other techniques,

CT scans (and MRI scans) can show the inside of the head, including soft tissue, bones, brains, and blood vessels. CT scans can often show the size and locations of brain abnormalities caused by tumors, blood vessel defects, blood clots, and other problems. CT scans are a primary method of determining whether a stroke is ischemic or hemorrhagic.

### Does a CT Scan Always Diagnose a Stroke?

No. Even if you are having a stroke, it might not be seen on CT scan for several reasons. In many cases, the involved area of the brain does not appear abnormal for the first several hours after the onset of stroke. Also, the stroke region may be too small to be seen on CT scan, or it may be in a part of the brain (brainstem or cerebellum) which the CT scan does not image well. Depending on the results of the CT scan, your doctor may wish to obtain additional testing, including an MRI scan. MRI can be more accurate for stroke and other conditions, but it takes longer and is often not available under emergency conditions.

### What Happens during a CT Scan?

You will remove any metallic objects which could diminish the quality of the images (this includes jewelry, glasses, dentures, and hair clips). You may also be asked remove your clothing and put on a patient gown. A technologist will help you to lie face up on the scanner table, with your head toward the "donut hole" of the CT scanner. The technologist will position you on the table, and a device to hold your head in place may be used. Then he or she leaves the exam room and goes to the control room, where you can still communicate by intercom.

An intravenous dye (contrast dye) may be given, through injection. This can help to highlight any areas of abnormality in the scan.

While CT images are being taken, it is important to lie still on the table, which will be moving very slowly in order to image the brain. It is normal for the CT scanner to make a whirring noise during the exam, so you should not be alarmed. The table will be moving a few millimeters at a time in order to obtain images of small slices of the brain, until the exam is finished. The procedure usually takes between 20 minutes and an hour.

### What Are the Risks of CT Scans?

The test is painless and there are few side effects. The CAT scan uses very little x-ray radiation. If you receive contrast dye, there is a chance of an allergic reaction. This reaction can be serious, and may require treatment with appropriate medication. If you have allergies to any foods or medicines, particularly seafood or iodine, it is important to inform the technologist before the procedure. You should also tell the technologist if you could be pregnant.

### How Does a CT Scan Work?

CT is based on the same principles as regular x-ray. The x-rays are absorbed differently by the different parts of the body. Bone absorbs the most x-rays, so the skull appears white on the image. Water (in the cerebral ventricles, fluid-filled cavities in the middle of the brain) absorbs little, and appears black. The brain has intermediate density and appears grey. Most ischemic strokes are less dense (darker) than normal brain, whereas blood in hemorrhage is denser and looks white on CT.

In brain CT imaging, a fan beam of x-rays is sent out through the skull, and a device on the other side of the scanner picks up the different strengths of the x-rays. After the x-ray tube and detector have made one 360° rotation, the image of one cross-section (a few millimeters in width) has been taken. During this rotation, hundreds of snapshots are taken, which are later used by a computer to make the final image.

## Magnetic Resonance Imaging (MRI, MR)

MRI is a test that produces very accurate pictures of the brain and its arteries without x-rays or dyes. This test is useful for detecting a wide variety of brain and blood vessel abnormalities, and can usually determine the area of the brain that is damaged by an ischemic stroke. During this painless test, you lie on a table that moves into the opening of the MRI machine. The machine creates a magnetic field which briefly alters the water molecules in your brain cells. The response to this magnetic field is then detected and used to create an image of the brain. Although MRI scans can be used on any part of the body, the following description applies only to MRI of the head.

### Why Do Doctors Use MRI?

MRI is useful for imaging soft tissues such as the brain because it shows great detail. It can detect minute differences, even between areas that are similar (unlike CAT scans, which are useful in imaging bone and soft tissue, but with less detail). MRI can often demonstrate brain abnormalities which are too small or located in regions of the brain that cannot be seen well by CAT scans. Another benefit of MRI is that it can be performed without x-rays or dyes (although many times, an intravenous dye called gadolinium is used to image the brain and its blood vessels). Brain MRI is commonly used to detect and diagnose many kinds of abnormalities of the skull, brain, and spinal cord. In addition to stroke, MRI is used to diagnose abnormal growths such as tumors, blood vessel abnormalities, infections, or disorders such as multiple sclerosis. MRI can provide direct views of the body from almost any direction, while CAT scans only provide images in an axial orientation. Medical images taken of the human body are usually displayed in three orientations:

- Coronal orientation: in a slice dividing the head into front and back halves.

- Sagittal orientation: in a slice dividing the head into left and right halves.

- Axial orientation: in a slice dividing the head into upper and lower halves.

There are several different kinds of MRI scan (called image sequences). Each sequence highlights different aspects of brain tissue, and may be used to answer specific questions. Some sequences (for example, diffusion-weighted MR) are particularly useful for detecting abnormalities in the first few hours after ischemic stroke. MRI can also be used to obtain an image of the blood vessels which supply the brain (magnetic resonance angiography or MRA).

### What Happens during an MRI?

Before the test, you will be asked a number of questions about previous operations or the presence of any metallic objects in your body. If you have artificial joints, a pacemaker, aneurysm clips, or other metal in your body, consult your doctor before having an MRI. You will be asked to remove all jewelry and metallic objects, and you may be asked to change into a patient gown. The technologist will help you lie down on the scanner table. After you are in the proper place, your head will be put in position and a special radio antenna (called a surface coil) will be placed around your head. The technologist will leave the exam room and go to the control room, where you can still communicate with him or her by intercom. You may have the option of listening to music during the test. While the MR images are being taken, it is important for you to lie still on the table, which will be moving very slowly to image the brain. It is normal for the MRI machine to make a loud knocking noise during the exam, so you should not be alarmed. The table will be moving a few millimeters at a time to obtain images of each "slice" of the brain, until the exam is finished. The test takes between 30 and 90 minutes to complete. A dye (contrast medium) may be given, through intravenous injection, to highlight the area being studied.

### What Are the Risks of an MRI Scan?

The MRI does not involve x-rays and there are no side effects. However, if you have any metallic objects in your body, the magnetic field can cause dangerous interactions. It is essential that you tell your doctor or the technologist about any previous surgery, implanted devices such as pacemakers, bullets or shrapnel wounds. You will have to lie flat within a relatively small space for as long as an hour. If you think this may be a problem for you (for example, if you are claustrophobic), you should discuss this with your doctor before you schedule the test. If the MRI test involves contrast dye, you will have an injection by vein (usually in your arm).

### How Does MRI Work?

During the exam, a radio signal is turned on in bursts, and the energy is absorbed differently by the different atoms in the body. This energy is reflected out of the body and detected by the MRI scanner. A digital computer constructs these reflections into a picture of the brain. The switching on and off of the device that measures the reflected MR signals (called the gradient coils) produces the knocking sound heard during the exam.

## American Stroke Association Reports that Backpack-Sized Ultrasound Device Detects Neck Artery Blockages

A low-cost portable device detected blockages in carotid (neck) arteries in less than half the time required for a standard laboratory ultrasound, according to research presented February 7, 2002 at the American Stroke Association's 27th International Stroke Conference. The American Stroke Association is a division of the American Heart Association.

This device could one day become a quick neighborhood stroke prevention screening tool and be added to the protocol for mobile programs that screen for other risk factors such as high cholesterol or high blood pressure. Ultrasonography has not been considered a cost-effective stroke-screening tool because of expensive equipment costs and lengthy screening times.

"Most standard ultrasound machines are at hospitals or a lab, and they are expensive to operate," says Ulf Schminke, M.D., lead author of the study and research fellow at Wake Forest University in Winston-Salem, North Carolina. "So it's not a convenient screening tool if you have to send patients to a private laboratory or a hospital for an examination."

The portable device Schminke's team used, SonoSite 180, is commercially available and costs about $18,000 to $20,000. Schminke estimates that stationary laboratory ultrasound machines cost more than $100,000. Researchers investigated how to make ultrasonography cheaper and faster to screen carotid arteries with ultrasound for stroke prevention. The lightweight ultrasound is commonly used for abdominal examinations rather than vascular screening.

Researchers screened 102 carotid arteries in 51 patients. While a normal laboratory ultrasound measured the speed of blood flow in the arteries, the portable device was used to take two different views of the arteries: a diameter measurement and a cross-sectional view. The average examination time with the portable device was 8.8 minutes. A standard laboratory ultrasound may take 30 minutes or longer, says Schminke.

They compared the accuracy of the portable device to that of a laboratory ultrasound and found that the portable ultrasound was 89.7 percent accurate in detecting stenoses (blockages) greater than 75 percent of the vessel. The portable device was also accurate (83.8 percent) at detecting stenoses of 50 percent or greater. Overall, the device's accuracy was considered excellent for use as a primary prevention tool.

"If a patient is determined to have a high degree of stenosis with this device, they could then be referred for further testing and possibly surgery to unclog their carotid arteries," says Schminke. "The idea of this type of screening is to find out which people are normal and which people may need a further work-up."

## Spiral Scan Sees Stroke Blockage More Clearly Reports Stroke: Journal of the American Heart Association

The accuracy of diagnosing a blocked brain vessel in an emergency setting improved nearly 100 percent when physicians used a high-speed

CT scanner, researchers report in the April 2002 *Stroke: Journal of the American Heart Association.*

Physicians working in emergency rooms typically do a physical examination of stroke patients, including a standard CT scan of the head. They also ask them or their families a series of questions about symptoms to assess the location and nature of the stroke. A standard CT scan can quickly determine whether the stroke is ischemic or hemorrhagic.

However, high-speed helical CT scans (sometimes called spiral CT), which use a contrast dye, give physicians a view of blood flow inside vessels and the pattern of blood distribution throughout the brain. Helical scanners also allow them to quickly determine if a stroke is ischemic and find where a blockage exists, says study author Michael H. Lev, M.D. The scan can also show the doctor if the vessel is partially or completely blocked, and can show which areas of the brain are not getting enough blood.

"The bottom line is that this is a convenient, cost-effective, minimally invasive way to rapidly get more information that can help acute stroke patients," says Lev. "Most emergency departments in the U.S. have a CT scanner, and the majority are helical scanners. Our study shows they can be used for the brain."

Information from these scans could help physicians assess how best to treat ischemic stroke patients.

"It may turn out that the patient isn't having a stroke at all, as happened with four of our patients," says Lev, who is director of the neurovascular laboratory at Massachusetts General Hospital and an assistant professor of radiology at Harvard Medical School in Boston. "It may be a seizure, a migraine headache, or a drastic drop in blood sugar mimicking a stroke."

About 600,000 Americans suffer a first or recurrent stroke each year and about 167,000 of them die. The two major types of stroke are ischemic, caused by a blood clot that blocks a vessel and prevents oxygen-rich blood from reaching a portion of the brain, and hemorrhagic, which occurs when a blood vessel leaks or ruptures.

The only approved therapy for acute ischemic stroke is a clot-busting (thrombolytic) drug either through the veins within three hours after the onset of symptoms, or by infusing it directly into a brain artery, usually within six hours. Thrombolytic drugs do not benefit people with hemorrhagic strokes, and can worsen the bleeding in the brain.

At Massachusetts General, helical CT scans are standard for stroke patients brought to the emergency room. "We had established helical

CT as an accurate technique for determining where the damage occurs," says Lev. "The question for our study was to find out how useful it is in diagnosing stroke in addition to what we were using already."

He and his colleagues selected the medical records of 40 acute stroke patients (23 men and 17 women) who had received helical CT scans. Neurologists on the hospital's stroke team reviewed each case. They answered a series of questions at five points in the patients' assessments.

The first point was when the patient's physical examination, symptoms, and initial CT scan without the contrast dye were completed. The last was when all the data, including results from the helical CT scan, was available.

At each point the neurologists were asked to give the stroke location, how much brain tissue was affected, which blood vessel was obstructed, and the severity of the stroke. Their answers were compared to the final assessment made after the patient had been released from the hospital.

The average accuracy of the neurologists' answers between their first and final stroke assessments rose from 40 percent to 80 percent for stroke location and from 40 percent to 78 percent in identifying the blocked vessel. Determining the brain area affected by the stroke rose from 55 percent to 83 percent and the accuracy of their classification increased from 55 percent to 88 percent.

"As the neurologists gained information about the patients, their assessment of the stroke became more accurate," says Lev. "The difference in stroke assessment was substantial after doctors saw results from the helical CT."

# Chapter 21

# Stroke Victims Need Drugs Fast

Speeding up delivery of clot-busting drugs to stroke victims could greatly improve their chances of recovery, even if doctors manage to shave off just a few minutes, a new analysis shows. Medicines that break up clots are the only effective treatment in the hours after a stroke. To do any good, however, they must be administered before brain cells die.

The current standard requires that treatment begin within three hours of the onset of the stroke, and most patients who make it to the hospital in time get the drugs within the last half hour before that deadline. Now, a new report finds that earlier treatment—in the first 90 minutes after symptoms begin—doubles the chances of full recovery compared with treatment that starts later.

"If we can convince people that every minute counts, it could be a big boost," said Dr. Thomas G. Brott of the Mayo Clinic in Jacksonville, FL. "We can't relax for one minute. With every minute, brain cells

This chapter includes "Study: Stroke Victims Need Drugs Fast," by Daniel Q. Haney, AP Medical Editor, Saturday, February 9, 2002, reprinted with permission of the Associated Press; "Thrombolytic Therapy (Tissue Plasminogen Activator—tPA)," Updated 9/04/01 by Victoria Kennedy, RN, © 2000 A.D.A.M., Inc., reprinted with permission; "NIH Experts Say Few Eligible Stroke Patients Receive Treatments that Save Lives and Reduce Disability," NIH News Release 05/15/2000, National Institute of Neurological Disorders and Stroke (NINDS); and "Ultrasound Aids Stroke Treatment," by Peggy Peck, UPI Science News, Published 2/8/2002, © 2002 United Press International, reprinted with permission.

are dying by the tens of thousands." Brott presented his findings Saturday, February 9, 2002 at the annual meeting of the American Stroke Association in San Antonio.

TPA—tissue plasminogen activator—can dissolve clots that block arteries and has long been the mainstay of heart attack treatment. In 1995, a federally-funded study showed it could reverse strokes the same way if given within three hours of symptom onset. As a result of that study, the three-hour time window became standard. But some specialists say that isn't good enough. Faster treatment will better the odds that patients will escape with their thinking power and other functions intact, they say, and the latest analysis supports that belief.

Brott and colleagues combined data from six studies of clot-dissolving drugs involving 2,776 patients in 18 countries. They found that those treated within the first 90 minutes after the start of symptoms have almost three times the chance of a full recovery compared to people who are not treated. However, those treated in the second 90 minutes have only a 1.5 times greater chance of recovery.

"We conclude that time in fact is brain," he said. "The earlier the treatment, the more the benefit." Brott said hospitals should strive to start treatment—the so-called door-to-needle time—within an hour of the patient's arrival.

Dr. Joseph Broderick of the University of Cincinnati said hospitals need to work out systems to coordinate treatment to shave off delays. "Hospitals that won't do it right should not be taking stroke patients, but most community hospitals can do this, he said. "It's not rocket science, but it has to be organized properly."

Currently only about 2 percent of stroke patients end up getting TPA. The biggest barrier is that they arrive at the hospital too late. Many ignore their symptoms or don't realize anything is wrong.

Once at a hospital, doctors must make sure the stroke is actually caused by a clot in the brain. Broken blood vessels can also cause strokes, and giving TPA to those people makes the situation worse.

Hospitals must give patients CT scans, have them read by a neurologist to make sure there is no bleeding, and then begin administering TPA through a catheter. Small delays quickly add up, especially if hospitals work step by step rather than getting everyone involved in the treatment moving simultaneously.

"You have to take a drop everything approach," said Brott. "That is difficult for a neurologist who has an office full of patients or is home 15 miles away from the hospital."

Dr. Robert Hobson of the New Jersey Medical School in Newark said new technology can help. For instance, neurologists reached at night can receive digital CT images over phone lines and make a treatment decision without leaving home.

## Thrombolytic Therapy (Tissue Plasminogen Activator—tPA)

### Alternative Names

TPA; Alteplase; Activase thrombolytic agent; Clot-dissolving agents; Reperfusion therapy

### Definition

Tissue plasminogen activator (tPA) is a drug that break ups or dissolves blood clots. Blood clots are the main cause of both heart attacks and stroke. The best results occur if this medicine is given within 3 hours of a heart attack or stroke.

### Information

Since 1996, tPA has been approved by the Food and Drug Administration (FDA) for the treatment of stroke and heart attack. According to the American Heart Association (AHA), if tPA is given within the first 3 hours of a stroke, it may reduce permanent disability. If given within the first 3 hours of a heart attack, the person has a better chance for recovery.

There are various drugs that dissolve clots, but tPA is currently used most often. Others include Streptokinase (SK), Reteplase, Tenecteplase, Urokinase, Lanoteplase, and Staphylokinase.

### Heart Attack

Guidelines are used to determine if someone is a good candidate for using tPA. According to the American College of Cardiology (ACC), each year 800,000 persons in the United States have acute heart attacks and 213,000 die. Those who die from heart attacks generally die within 1 hour from the initial onset of symptoms and sometimes before they get to the hospital. Many national groups are working together to decrease the time it takes to get people having a heart attack to facilities where tPA can be given. The sooner thrombolysis therapy is given, the better the outcome. The window of opportunity is a very short amount of time.

For a person having an acute heart attack, tPA works by dissolving a major clot quickly. The clot is most likely blocking one of the coronary arteries that normally allows blood and oxygen get to the heart muscle. By dissolving the clot, the blood is able to start flowing again to that area of the heart. If the blood flow to the heart is started again rapidly, it may prevent long-term damage to the heart muscle and may even stop an event that could have been fatal.

Physicians base their decisions about whether to give tPA for a heart attack on many factors, including results of an ECG test. Other factors used to determine if someone is a good candidate for tPA include age, medical history, gender, history of previous heart attack, history of diabetes, history of low blood pressure or increased heart rate, and if the person is elderly (older than 70 years).

Generally, tPA will not given if the person has had a recent head injury, trauma, surgery, bleeding problems, uncontrolled high blood pressure, bleeding ulcers, or pregnancy.

### *Stroke*

Close to 80% of all strokes are ischemic strokes, caused when blood clots form in one place in the body then travel to a smaller blood vessel in the brain, blocking the blood flow to that part of the brain. For strokes of this nature, tPA can help dissolve the clot quickly. Often, tPA can limit the amount of permanent disability that can result from an ischemic stroke, especially if given within 3 hours of the initial symptoms of the stroke.

tPA is not given if someone is having a hemorrhagic stroke or a stroke caused by bleeding in the brain, because this could worsen the stroke by causing increased bleeding. Ischemic strokes often occur when a person is relatively tranquil or calm. Hemorrhagic strokes often occur during some sort of physical exertion. Hemorrhagic strokes generally have more profound symptoms at the very beginning of the stroke, whereas the symptoms with an ischemic stroke sometimes develop over a longer period of time and may not be as severe.

In some cases the diagnosis of the actual type of stroke may be difficult and the risk of bleeding from tPA is a concern. Generally, the benefits of receiving it outweigh the risks.

### *Risks*

Hemorrhage or bleeding is the most common risk associated with the administration of tPA therapy. This is true for both stroke and heart attack patients. When given to patients who have been diagnosed with a heart attack, there is a risk that they could have a stroke or an intracranial hemorrhage as a complication of the therapy. With stroke patients, there is also a possibility of intracranial hemorrhage.

## Contact a Healthcare Provider or Call 911 Emergency Service

The key for people suffering from a heart attack or a stroke is recognizing that both conditions are medical emergencies. The sooner transportation and treatment with tPA takes place for acceptable candidates, the better the chance that person has for a good outcome. If you suspect you or someone you know is suffering from symptoms of a heart attack or stroke, you should seek help immediately.

## NIH Experts Say Few Eligible Stroke Patients Receive Treatments That Save Lives and Reduce Disability

The National Institute of Neurological Disorders and Stroke, a component of the National Institutes of Health, said that few eligible stroke patients receive treatments that can significantly reduce disability and save lives. Gerald D. Fischbach, MD, director of NINDS, said that nearly five years after a NINDS clinical trial found that clot busting treatments can reduce or even reverse the symptoms of ischemic stroke, the treatment's promise is unfulfilled. The vast majority of patients who might benefit from it do not receive it.

"Again and again we see in research studies that patients do not recognize symptoms as stroke and get to the hospital in time," Dr. Fischbach said. "This is a crisis of under-utilization that causes unnecessary disability and costs millions extra in health care costs."

Patients who suffer from ischemic strokes, those that cause blood clots in the brain, have the most potential of receiving treatments that can reduce deaths and disability. One of the most effective ischemic stroke treatments is tissue plasminogen activator (tPA). Nearly five years ago, a NINDS clinical trial found that patients who received tPA treatment within three hours of their initial stroke symptoms were at least 30 percent more likely than untreated patients to recover from their stroke with little or no disability after three months.

Currently, there is no official national estimate of the percentage of ischemic stroke patients who receive thrombolytic treatments. However, numerous research studies in individual communities have concluded that about 10 percent or less of eligible stroke patients receive tPA or other treatments, primarily because they arrive at the hospital after the three-hour window has closed. For example, a Cleveland-area study published in the March 1, 2000, issue of the *Journal of the American Medical Association*, found that "the rate of IV tPA use among hospitals varied from 0 percent to 10.2 percent of stroke admissions."[1]

"Two things need to happen in order to ensure that more stroke patients benefit from treatments that dissolve blood clots in the brain," said John R. Marler, MD, associate director for clinical trials at NINDS. "First, people at risk for stroke and the people around them must know the signs of stroke. Then, they must call 911 and get to a hospital quickly. The sooner they begin receiving treatment, the better their chances for a complete recovery."

The main symptoms of stroke are:

- Sudden numbness or weakness of face, arm, or leg—especially on one side of the body

- Sudden confusion or trouble speaking or understanding

- Sudden trouble seeing in one or both eyes

- Sudden trouble walking, dizziness, loss of balance or coordination.

- Sudden severe headache with no known cause

NINDS researchers encourage people at risk for stroke and their family members, friends, and caregivers to learn the signs of stroke. In many cases, because stroke attacks the brain, a person experiencing stroke will not realize a stroke is occurring. But the people around them can recognize the symptoms and act fast. Candidates can receive certain stroke therapies only if they can verify the onset of their symptoms to within three hours of arriving at the hospital.

"Stroke is a condition that is easy to see," said Dr. Marler. "There are few other medical conditions that come on so suddenly and that are so noticeable to a bystander. Many people avoid stroke because they treat their high blood pressure and stop smoking. But of those who do have strokes, few receive treatment."

### References

1. Katzan, et.al., Use of Tissue-Type Plasminogen Activator for Acute Ischemic Stroke: The Cleveland Area Experience. *JAMA*, March 1, 2000. Vol 283, No. 9. Pp. 1151-1158.

## Ultrasound Aids Stroke Treatment

Surgeons use sound waves to pulverize gallstones and now stroke experts are trying to determine if less powerful ultrasound can improve the efficacy of the clot-busting drugs used to restore blood flow to the brain.

Dr. Andrei Alexandrov, of the University of Texas Houston, said he was using intracranial ultrasound to track the efficacy of the clot-busting drug called tPA or alteplase.

Shortly after initiating the ultrasound monitoring, emergency room nurses told him patients "were getting better really fast." At that point, he decided to initiate a pilot study to determine if ultrasound could boost the clot-busting or thrombolysis ability of tPA, he explained Friday, February 8, 2002 during a news briefing at the 27th International Stroke Conference in San Antonio.

Alexandrov uses a hand-held ultrasound device fitted into a frame "like the frame inside a construction worker's hard hat," he said. Using a Food and Drug Administration-approved diagnostic frequency setting of 2 megahertz, the device focuses on the clot while the tPA is infused over a period of about an hour and then continues to track the clot for an hour after infusion.

Alexandrov said sound waves are very powerful and a low thumping "could mechanically shake apart a clot." But that approach would be dangerous because it would be difficult to control. The FDA approved diagnostic frequency is "faster but gentler. It creates microvibrations that work on the surface of the clot to open up more surface that the tPA can then bind to and penetrate," he said.

The pilot study enrolled 55 patients, average age 69. Thirty-seven percent had complete clearance of clots, called recanalization, within two hours of treatment initiation and "70 percent had a partial clearance of clots," Alexandrov said in an interview with United Press International. He cautioned, however, the pilot study was designed to test the safety not efficacy of the approach. "We did prove that ultrasound is safe when used in this way," he said.

Dr. Gregory del Zoppo, of Scripps Research Institute in La Jolla, Calif., and a member of the American Stroke Association's executive committee told UPI ultrasound "has been looked at by a number of investigators. There is no doubt that sound waves can (break-up) clots, but safety is a concern."

While Alexandrov's study, which was designed as a safety trial, found no safety problems using the diagnostic ultrasound devices, del Zoppo said he doubts such low power devices actually improve the recanalization rate of clot-busting drugs. The temptation, he said, will be to use more powerful devices "and that's where safety becomes an issue."

He noted researchers in Germany and in Oregon tried putting ultrasound clot-busting probes on catheters that were guided to the clot site but those studies were halted when the sound waves not only dissolved the clots but also damaged artery walls. Moreover, del Zoppo said the recanalization rates cited by Alexandrov are not especially high. But Alexandrov said his early results are so promising a new phase II study aimed at determining the most effective frequency has already begun. So far 41 patients have been treated and the goal is to enroll 136 patients.

"We will evaluate the findings half-way through and may at that point move directly to a phase III trial," he said. Phase III trials are the final studies required before FDA approval.

## Additional Information

### NIH Neurological Institute
P.O. Box 5801
Bethesda, MD 20824
Toll-Free: 800-352-9424
Tel: 301-496-5751
TTY: 301-468-5981
Website: www.ninds.nih.gov

# Chapter 22

# Acute Stroke Management

## Principles of Effective Management of Acute Stroke

From Shakespearean times and beyond, stroke has aged our youth, destroyed the autumn of our life, and chilled the winter of our discontent. But in more recent times, there has been a major change in the effect stroke has had on our lives and we are hopeful that there will be future changes as well.

Over the last few years we have reached a number of milestones in the management of stroke. The list of milestones begins with the development of arteriography and echocardiography, procedures that were first used in the early 1950s. Another major advance was the identification of risk factors for stroke and the discovery that these risk factors could be manipulated to reduce the incidence and prevalence of stroke.

The introduction of randomized clinical trials by the National Institute of Neurological Disorders and Stroke was a particularly notable step forward. These trials included not only trials for drugs like platelet inhibitors and anticoagulants, but also surgical trials. This was an extraordinary achievement for stroke research and major

"Keynote Address: Principles of Effective Management of Acute Stroke," by K.M.A. Welch M.D., Henry Ford Hospital and Health Sciences Center, Detroit, Michigan, National Institute of Neurological Disorders and Stroke (NINDS), reviewed July 1, 2001; and "Recommendations: Prehospital Emergency Medical Care Systems Panel," National Institute on Neurological Disease and Stroke (NINDS), reviewed July 1, 2001.

credit goes to the clinical scientists, particularly the surgeons, who provided the skills to conduct and design these trials. When we look back over the last 15 years at the results and changes brought about by these studies—the NASCET,[1] the SPAF trials,[2-4] the ACAS,[5] and now the NINDS tPA Stroke Study[6]—we can see just how extraordinary these programs are. They reflect clear planning and a great deal of foresight, and have had a major impact on the health of our society. We entered another major technological era with the introduction of CT scanning and MRI/MRA, tools that will help us further define the progression of stroke in our patients.

But now we come to a new milestone in stroke management: advances in acute stroke treatment. The spotlight has been on tPA and indeed this drug did precipitate the need for new strategies in acute stroke management. But our focus during this symposium has been not only on this new drug treatment, but also on how we manage acute stroke and the strategies we can use in the future to manage it more effectively. In addition, we hope that a number of other new brain protective drugs will be available soon and for which we will be prepared because of the new systems we develop as a result of this symposium.

This monograph outlines a number of underlying general principles of effective stroke management. The first is that the interests and needs of patients with stroke and their families should be the primary concern of all stroke care professionals. Progress in acute stroke management will only be achieved if stroke is considered a medical emergency and that means that all stroke patients must receive immediate evaluation at hospitals. Support by self-help and voluntary patient associations must be encouraged to educate the public about the symptoms of stroke so that care providers have the opportunity to deliver this immediate evaluation.

A second principle is that all current and future therapies for stroke should be based on scientific evidence, and treatments of unproved value should not be used routinely in stroke patients. Management of all aspects of disability should be planned in close collaboration with patients and their families. And collaboration in stroke research—including prevention, acute management, nursing care and rehabilitation, and education—should be promoted at local, national, and international levels taking into account the needs and contributions of all professional groups and patient associations.

These principles reflect the same essential principles for good practice that have been outlined by the Europeans in the Helsingborg Declaration of stroke management.[7] The European community recently recognized the need for community strategies in the management of acute stroke and put this recognition on record. And now this monograph presents the generalized recommendations for changes in stroke management in the United States. The specific details of how this is carried out should be determined by organizations at the local level, and we recognize that regional implementation will vary widely.

Conclusions from this conference that all participants can agree on are summarized as follows:

- **Prehospital care:** This part of our community is already willing to change and be flexible. In fact, the system needs only minor modifications to achieve the goals we have established of more rapid response to acute stroke. Perhaps more important is to establish that research is needed to continue to make improvements in our prehospital care of patients.

- **Emergency department care:** For stroke, just as for myocardial infarction and trauma, it is essential that emergency departments be reorganized and realigned to work in concert with prehospital care providers and then to move carefully selected patients into acute hospital care departments.

- **Acute hospital care:** This critical link in the management of stroke may be the most challenging in terms of making changes to accommodate the movement toward rapid treatment. But changes can and will occur, as was demonstrated in the NINDS tPA Stroke Study. That study showed that, with proper management of the systems, we can indeed recruit patients within the 3-hour time-frame. We must work, however, to extend that therapeutic window, perhaps through the use of newer, sophisticated imaging techniques or with enhancement of CT scan diagnostic potential. Questions we should answer include: "Is reperfusion safe?" "Will treatment cause hemorrhage?" "What are the issues we should consider in predicting hemorrhagic conversion, staging of stroke, identifying viable tissue, predicting cell death, and identifying creative ways to extend the therapeutic window?"

- **Health care systems:** We must work to continually improve integrated stroke management delivery systems. It is vital for us to create a system of care that responds appropriately to the needs of our patients while considering also the larger societal need to control costs.

- **Public education:** The final domain is public education, that which is most essential if we are to deliver acute treatment strategies to patients. This is clearly the most difficult challenge—changing the behavior of our patients—and we will need to develop innovative processes to accomplish this goal.

## *Conclusion*

A final observation is that we should set targets for ourselves: these targets should include establishing systems of organized management of acute stroke, providing access to specialized assessment and treatment at stroke centers, providing access to specialty stroke rehabilitation, and providing access to information on stroke prevention. We can never forget the importance of continuous improvements of our systems and quality assessment programs.

What rigorous targets can we set for ourselves? Suggestions include reducing the 1-month death rate to below 20%, reducing the 2-year recurrent fatal and nonfatal stroke rate to below 20%, reducing vascular death overall to less than 40%, and having 70% of our stroke patients engaged in activities of daily living at 3 months after stroke.[7]

All of us involved in this effort should move forward with optimism to achieve these targeted goals and make successful management of acute stroke a reality for all communities.

## *References*

1. North American Symptomatic Carotid Endarterectomy Trial (NASCET) Investigators. Beneficial effect of carotid endarterectomy in symptomatic patients with high-grade carotid stenosis. *N Engl J Med* 1991;325(7):445-453.

2. Stroke Prevention in Atrial Fibrillation (SPAF I) Investigators. The Stroke Prevention in Atrial Fibrillation study: Final results. *Circulation* 1991;84:527-539.

3. Stroke Prevention in Atrial Fibrillation (SPAF II) Investigators. Aspirin versus warfarin for prevention of thromboembolism in atrial fibrillation: Stroke Prevention in Atrial Fibrillation II study. *Lancet* 1994;343:687-691.

4. Stroke Prevention in Atrial Fibrillation (SPAF III) Investigators. Adjusted dose warfarin versus low-intensity, fixed-dose warfarin plus aspirin for high-risk patients with atrial fibrillation:

Stroke Prevention in Atrial Fibrillation III randomised clinical trial. *Lancet* 1996;348:633-638.

5. Executive Committee for the Asymptomatic Carotid Atherosclerosis Study. Endarterectomy for asymptomatic carotid artery stenosis. *JAMA* 1995;273(18):1421-1428.

6. The National Institute of Neurological Disorders and Stroke rt-PA Stroke Study Group. Tissue plasminogen activator for acute ischemic stroke. *N Engl J Med* 1995;333:1581-1587.

7. Adams HP Jr. Editorial: Stroke management in Europe. *J Intern Med* 1996;240:169-171.

# Recommendations: Prehospital Emergency Medical Care Systems Panel

The Prehospital Emergency Medical Care Systems Panel addressed the early needs of the stroke patient in the prehospital setting. The panel, consisting of invited acknowledged specialists in emergency medical services (EMS) systems, took commentary from invited organizations and audience members at large. The assimilated summary recommendations are as follows:

## Overall Recommendations

1. Stroke management should be re-prioritized in EMS systems as a time-dependent, urgent medical emergency, just as is currently stressed for major trauma and acute myocardial infarction.

2. A Chain of Recovery should be ensured in each community and emphasized with educational initiatives in order to optimize the chances of recovery for stroke patients.

3. New educational initiatives should be developed and widely promulgated, as applicable, for each of the various persons constituting the respective links in the Chain of Recovery: (a) the public at large; (b) EMS dispatchers; (c) first-responder crews; (d) basic and advanced life-support ambulance/response crews; and (e) receiving facility personnel, including emergency department (ED) staff members and neurological disease specialists.

4.  Task forces should be created to: (a) help develop model educational initiatives for each of the respective links; and (b) develop standardized data sets to help ensure more effective research and outcomes analyses.

### Specific Subpanel Recommendations

Three subpanels were organized to specifically address issues related to: (a) EMS dispatch activities; (b) procedures and medical care that should be performed on the scene and en route to the hospital; and (c) special considerations in terms of access to care. The specific subpanel recommendations are detailed in separate sections, but can be summarized as follows:

- Dispatch Issues

- Prehospital Medical Care Issues

- Special Considerations in Access to Care

- Research Recommendations

### Dispatch Issues

1.  The public at large should be educated about how to "make the right call."

2.  Enhanced 911 systems (that automatically display the caller's address and telephone number) are strongly encouraged.

3.  Dispatchers and dispatching systems should have medical (as well as administrative) supervision that provides medical oversight and continuing medical education.

4.  New educational initiatives for dispatchers should emphasize stroke as a time-dependent, urgent medical emergency.

5.  Even with the emphasis on re-prioritizing stroke patients, dispatch protocols should still consider sending the closest available transport unit, basic or advanced, in tiered ambulance systems.

6.  Additional information should be elicited from the callers regarding relevant medical conditions (such as history of diabetes and current medications) and, also, certain basic medical care instructions should be provided prior to arrival of the EMS crews (i.e., "prearrival instructions").

7. Like all other rescuers in the Chain of Recovery, dispatchers should receive feedback and additional reinforcement regarding their actions in stroke cases.

8. Policies regarding stroke patients should be re-evaluated by managed care organizations to ensure that stroke patients receive timely and appropriate care.

## *Prehospital Medical Care Issues*

1. It should be recognized that most texts currently utilized by EMS personnel are lacking in terms of stroke management.

2. Simple, directed assessments should be emphasized in training of EMS personnel regarding stroke management.

3. Except for patients with respiratory distress or insufficiency, low-flow oxygen (1-2 liters/minute) should be administered and, if the tools are readily available, serum glucose levels should be measured.

4. Respiratory efforts and airway patency should be continuously monitored.

5. Although intravenous catheter placement and 12-lead electrocardiographic tracings are preferable, performing these procedures in the prehospital setting should not significantly delay transport to definitive care facilities. Therefore their performance may be venue-dependent (e.g., there is more help available in the prehospital setting than in the ED).

6. In general, hypertension should not be treated in the prehospital setting; hypotension should be treated aggressively (in accordance with the underlying etiology for the hypotension).

7. More data on neuroprotective agents are needed and future prehospital research is recommended.

8. EMS personnel should gather applicable onset information, including telephone access to witnesses/bystanders, and they should collect and/or document all medications (particularly aspirin, warfarin, insulin, and antihypertensives).

9. Systems for prealerting receiving facilities should be established so that ED staff members, imaging technicians, and

stroke specialists can be readied for the arriving stroke patient.

10. As in the case of dispatchers, EMS crews should receive more feedback and training opportunities that emphasize the urgency of both stroke and transient ischemic attacks (TIAs).

## Special Considerations in Access to Care

1. In those venues with multiple medical facilities, it is advised to bypass those facilities not capable of providing appropriate care for the stroke patient.
2. In those venues without nearby definitive stroke care capabilities, it is advised, in general, that EMS providers immediately transport patients to the closest appropriate emergency facility where rapid evaluation and transfer (if appropriate) can be performed.
3. In remote areas without nearby facilities, direct on-scene rescue by air medical services can be considered if: (a) the closest emergency facility is more than an hour away; (b) the closest facility is not capable of providing definitive diagnosis and care; and (c) the patient can reach the definitive care facility within the agreed upon therapeutic time window for stroke.

## Research Recommendations

Several recurring questions were asked during the panel sessions. These questions include the following potential research issues:

1. What are the sensitivities and specifics of various dispatch triage algorithms for stroke patients, particularly those evaluating "hot" and "cold" responses or advanced versus basic life-support ambulance dispatches in tiered systems?

2. What are optimal inspired oxygen fractions for stroke patients?

3. Are 12-lead electrocardiographs or glucose measurements of discernible value in any given stroke patient?

4. Is the prehospital administration of any neuroprotective agent of value?

5. Are designated stroke centers demonstrably efficacious in altering outcome?

6. What is the safety of air medical transport after treatment (e.g., thrombolytic therapy for stroke)?

## *Conclusions*

The Prehospital Emergency Medical Care Systems Panel delineated a roadmap for improving stroke management through an intensive and well-represented consensus process. It is anticipated that this plan will need further refinements, but for now, the document provides a significant advance in terms of the educational awareness needs as well as a global strategy for improving the chain of recovery for stroke patients.

# Chapter 23

# *Tool Allows Early Prediction of Patient's Stroke Outcome*

Scientists have developed a new tool that may help physicians predict, during the first several hours a stroke patient is in the hospital, the degree of recovery the patient will eventually experience. The tool uses three factors for the accurate prediction of stroke outcome: measurement of brain injury using magnetic resonance imaging (MRI); the patient's score on the NIH stroke scale; and the time in hours from the onset of symptoms until the MRI brain scan is performed.

Alison E. Baird, M.D., Ph.D., of the National Institute of Neurological Disorders and Stroke (NINDS), and colleagues published their findings in the June 30, 2001 issue of *Lancet*.[1] "We hope this new tool will not only help physicians manage their patients more efficiently, but also will alleviate the distress and anxiety about prognosis that patients and their families suffer in the first days after stroke," said Dr. Baird.

The researchers set out to see if a new type of brain imaging technology called magnetic resonance diffusion-weighted imaging (MR-DWI), in addition to standard clinical assessments, could yield prognostic information about a stroke. The MR-DWI can measure the volume of the lesions that appear during the first few hours after an ischemic stroke, which is caused by a clot obstructing blood flow to the brain. The study results showed that this measurement correlates

"New Tool Allows Early Prediction of Patient's Stroke Outcome," NIH News Release, 06/28/2001, National Institute of Neurological Disorders and Stroke (NINDS).

with the severity of the stroke as well as the patient's outcome. Patients with small lesion volumes (less than 14.1 milliliters) were five times more likely to recover from their strokes than patients with larger lesion volumes.

Another important prognostic tool that has been used widely for many years is the National Institutes of Health Stroke Scale (NIHSS), used to measure the severity of neurological dysfunction at the time of a stroke. In the study reported in *Lancet*, the Stroke Scale was measured within 1 hour of the MRI scan. A score greater than 25 indicates very severe neurological impairment; a score between 15 and 25 indicates severe impairment, while a score between 5 and 15 mild to moderately severe impairment, and a score less than 5 mild impairment. The mean score of the patients in this study was 11.

The third measurement in the scale is the time from the onset of the patient's symptoms to the time of the brain scan. If a patient suffered the stroke while asleep, the time was backdated to the last time the patient was known to have no stroke symptoms. Surprisingly, the patients who waited the longest before receiving their scans were more likely to recover. The investigators speculate that this time relationship may reflect an "instability" factor in the earliest hours of stroke. There may be more certainty of a good outcome when the patient is assessed beyond the first 6 hours, by which time the most critical changes in blood flow in the brain have occurred.

The NINDS study involved looking at the data from a total of 129 stroke patients—66 at the Beth Israel Deaconess Medical Center in Boston and 63 at the Royal Melbourne Hospital in Australia—and then developing a three-item scale for early prediction of stroke recovery. (Good stroke recovery in this study was defined as a score of greater than 90 on the Barthel Index, indicating a patient who has nearly full functional independence.)

Using the three-item scale the researchers assigned points (with a maximum score of 7) based on the brain lesion volume, the patient's score on the NIHSS, and the time from symptoms to scanning. The clinicians rated a patient's likelihood of recovery using categories of low (total score 0-2), medium (total score 3-4), or high (total score 5-7).

The new scale proved to be a very accurate predictor of stroke recovery with high sensitivity and specificity. In the Boston group, only 6 percent of the patients who had a low score (0-2) recovered. Forty-seven percent of the patients with a medium range score recovered, and 93 percent of those with a high score recovered. In the Australian group, 8 percent of patients with a low score recovered, 57 percent of patients with a medium score recovered, and 78 percent of patients with a high score recovered.

The researchers concluded that the combination of clinical and imaging data allowed more reliable early prediction of stroke recovery than any single factor alone.

Future studies will focus on evaluating the potential of CT scanning in the prediction of recovery from stroke. CT scanning is the standard imaging tool for stroke patients and, unlike MRI, is available in nearly every hospital. "This would allow us to make a prognostic stroke scale more widely available for clinical use," said Dr. Baird. Dr. Baird is a member of the NIH Stroke Team at Suburban Hospital in Bethesda, Maryland. The NIH Stroke Team is headed by Steven Warach, M.D., Ph.D., of NINDS, who is senior author on the *Lancet* paper.

## *References*

1. Baird, A.E., Dambrosia, J., Janket, S., Eichbaum, Q., Chaves, C., Silver, B., Barber, P.A., Parsons, M., Darby, D., Davis, S., Caplan, L.R., Edelman, R.R., Warach, S. "A Three-Item Scale for the Early Prediction of Stroke Recovery." *Lancet*, June 30, 2001, Vol. 357, No. 9274, pp. 2095-2099.

# Chapter 24

# *Stroke Scales—*
# *Evaluating Effects of Stroke*

## *National Institutes of Health (NIH) Stroke Scale*

### *NIH Stroke Scale Definitions*

- Each examination is assessed independently from previous examinations.

- A response must be checked for each item, using the following definitions.

### *1.a. Level of Consciousness*

This global measure of responsiveness is assessed by the patient's interactions with the physician at the bedside when the patient is first examined. The physician should stimulate the patient (by patting or tapping the patient) to determine the best level of consciousness. On occasion, more noxious stimuli, such as pinching, may be required to check the level of consciousness.

This chapter includes "The NIH Stroke Scale," and "NIH Stroke Scale Definitions," National Institutes of Health (NIH), 1989, available from the Brain Attack Coalition, National Institute of Neurological Disorders and Stroke (NINDS), reviewed in November 2002 by David A. Cooke, MD, Diplomate, American Board of Internal Medicine; and "Barthel Index," Mahoney FI, Barthel DW: Functional evaluation: the Barthel Index. *Maryland State Medical Journal*, 14 (2), 61-65, 1965 © Maryland State Medical Society, used with permission, reviewed in October 2002 by David A. Cooke, MD, Diplomate, American Board of Internal Medicine.

**0 = Alert**—Patient is fully alert and keenly responsive

**1 = Drowsy**—Patient is drowsy but can be aroused with minor stimulation. The patient obeys, answers, and responds to commands.

**2 = Stuporous**—Patient is lethargic but requires repeated stimulation to attend. The patient may need painful or strong stimuli to respond to or follow commands.

**3 = Coma**—Patient is comatose and responds only with reflexive motor or automatic responses. Otherwise, the patient is unresponsive.

### 1.b. Level of Consciousness (LOC): Questions

Level of Consciousness: Questions is checked by asking the patient to respond to two questions. The patient is asked the month of the year and his/her age. The answer must be correct—there is no partial credit for being close (for example, being off by one year in age). If the patient gives the wrong initial answer but then corrects it, the answer should still be scored as incorrect. Other measures of orientation such as time of day, location, etc. are not asked as part of this examination. If the patient has aphasia, the physician should judge the responses to questions in light of the language impairment.

**0 = Answers both correctly**

**1 = Answers one correctly**

**2 = Both incorrect**

### 1.c. LOC: Commands

The Level of Consciousness: Commands is checked by asking the patient to follow two commands. The patient is asked to open and close his/her eyes and then is asked to make a grip (close and open his/her hand). Only the initial response is scored. If a patient is aphasic and unable to follow verbal commands, the patient may imitate these movements (pantomime). For a patient who has hemiparesis, the response in the unaffected limb should be measured. For example, if the patient has a left hemiparesis, making a fist with the right hand is a normal response to the command. If a paralyzed patient does try to move the limb in response to a command but is unable to form a fist, it is counted as a normal response.

**0 = Obeys both correctly**

**1 = Obeys one correctly**

**2 = Both incorrect**

## 2. Gaze

The position of the eyes at rest and movement of the eyes to command are tested. First look at the position of the eyes at rest. Spontaneous eye movements to the left and right should be noted. The patient is then asked to look to the left or right. Only horizontal eye movements are tested. Disorders of vertical gaze, nystagmus, or skew deviation are not measured. Reflexive eye movements (oculocephalic or oculovestibular) should be tested in patients who are unable to respond to commands. If a patient has ocular rotatory problems, such as a strabismus, but leaves the midline and attempts to look both right and left, he/she should be considered to have a normal response. If a patient has an isolated oculorotatory problem, such as an oculomotor (CN III) or abducens (CN IV) palsy, the score should be 1. If the patient has a conjugate deviation of the eyes that can be overcome by voluntary or reflexive activity, the score should be 1. If there is a conjugate lateral deviation that is not overcome with reflexive movements, the score should be 2.

**0 = Normal**—The patient has normal lateral eye movements.

**1 = Partial Gaze Palsy**—Patient is unable to move one or both eyes completely to both directions.

**2 = Forced Deviation**—The patient has conjugate deviation of the eyes to the right or left, even with reflexive movements.

## 3. Visual Fields

Visual fields of both eyes are examined. In most cases, the physician asks the patient to count fingers in all four quadrants. Each eye is independently tested. If a patient is unable to respond verbally, the physician should check responses (attending) to visual stimuli in the quadrants or have the patient hold up the number of fingers seen. A quadrantic field cut should be scored 1. The entire half field (both upper and lower quadrants) should be involved with a dense field loss to be scored 2. If a patient has severe monocular visual loss due to intrinsic eye disease and the visual fields in the other eye are normal, the physician should score the visual fields are normal. If the patient has monocular blindness due to primary eye disease and the visual fields in the other, normal eye demonstrate a partial or dense visual field defect, the visual loss should be scored as 1, 2, or 3 as appropriate.

**0 = No visual loss**

**1 = Partial hemianopia**—There is a partial visual field defect in both eyes. Included is a quadrantic field defect or sector field defect.

**2 = Complete hemianopia**—There is dense visual field defect in both eyes. A homonymous hemianopia is included.

**3 = Bilateral hemianopia**—There are bilateral visual field defects in both eyes. Cortical blindness is included.

## 4. Facial Movement (Facial Paresis)

The patient is examined by looking at the patient's face and noting any spontaneous facial movements. The facial movements in response to commands are also tested. Such commands may include asking the patient to grimace or smile, to puff out his/her cheeks, to pucker, and to close his/her eyes forcefully. If the patient is aphasic and is unable to follow commands, the physician should have the patient attempt imitative (pantomime) responses. The facial responses to painful stimuli (grimace) may substitute for responses to commands in a patient who has decreased levels of alertness.

**0 = Normal facial movements.** No asymmetry.

**1 = Minor paresis.** Asymmetrical facial movements or facial asymmetry at rest. This response may be noted with a spontaneous smile but not with forced facial movements.

**2 = Partial paresis.** Unilateral central facial paresis. Decreased spontaneous and forced facial movements with changes most prominent at the mouth. Orbital and forehead musculature movements are normal.

**3 = Complete palsy.** Dysfunction involves forehead, orbital, and circumoral muscles (the entire distribution of the facial nerve). Deficits may be unilateral or bilateral (facial diplegia) complete facial paresis.

## 5. Motor Function: Arms (Left and Right)

The patient is asked to extend his arm outstretched in front of the body at 90 degrees (if sitting) or at 45 degrees (if supine). The effort is for a full 10 seconds. The physician should count to ten aloud to encourage the patient to maintain the limb's position. If a limb is paralyzed, the physician may wish to test any normal limb first. If a patient is aphasic, directions may be achieved by non-verbal cues or pantomime. Patients may be helped by the physician by placing the limb in the desired position. If the patient has restricted limb function due to arthritis or non-stroke related limitations, the physician should attempt to judge the best motor response. If the patient has decreased level of consciousness, an estimate of response to noxious stimuli should be measured. Volitional motor responses that are performed well should be graded as 0. If the patient has reflexive responses, such as flexor or extensor posturing, the response should be scored as 4. The only indication for scoring this item as 9—untestable, is if the limb is missing or amputated, or if the shoulder joint is fused. A patient with a partial limb amputation should be tested.

**0 = No drift.** The patient is able to hold the outstretched limb for 10 seconds.

**1 = Drift.** The patient is able to hold the outstretched limb for 10 seconds but there is some fluttering or drift of the limb. If the limb falls to an intermediate position, the score is 1.

**2 = Some effort against gravity.** The patient is not able to hold the outstretched limb for 10 seconds but there is some effort against gravity.

**3 = No effort against gravity.** The patient is not able to bring the limb off the bed but there is some effort against gravity. If the limb is raised in the correct position by the examiner, the patient is unable to sustain the position.

**4 = No movement.** The patient is unable to move the limb. There is no effort against gravity.

**9 = Untestable.** May be used only if the limb is missing or amputated, or if the shoulder joint is fused.

**Table 24.1.** NIH Stroke Scale Questionnaire

| | |
|---|---|
| 1.a. Level of Consciousness | 0 Alert<br>1 Not alert, but arousable with minimal stimulation<br>2 Not alert, requires repeated stimulation to attend<br>3 Coma |
| 1.b. Ask patient the month and their age | 0 Answers both correctly<br>1 Answers one correctly<br>2 Both incorrect |
| 1.c. Ask patient to open and close eyes and (one other command) | 0 Obeys both correctly<br>1 Obeys one correctly<br>2 Both incorrect |
| 2. Best gaze (only horizontal eye movement) | 0 Normal<br>1 Partial gaze palsy<br>2 Forced deviation |
| 3. Visual Field testing | 0 No visual field loss<br>1 Partial hemianopia<br>2 Complete hemianopia<br>3 Bilateral hemianopia (blind including cortical blindness) |
| 4. Facial Paresis (Ask patient to show teeth or raise eye brows and close eyes tightly) | 0 Normal symmetrical movement<br>1 Minor paralysis (flattened nasolabial fold, asymmetry on smiling)<br>2 Partial paralysis (total or near total paralysis of lower face)<br>3 Complete paralysis of one or both sides (absence of facial movement in the upper and lower face) |
| 5. Motor Function—Arm (right and left)<br><br>Right arm ____<br>Left arm ____ | 0 Normal (extends arms 90 (or 45) degrees for 10 seconds without drift)<br>1 Drift<br>2 Some effort against gravity<br>3 No effort against gravity<br>4 No movement<br>9 Untestable (Joint fused or limb amputated) |

**Table 24.1.** NIH Stroke Scale Questionnaire, continued

6. Motor Function—
   Leg (right and left)

   Right leg ____
   Left leg ____

0 Normal (hold leg 30 degrees position for 5
   seconds)
1 Drift
2 Some effort against gravity
3 No effort against gravity
4 No movement
9 Untestable (Joint fused or limb amputated)

7. Limb Ataxia

0 No ataxia
1 Present in one limb
2 Present in two limbs

8. Sensory (Use
   pinprick to test
   arms, legs, trunk,
   and face—
   compare side
   to side)

0 Normal
1 Mild to moderate decrease in sensation
2 Severe to total sensory loss

9. Best Language
   (describe picture,
   name items, read
   sentences)

0 No aphasia
1 Mild to moderate aphasia
2 Severe aphasia
3 Mute

10. Dysarthria
    (read several
    words)

0 Normal articulation
1 Mild to moderate slurring of words
2 Near unintelligible or unable to speak
9 Intubated or other physical barrier

11. Extinction and
    inattention

0 Normal
1 Inattention or extinction to bilateral simultaneous
   stimulation in one of the sensory modalities
2 Severe hemi-inattention or hemi-inattention to
   more than one modality

### 6. Motor Function: Leg (Right and Left)

The supine patient is asked to hold the outstretched leg 30 degrees above the bed. The limb should be held in this position for 5 seconds. The physician should count to 5 aloud to encourage the patient to maintain the limb's position. If the right leg is paralyzed, the examiner may wish to examine the normal left leg first. If a patient is unable to follow verbal commands, nonverbal cues may be used, or the limb may be placed in the desired position. If the patient has a decreased level of consciousness, an estimate of response to noxious stimuli should be measured. Volitional motor responses that are performed well should be scored 0. If the patient has reflexive responses, such as flexor or extensor posturing, the response should be scored 4. The only indication for scoring this item as 9—untestable is if the limb is missing or if the hip joint is fused. Patients with artificial joints or partial limb amputations should be tested.

**0 = No drift.** The patient is able to hold the outstretched limb for 5 seconds.

**1 = Drift.** The patient is able to hold the outstretched limb for 5 seconds but there is unsteadiness, fluttering, or drift of the limb.

**2 = Some effort against gravity.** The patient is unable to hold the outstretched limb for 5 seconds but there is some effort against gravity.

**3 = No effort against gravity.** The patient is not able to bring the limb off the bed but there is effort against gravity. If the limb is placed in the correct position, the patient is unable to sustain the position.

**4 = No movement.** The patient is unable to move the limb. There is no effort against gravity.

**9 = Untestable.** May be used only if limb is missing or hip joint is fused.

### 7. Limb Ataxia

This item is aimed at examining the patient for evidence of a unilateral cerebellar lesion. It will also detect limb movement abnormalities related to sensory or motor dysfunction. Limb ataxia is checked by the finger-to-nose and heel-to-shin tests. The physician should test the normal side first. The movements should be well performed, smooth, accurate, and non-clumsy. There should not be any dysmetria or dyssynergia. Non-verbal cues may be given to the patient. If a patient has dysmetria or dyssynergia in one limb, the score should be 1. If a patient has dysmetria or dyssynergia in both the arm and leg on one side, or if there are bilateral signs, the score should be 2. If limb ataxia is present, the ataxia should be rated as present regardless of the possible etiology. This item may be scored 9—untestable only if there is complete paralysis of the limbs (All Motor Function scores = 4), if the limb is missing, amputated, or fused, or if the patient is comatose (item 1.a., LOC = 3).

**0 = Absent.** The patient is able to perform both the finger-to-nose and heel-to-shin tasks well. The movements are smooth and accurate.

**1 = Present unilaterally in either arm or leg.** The patient is able to perform one of the two required tasks well.

**2 = Present unilaterally in both arm and leg or bilaterally.** The patient is unable to perform either task well. Movements are inaccurate, clumsy, or poorly done.

**9 = Untestable.** May be used only if all Motor Function Scores = 4, limb is missing, amputated, or fused, or if item 1.a., LOC = 3.

## 8. Sensory

The patient is examined with a pin in the proximal portions of all four limbs and asked how the stimulus feels. The patient's eyes do not need to be closed. The patient is asked if the stimulus is sharp or dull and if there is any asymmetry between the right and left sides. Only sensory loss that can be attributed to stroke should be counted as abnormal—usually this will be a hemisensory loss. Sensory loss due to a non-stroke-related condition, such as a neuropathy, should not be graded as abnormal. If a patient has depressed level of consciousness, neglect, aphasia, or is unable to describe the sensory perception, the patient's non-verbal responses, such as a grimace or withdrawal, should be graded. If the patient responds to the stimulus, it should be scored 0. The response to the stimulus on the right and left sides should be compared. If the patient does not respond to a noxious stimulus on one side, the score should be 2. Patients with severe depression of consciousness should be examined.

249

**0 = Normal.** No sensory loss to pin is detected.

**1 = Partial loss.** Mild to moderate diminution in perception to pin stimulation is recognized. This may involve more than one limb.

**2 = Dense loss.** Severe sensory loss so that the patient is not aware of being touched. Patient does not respond to noxious stimuli applied to that side of the body.

### 9. Best Language

The patient's language will be tested by having the patient identify standard groups of objects and by reading a series of sentences. Comprehension of language should be judged as the physician performs the entire neurologic examination. The physician should give the patient adequate time to identify the objects on the sheet of paper. Only the first response is measured. If the patient misidentifies the object and later corrects himself, the response is still considered abnormal. The physician should then give the patient a sheet of paper with the series of sentences. The examiner should ask the patient to read at least three sentences. The first attempt to read the sentence is measured. If the patient misreads the sentence and later corrects himself, the response is still considered abnormal. If the patient's visual loss precludes visual identification of objects or reading, the examiner should ask the patient to identify objects placed in his/her hand and the examiner should judge the patient's spontaneous speech and ability to repeat sentences. If the examiner judges these responses as normal, the score should be 0. If the patient is intubated or is unable to speak, the examiner should check the patient's writing.

**0 = No aphasia.** The patient is able to read the sentences well and is able to correctly name the objects on the sheet of paper.

**1 = Mild to moderate aphasia.** The patient has mild to moderate naming errors, word finding errors, paraphasias, or mild impairment in comprehension or expression.

**2 = Severe aphasia.** The patient has severe aphasia with difficulty in reading as well as naming objects. Patient with either Broca's or Wernicke's aphasia is included here.

**3 = Mute**

## 10. Dysarthria

The primary method of examination is to ask the patient to read and pronounce a standard list of words from a sheet of paper. If the patient is unable to read the words because of visual loss, the physician may say the word and ask the patient to repeat it. If the patient has severe aphasia, the clarity of articulation of spontaneous speech should be rated. If the patient is mute or comatose (item 9, Best Language = 3 ) or has an endotracheal tube, this item can be rated as 9—untestable.

**0 = Normal articulation.** Patient is able to pronounce the words clearly and without any problem in articulation.

**1 = Mild to moderate dysarthria.** Patient has problems in articulation. Mild to moderate slurring of words is noted. The patient can be understood but with some difficulty.

**2 = Near unintelligible or worse.** Patient's speech is so slurred that it is unintelligible.

**9 = Untestable.** May be used only if item 9, Best Language = 3, or if the patient has an endotracheal tube.

## 11. Neglect (Extinction and Inattention)

The presence of neglect is examined by the patient's ability to recognize simultaneous cutaneous sensory and visual stimuli from the right and left sides. The visual stimulus is a standard picture. The picture is shown to the patient and s/he is asked to describe it. The physician should encourage the patient to scan the picture and identify features on both the right and left sides of the picture. The physician should encourage the patient to compensate for any visual loss. If the patient does not identify parts of the picture on one side, the result should be considered abnormal. The physician then assesses the ability to recognize bilateral simultaneous touch to upper or lower limbs. The test is done by touching the patient with the patient's eyes closed. The test should be considered abnormal if the patient ignores sensory stimuli from one side of the body. If the patient has a severe visual loss and the cutaneous stimuli are normal, the score should be 0. If the patient has aphasia and is unable to describe the picture, but does attend to both sides, the score should be 0.

**0 = No neglect.** The patient is able to recognize bilateral simultaneous cutaneous stimuli on the right and left sides of the body and is able to identify images on the right and left sides of the picture.

**1 = Partial neglect.** The patient is able to recognize either cutaneous or visual stimuli on both the left and right, but is unable to do both successfully (unless severe visual loss or aphasia is present).

**2 = Complete neglect.** The patient is unable to recognize either bilateral cutaneous sensory or visual stimuli.

**Table 24.2.** Barthel Index/Stroke Scale

| Item | Factor | Score |
|---|---|---|
| All categories | Unable to perform task | 0 |
| Feeding | Independent | 10 |
| | Needs help | 5 |
| Bathing | Performs without assistance | 5 |
| Personal toilet (grooming) | Independent | 10 |
| | Needs help | 5 |
| Dressing | Independent | 10 |
| | Needs help | 5 |
| Bowel control | No accidents | 10 |
| | Occasional accidents | 5 |
| Bladder control | Independent | 10 |
| | Occasional accidents | 5 |
| Toilet | Independent | 10 |
| | Needs help | 5 |
| Chair/bed transfers | Independent | 15 |
| | Minimum assistance | 10 |
| | Able to sit but needs maximum assistance to transfer | 5 |
| Ambulation | Independent for 45 meters | 15 |
| | With help for 45 meters | 10 |
| | Wheelchair for 45 meters | 5 |
| Stair climbing | Independent | 10 |
| | Needs help | 5 |

# Chapter 25

# *Surgical Treatments for Stroke*

## *Neurons Implanted in Stroke-Damaged Brain Tissue Show Function*

An imaging study of neurons implanted in damaged areas of the brains of stroke patients in the hopes of restoring function has shown the first signs of cellular growth, say University of Pittsburgh researchers.

Positron Emission Tomography (PET) scans taken six months after surgery to implant Layton BioScience (LBS)-neurons showed a greater than 10 percent increase in metabolic activity in the damaged parts of some patients' brains compared to scans taken just a week prior to surgery. The increased metabolism corresponds with better performance on standardized stroke tests for behavioral and motor function.

While PET scans taken at 12 months post-surgery showed that metabolism in the implanted area itself had lessened to baseline, the surrounding area in some patients showed maintained or even improved function—perhaps evidence that the LBS-neurons were becoming integrated into the brain.

This chapter includes "Neurons Implanted in Stroke-Damaged Brain Tissue Show Function Say University of Pittsburgh Researchers," University of Pittsburgh Medical Center News Bureau, © 2001 UPMC Health System, reprinted with permission; and "Medicine Implants Drastically Reduce Stroke Complications," *Stroke News* 04/05/2002. Reprinted with permission from the American Heart Association World Wide Web Site, www.americanheart.org. © Copyright American Heart Association.

Results of the study from the first human neuroimplantation trial for chronic stroke appeared in the September 2001 issue of *Neurosurgery*.

"These changes in glucose metabolism in the stroke and surrounding brain tissue may represent cellular activity or grafting of the implanted neurons," said Carolyn Cidis Meltzer, M.D., associate professor of radiology and psychiatry and medical director of the University of Pittsburgh Medical Center's PET facility and principal author of the study. "Although this is not direct evidence of synapse formation, it does suggest that the new neurons are being wired into the brain."

Dr. Meltzer and her colleagues performed PET imaging on 11 patients who suffered strokes resulting in persistent motor deficits at least a week before, then six months after implantation surgery. Nine of the original group went through the scans again at 12 months. Metabolism was measured by the uptake of a glucose analog called fluorodeoxyglucose (FDG) by the cells.

After six months, increases of FDG greater than 10 percent were observed in seven of 11 patients. After 12 months, the increase was sustained by three of the 11. In the areas surrounding the stroke, only two of 11 patients showed a greater than 10 percent increase in metabolism at six months, but after a year, five of 11 patients had at least one scan demonstrating a rise in relative metabolism over baseline.

The increased metabolism correlated with positive changes in neurological evaluations (National Institutes of Health stroke scale, European stroke scale) given to the patients during a 52-week period following transplant.

Patients are all part of the first human trial of the effectiveness of neuroimplantation to repair damage caused by stroke. Principal investigators in the trial are Douglas Kondziolka, M.D., professor of neurological surgery and radiation oncology and Lawrence Wechsler, M.D., professor of neurology and neurosurgery, both of the University of Pittsburgh School of Medicine.

LBS-neurons originated from a human teratocarcinoma, a tumor of the reproductive organs that is composed of embryonic-like cells, which was removed from a 22-year-old cancer patient in the early 1980s. Layton BioScience Inc. has licensed a patented process that uses several chemicals to transform this cell line into fully differentiated non-dividing human neuronal cells that can be used in clinical applications. In extensive pre-clinical testing, implants of LBS-neurons reversed cognitive and motor deficits in animals in which stroke had been induced.

The implantation procedure begins with the placement of a stereotactic frame on the head of the patient. The frame is a standard tool in neurosurgery to provide a fixed way to find specific locations within the brain. The patient then receives a computed tomography (CT) or magnetic resonance imaging (MRI) scan of the brain and the surgical team makes its final decision for location of cell implantation.

Concurrently, the University of Pittsburgh Immunologic Monitoring and Diagnostic Laboratory team thaws the human neuronal cells that were frozen by and transported from Layton BioScience Inc.

After the cells are transferred to a long-needled syringe, the surgeon uses CT to guide their injection at multiple sites. The surgeon injects these cells through a small opening in the skull and patients leave the hospital the next day.

Stroke affects approximately 750,000 people in the United States each year and is the third leading cause of death and most common cause of disability.

There are no known effective treatments for chronic stroke with fixed neurological deficit.

## The American Heart Association Reports That Medicine Implants Drastically Reduce Stroke Complications

Implanting tiny rods containing a calcium-channel blocker in brain vessels prevented vasospasm, a complication that can occur after surgical repair of a brain hemorrhage, according to a report in the April 5, 2002 *Stroke: Journal of the American Heart Association*.

A subarachnoid hemorrhage (SAH) is a type of stroke. It occurs when an aneurysm, a blood-filled pouch, balloons out from a weak spot in the artery wall and bursts. Then the vessel bleeds into the space that covers the surface of the brain with spinal fluid. Surgery is required to repair the vessel. A patch or artificial piece of blood vessel is sewn over the rupture.

A major complication of SAH is vasospasm, a prolonged contraction of the artery walls. "Vasospasm is a major cause of death and disability because it can reduce blood flow enough to kill brain tissue," says Hidetoshi Kasuya, M.D., lead author of the study and a senior lecturer in the department of neurosurgery at Tokyo Women's Medical University. "In this study, vasospasm was completely prevented by inserting the pellets of the medication next to the arteries where vasospasm was most likely to occur."

The new drug delivery system, implanted during surgery, uses a calcium-channel blocker, which dilates the blood vessel.

The 20 patients in this study had SAH. "Aneurysmal SAH accounts for approximately 6 percent to 8 percent of all strokes and affects more than 28,000 individuals in North America each year," he says.

In the current study, two to 10 pellets of nicardipine—a common calcium-channel blocker used to treat high blood pressure—were implanted during brain surgery. They were placed parallel to the arteries and adjacent to thick clots identified during the surgery. The drug has a localized effect in the brain, so the patients' own blood vessels in distant parts of the brain were used as controls in the current study, he explains.

In the first three days, about 7 percent of the nicardipine was released with 46 percent after the next three days. The amount of nicardipine released within the first nine days was 62 percent of the total amount.

The risk of vasospasm is rarely significant before the fourth day following the initial hemorrhage. It reaches a peak around the eighth day, when about 70 percent of patients have some narrowing in one or more arteries, Kasuya says. The risk of vasospasms decreases substantially two weeks after a SAH.

The subjects' vessels were examined using angiography at seven and 12 days after surgery. All vessels adjacent to the medication pellets remained free of vasospasm. Eight of the 20 patients experienced vasospasm in arteries remote from the medication site. The contraction was mild in six patients, moderate in one, and severe enough to cause disability in one patient. This is far below the rates seen in untreated SAH patients.

No side effects were reported, possibly because such focused, time-released treatment allows doctors to drastically reduce the dose, says Kasuya.

"This drug system is the most promising approach for preventing vasospasm," he says. The next step would be to develop a treatment based on this technology.

Even when aneurysms are found early and treated with surgery the outlook is cloudy because of vasospasm. The reduced blood flow from a vasospasm can cause an ischemic stroke, he adds.

Physicians don't know what causes vasospasm, but it seems related to blood clots in the large vessels that run between the two sides of the brain. Current treatments to reduce or prevent vasospasm are either difficult to administer, prone to complications or both, the researcher explains.

"Our results suggest that nicardipine can prevent vasospasm completely if appropriate concentrations are maintained around the broken vessel using the newly-developed drug delivery system," says Kasuya. "We show that this system is an effective, simple, and safe treatment for preventing vasospasm."

Chapter 26

# Do You Have Access to the Best Treatment for Stroke?

## A Checklist for Communities

- Does the hospital have a Stroke Team led by a health care professional with training and expertise in stroke? A Stroke Team is a professional staff available around the clock, seven days a week to evaluate the patient within 15 minutes of arrival.

- Does the hospital have written guidelines for emergency treatment for stroke patients?

- Does the city's emergency medical system transport patients with suspected strokes as rapidly as possible to the hospital?

- Are the hospital's emergency department physicians trained to rapidly diagnose and treat acute stroke?

- Does the hospital provide coordinated stroke care beyond the emergency department physician's evaluation? If not, is the hospital prepared to transfer the patient to a hospital that does?

- Does the hospital have a neurosurgeon available around the clock, seven days a week? If not, is the hospital prepared to transfer the patient to a hospital that does?

- Is the hospital administration committed to the Stroke Center?

"Establishing a Stroke Center," The Brain Attack Coalition, July 2001.

- Does the hospital have capability around the clock, seven days a week to perform and interpret either a head CT scan or a brain MRI scan within 45 minutes of the stroke patient being admitted?

- Is the hospital lab open around the clock, seven days a week?

- Does the hospital track patient outcomes, perform ongoing program evaluation, and strive for improvements?

- Does the hospital staff of the Stroke Center receive at least eight hours per year of continuing medical education?

- Does the hospital have at least two annual programs to educate the public about stroke prevention, diagnosis, and the availability of acute therapies?

# Part Four

# Stroke Recovery and Rehabilitation

Chapter 27

# Family Plays Critical Role in Stroke Recovery

Many high profile Americans have experienced stroke episodes—actors Kirk Douglas, Robert Guillaume, and Patricia Neal; entertainers Quincy Jones and Gene Kelly; Hugh Hefner; and writer Ray Bradbury. Quick medical intervention and rigorous rehabilitation helped these people and many more to return to their chosen professions.

For the 700,000 Americans who experience strokes each year, time is of the essence when it comes to treatment—so much so that health practitioners are now referring to strokes as "brain attacks" to emphasize the importance of getting medical help right away. Recent research has shown that quick intervention dramatically improves a patient's recovery.

But equally important in a stroke patient's recovery is early rehabilitation and a complete understanding of and commitment to the rehabilitation process. Ideally, this means working with a physical medicine and rehabilitation (PM&R) physician, also called a physiatrist, to design an individualized recovery program.

## Early Rehabilitation

"Stroke recovery begins immediately and takes place over a long time—not just during a hospital stay or physical rehabilitation session," says Dr. Steven Flanagan, vice chairman, department of rehabilitation

"Family Plays Critical Role in Stroke Recovery," © 9/2000 American Academy of Physical Medicine and Rehabilitation (AAPM&R), reprinted with permission.

medicine at The Mount Sinai School of Medicine. "It is extremely important for people to begin as soon as possible and to then continue exercising beyond their rehabilitation stay."

After patients are treated for a stroke, their typical initial rehabilitation program will last 2-3 weeks depending on how severely the stroke disabled them. This program is critical to the patient's long-term recovery and well being.

A PM&R physician will evaluate not only the negative effects of the stroke but also the patient's pre-attack status taking into account their physical abilities, emotional state, family support, education, and even spiritual resources. This in-depth personal understanding allows the PM&R physician to create a comprehensive recovery program with physical therapists, speech therapists, psychologists, and social workers.

"PM&R specialists provide the overview. Rehabilitation is a team sport with the patient and family included first and foremost. The team may also include physical, occupational, and recreational therapists, speech language pathologists, psychologists, and social workers. The physiatrist has the responsibility to direct and coordinate the team," says Dr. Charles E. Levy, system chief of physical medicine and rehabilitation services for the North Florida/South Georgia Veterans Health System. "In this active partnership we strive to find out what motivates the patient and how we can use this to his or her benefit."

## Different Strokes

Flanagan stresses that every stroke patient is unique as is every brain attack and the resulting deficits that occur. Therefore every recovery is unique. Typically, after a PM&R physician evaluates a patient, the goal is to help clear as many of the obstacles as possible to his or her recovery so the patient can focus on returning to the daily activities that he or she is able to perform.

"Stroke happens. That's the bad news," says Levy who is also an assistant professor in the department of orthopaedics and rehabilitation at the University of Florida College of Medicine. "The good news is there is great potential for the brain to recover from stroke. With diligent rehabilitation, those prospects improve."

## Family Support

Both specialists quickly point out that one of the most critical elements in a patient's rehabilitation from stroke is the strength and commitment of their primary support system—usually their family.

"Stroke often threatens our definition of ourselves by forcing us to rely on others to complete everyday activities. Family acceptance is crucial in helping a person understand that just because he or she needs assistance is no reason to feel ashamed or unworthy. If we live long enough, all of us can expect that our skills will diminish. Ultimately it is who we are, not what we can do that is important," explains Levy.

According to Levy, family members can be particularly helpful when it comes to identifying the best ways to psychologically motivate the patient. Family members may also be particularly adept at interpreting communications and signs when speech impairments are present. "Family members know the patient better than we ever can. We try to involve them as much as possible. Their commitment often makes a world of difference in terms of recovery."

## A Helping Hand

Since the vast majority of people recovering from stroke will be cared for by family or loved ones, part of the rehabilitation program requires educating those caregivers on how to assist with necessary tasks, such as:

- Transfers—from bed to wheelchair, wheelchair to car, etc.

- Rehabilitation exercises to strengthen and stretch weakened muscles.

- Organizational strategies—such as laying clothes out in order.

- Empowerment tips—such as verbal cues, a gentle inquiry rather than an order.

- Food preparation—because swallowing problems are common.

Depression is more common in patients recovering from a stroke than many other diseases with similar deficits, although it is not completely clear why this happens. Depression can rob a person of their willingness to work towards recovery. This can be very damaging. Motivation and a positive attitude are key to obtaining an optimal level of recovery. "Obviously family are a great resource," reports Levy. "It is not uncommon for the patient to report that everything is fine only to have the spouse vigorously nod her head 'No!' It may the spouse who alerts us to the real problems at home. Together we can begin to address the physical, medical, thinking, and emotional problems so common to those living with the effects of stroke."

## Brighter Future

"This is a very exciting time for us—five to ten years ago the consensus was not much could be done to influence the limited natural recovery from stroke," says Levy. "Now we're making enormous strides in helping more and more people enjoy normal daily living." For example, one of the new treatments being investigated is constraint induced movement therapy where intensive training of the weak side (5-6 hours per day for two weeks) can result in dramatic recovery of arm and hand skills. Investigations of different medicines to encourage recovery are underway. New imaging techniques are allowing us to see how the brain reorganizes after a stroke to regain lost abilities. Promising new strategies using body-supported treadmill training are helping to restore walking.

## Additional Information

***American Academy of Physical Medicine and Rehabilitation (AAPM&R)***
One IBM Plaza, Suite 2500
Chicago, IL 60611-3604
Tel: 312-464-9700
Fax: 312-464-0227
Website: www.aapmr.org
E-mail: info@aapmr.org

Chapter 28

# Discharge Planning for Stroke Patients

## Discharge Planning

Discharge planning begins early during rehabilitation. It involves the patient, family, and rehabilitation staff. The purpose of discharge planning is to help maintain the benefits of rehabilitation after the patient has been discharged from the program. Patients are usually discharged from rehabilitation soon after their goals have been reached.

Some of the things discharge planning can include are to:

- Make sure that the stroke survivor has a safe place to live after discharge.

- Decide what care, assistance, or special equipment will be needed.

- Arrange for more rehabilitation services or for other services in the home (such as visits by a home health aide).

- Choose the health care provider who will monitor the person's health and medical needs.

- Determine the caregivers who will work as a partner with the patient to provide daily care and assistance at home and teach them the skills they will need.

"Recovering After a Stroke: A Patient and Family Guide," Agency for HealthCare Research and Quality (AHRQ), AHCPR Publication No. 95-0664, May 1995, reviewed in October 2002 by Dr. David A. Cooke, MD, Diplomate, American Board of Internal Medicine.

- Help the stroke survivor explore employment opportunities, volunteer activities, and driving a car (if able and interested).

- Discuss any sexual concerns the stroke survivor or husband/wife may have. Many people who have had strokes enjoy active sex lives.

## Preparing a Living Place

Many stroke survivors can return to their own homes after rehabilitation. Others need to live in a place with professional staff such as a nursing home or assisted living facility. An assisted living facility can provide residential living with a full range of services and staff. The choice usually depends on the person's needs for care and whether caregivers are available in the home. The stroke survivor needs a living place that supports continuing recovery.

It is important to choose a living place that is safe. If the person needs a new place to live, a social worker can help find the best place.

During discharge planning, program staff will ask about the home and may also visit it. They may suggest changes to make it safer. These might include changing rooms around so that a stroke survivor can stay on one floor, moving scatter rugs or small pieces of furniture that could cause falls, and putting grab bars and seats in tubs and showers.

It is a good idea for the stroke survivor to go home for a trial visit before discharge. This will help identify problems that need to be discussed or corrected before the patient returns.

## Deciding about Special Equipment

Even after rehabilitation, some stroke survivors have trouble walking, balancing, or performing certain activities of daily living. Special equipment can sometimes help. Here are some examples:

- **Cane.** Many people who have had strokes use a cane when walking. For people with balancing problems, special canes with three or four "feet" are available.

- **Walker.** A walker provides more support than a cane. Several designs are available for people who can only use one hand and for different problems with walking or balance.

- **Ankle-foot orthotic devices (braces).** Braces help a person to walk by keeping the ankle and foot in the correct position and providing support for the knee.

266

- **Wheelchair.** Some people will need a wheelchair. Wheelchairs come in many different designs. They can be customized to fit the user's needs and abilities. Find out which features are most important for the stroke survivor.

- **Aids for bathing, dressing, and eating.** Some of these are safety devices such as grab bars and nonskid tub and floor mats. Others make it easier to do things with one hand. Examples are Velcro fasteners on clothes and placemats that won't slide on the table.

- **Communication aids.** These range from small computers to homemade communication boards. The stroke survivor, family, and rehabilitation program staff should decide together what special equipment is needed. Program staff can help in making the best choices. Medicare or health insurance will often help pay for the equipment.

## Preparing Caregivers

Caregivers who help stroke survivors at home are usually family members such as a husband or wife or an adult son or daughter. They may also be friends or even professional home health aides. Usually, one person is the main caregiver, while others help from time to time. An important part of discharge planning is to make sure that caregivers understand the safety, physical, and emotional needs of the stroke survivor, and that they will be available to provide needed care.

Since every stroke is different, people have different needs for help from caregivers. Here are some of the things caregivers may do:

- Keep notes on discharge plans and instructions and ask about anything that is not clear.

- Help to make sure that the stroke survivor takes all prescribed medicines and follows suggestions from program staff about diet, exercise, rest, and other health practices.

- Encourage and help the person to practice skills learned in rehabilitation.

- Help the person solve problems and discover new ways to do things.

267

- Help the person with activities performed before the stroke. These could include using tools, buttoning a shirt, household tasks, and leisure or social activities.

- Help with personal care, if the person cannot manage alone.

- Help with communication, if the person has speech problems. Include the stroke survivor in conversations even when the person cannot actively participate.

- Arrange for needed community services.

- Stand up for the rights of the stroke survivor.

If you expect to be a caregiver, think carefully about this role ahead of time. Are you prepared to work with the patient on stroke recovery? Talk it over with other people who will share the caregiving job with you. What are the stroke survivor's needs? Who can best help meet each of them? Who will be the main caregiver? Does caregiving need to be scheduled around the caregivers' jobs or other activities? There is time during discharge planning to talk with program staff about caregiving and to develop a workable plan.

## Going Home

### Adjusting to the Change

Going home to the old home or a new one is a big adjustment. For the stroke survivor, it may be hard to transfer the skills learned during rehabilitation to a new location. Also, more problems caused by the stroke may appear as the person tries to go back to old activities. During this time, the stroke survivor and family learn how the stroke will affect daily life and can make the necessary adjustments.

These adjustments are a physical and emotional challenge for the main caregiver as well as the stroke survivor. The caregiver has many new responsibilities and may not have time for some favorite activities. The caregiver needs support, understanding, and some time to rest. Caregiving that falls too heavily on one person can be very stressful. Even when family members and friends are nearby and willing to help, conflicts over caregiving can cause stress.

A stroke is always stressful for the family, but it is especially hard if one family member is the only caregiver. Much time may be required to meet the needs of the stroke survivor. Therefore, the caregiver needs as much support as possible from others. Working together eases the stress on everyone.

## Tips for Reducing Stress

The following tips for reducing stress are for both caregivers and stroke survivors.

- Take stroke recovery and caregiving one day at a time and be hopeful.

- Remember that adjusting to the effects of stroke takes time. Appreciate each small gain as you discover better ways of doing things.

- Caregiving is learned. Expect that knowledge and skills will grow with experience.

- Experiment until you find what works for you. Try new ways of doing activities of daily living, communicating with each other, scheduling the day, and organizing your social life.

- Plan for breaks so that you are not together all the time. This is a good way for family and friends to help on occasion. You can also plan activities that get both of you out of the house.

- Ask family members and friends to help in specific ways and commit to certain times to help. This gives others a chance to help in useful ways.

- Read about the experiences of other people in similar situations. Your public library has life stories by people who have had a stroke as well as books for caregivers.

- Join or start a support group for stroke survivors or caregivers. You can work on problems together and develop new friendships.

- Be kind to each other. If you sometimes feel irritated, this is natural and you don't need to blame yourself. But don't take it out on the other person. It often helps to talk about these feelings with a friend, rehabilitation professional, or support group.

- Plan and enjoy new experiences and don't look back. Avoid comparing life as it is now with how it was before the stroke.

## Follow-Up Appointments

After a stroke survivor returns to the community, regular follow-up appointments are usually scheduled with the doctor and sometimes with rehabilitation professionals. The purpose of follow-up is to check on the stroke survivor's medical condition and ability to use the skills learned in rehabilitation. It is also important to check on how well the stroke survivor and family are adjusting. The stroke survivor and caregiver can be prepared for these visits with a list of questions or concerns.

## Where to Get Help

Many kinds of help are available for people who have had strokes and their families and caregivers. Some of the most important are:

- **Information about stroke.** A good place to start is with the books and pamphlets available from national organizations that provide information on this subject. Many of their materials are available free of charge.

- **Local stroke clubs or other support groups.** These are groups where stroke survivors and family members can share their experiences, help each other solve problems, and expand their social lives.

- **Home health services.** These are available from the Visiting Nurses Association (VNA), public health departments, hospital home care departments, and private home health agencies. Services may include nursing care, rehabilitation therapies, personal care (for example, help with bathing or dressing), respite care (staying with the stroke survivor so that the caregiver can take a vacation or short break), homemaker services, and other kinds of help.

- **Meals on Wheels.** Hot meals are delivered to the homes of people who cannot easily shop and cook.

- **Adult day care.** People who cannot be completely independent sometimes spend the day at an adult day care center. There they get meals, participate in social activities, and may also get some health care and rehabilitation services.

- **Friendly Visitor (or other companion services).** A paid or volunteer companion makes regular visits or phone calls to a person with disabilities.

- **Transportation services.** Most public transportation systems have buses that a person in a wheelchair can board. Some organizations and communities provide vans to take wheelchair users and others on errands such as shopping or doctor's visits.

Many communities have service organizations that can help. Some free services may be available or fees may be on a sliding scale based on income. It takes some work to find out what services and payment arrangements are available. A good way to start is to ask the social workers in the hospital or rehabilitation program where the stroke survivor was treated. Also, talk to the local United Way or places of worship. Another good place to look is the Yellow Pages of the telephone book, under "Health Services," "Home Health Care," "Senior Citizen Services," or "Social Service Organizations." Just asking friends may turn up useful information. The more you ask, the more you will learn.

## Additional Resources

### Administration on Aging
1 Massachusetts Ave., NW
Washington, DC 20001
Toll-Free: 800-677-1116 (call for list of community services for older Americans in your area)
Tel: 202-619-0724
Website: www.aoa.dhhs.gov
E-mail: aoainfo@aoa.gov

### AHA Stroke Connection
### (formerly the Courage Stroke Network)
American Heart Association
7272 Greenville Avenue
Dallas, TX 75231
Toll-Free: 800-4-STROKE
Website: www.strokeassociation.org
E-mail: strokeconnection@heart.org

Provides prevention, diagnosis, treatment, and rehabilitation information to stroke survivors and their families.

### American Dietetic Association/National Center for Nutrition and Dietetics
216 W. Jackson Blvd.
Chicago, IL 60606
Toll-Free: 800-366-1655 (Consumer Nutrition Hotline)
Tel: 312-899-0040
Website: www.eatright.org/nend.html

Consumers may speak to a registered dietitian for answers to nutrition questions, or obtain a referral to a local registered dietitian.

### American Self-Help Clearinghouse
St. Clares-Riverside Medical Center
Denville, NJ 07834
Tel: 973-625-3037
TTY: 973-625-9053
Website: www.mentalhelp.net/selfhelp

Provides information and assistance on local self-help groups.

### National Aphasia Association
P.O. Box 1887
Murray Hill Station
New York, NY 10156
Toll-Free: 800-922-4622
Website: www.aphasia.org
E-mail: naa@aphasia.org

Provides information on the partial or total loss of the ability to speak or comprehend speech, resulting from stroke or other causes.

### National Easter Seal Society
230 West Monroe Street, Suite 1800
Chicago, IL 60606
Toll-Free: 800-821-6827
Tel: 312-726-6200 (or check telephone book for local Easter Seal Society)
TTY: 312-726-4258
Fax: 312-726-1494
Website: www.easter-seals.org

Provides information and services to help people with disabilities.

## National Stroke Association
9707 E. Easter Lane
Englewood, CO 80112-3747
Toll-Free: 800-STROKES (787-6537)
Tel: 303-649-9299
Fax: 303-649-1328
Website: www.stroke.org

Serves as an information referral clearinghouse on stroke. Offers guidance on forming stroke support groups and clubs.

## Rosalynn Carter Institute
Georgia Southwestern College
800 Wheatley St.
Americus, GA 31709
Tel: 229-928-1234
Fax: 229-931-2663
Website: http://rci.gsw.edu
E-mail: rci@gsw.edu

Provides information on caregiving. Reading lists, video products, and other caregiver resources are available by writing to the address listed above.

## Stroke Clubs International
805 12th Street
Galveston, TX 77550
Tel: 409-762-1022 (call for the name of a stroke club located in your area)
E-mail: strokeclub@aol.com

Maintains a list of over 800 stroke clubs throughout the United States.

## The Well Spouse Foundation
63 West Main St., Suite H
Freehold, NJ 07728
Toll-Free: 800-838-0879
Tel: 732-577-8899
Fax: 732-577-8644
Website: www.wellspouse.org
E-mail: info@wellspouse.org

Provides support for the husbands, wives, and partners of people who are chronically ill or disabled.

Chapter 29

# Post-Stroke Rehabilitation

## Stroke Rehabilitation Information

Stroke is the third leading cause of death and the leading cause of long-term disability in the U.S. There are approximately 4 million Americans living with the effects of stroke. In addition, there are millions of husbands, wives, children, and friends who care for stroke survivors and whose own lives are personally affected. According to the National Stroke Association:

- 10% of stroke survivors recover almost completely

- 25% recover with minor impairments

- 40% experience moderate to severe impairments that require special care

- 10% require care in a nursing home or other long-term facility

- 15% die shortly after the stroke

- Approximately 14% of stroke survivors experience a second stroke in the first year following a stroke

Successful rehabilitation depends on:

"Stroke Rehabilitation Information," National Institute of Neurological Disorders and Stroke, (NINDS), reviewed July 1, 2001; and "Post-Stroke Rehabilitation," Fact Sheet, National Institute of Neurological Disorders and Stroke (NINDS), reviewed July 1, 2001.

- Amount of damage to the brain

- Skill on the part of the rehabilitation team

- Cooperation of family and friends. Caring family/friends can be one of the most important factors in rehabilitation

- Timing of rehabilitation—the earlier it begins the more likely survivors are to regain lost abilities and skills

The goal of rehabilitation is to enable an individual who has experienced a stroke to reach the highest possible level of independence and be as productive as possible. Because stroke survivors often have complex rehabilitation needs, progress and recovery are unique for each person. Although a majority of functional abilities may be restored soon after a stroke, recovery is an ongoing process.

### Effects of a Stroke

1. Weakness (hemiparesis) or paralysis (hemiplegia) on one side of the body that may affect the whole side or just the arm or leg. The weakness or paralysis is on the side of the body opposite the side of the brain affected by the stroke.

2. Spasticity, stiffness in muscles, painful muscle spasms

3. Problems with balance and/or coordination

4. Problems using language, including having difficulty understanding speech or writing (aphasia); and knowing the right words, but having trouble saying them clearly (dysarthria)

5. Being unaware of or ignoring sensations on one side of the body (bodily neglect or inattention)

6. Pain, numbness, or odd sensations

7. Problems with memory, thinking, attention, or learning

8. Being unaware of the effects of a stroke

9. Trouble swallowing (dysphagia)

10. Problems with bowel or bladder control

11. Fatigue

12. Difficulty controlling emotions (emotional lability)

13. Depression

14. Difficulties with daily tasks

## *Types of Rehabilitation Programs*

- Hospital programs: in an acute care facility or a rehabilitation hospital
- Long-term care facility with therapy and skilled nursing care
- Outpatient programs
- Home-based programs

## *Rehabilitation Specialists*

- Physicians: physiatrists (specialists in physical medicine and rehabilitation), neurologists, internists, geriatricians (specialists in the elderly), family practice
- Rehabilitation nurses: specialize in nursing care for people with disabilities
- Physical therapists: help to restore physical functioning by evaluating and treating problems with movement, balance, and coordination
- Occupational therapists: provide exercises and practice to help patient perform activities of daily living
- Speech-language pathologists: to help improve language skills
- Social workers: assist with financial decisions and plan the return to the home or a new living place
- Psychologists: concerned with the mental and emotional health of patients
- Therapeutic recreation specialists: help patients return to activities they enjoyed before the stroke.

## *Preventing Another Stroke*

People who have had a stroke are at an increased risk of having another one, especially during the first year following the original stroke. The following factors increase the risk of having another stroke:

- High blood pressure (hypertension)
- Cigarette smoking
- Diabetes

- Having had a TIA (transient ischemic attack)
- Heart disease
- Older age
- High cholesterol
- Obesity
- Sedentary lifestyle

Although some risk factors for stroke cannot be changed (e.g. age) others such as high blood pressure and smoking can be altered. Patients and families should seek guidance from their physician about lifestyle changes to help prevent another stroke.

## Post-Stroke Rehabilitation

In the United States more than 700,000 people suffer a stroke each year, and approximately two-thirds of these individuals survive and require rehabilitation. The goals of rehabilitation are to help survivors become as independent as possible and to attain the best possible quality of life. Even though rehabilitation does not cure stroke in that it does not reverse brain damage, rehabilitation can substantially help people achieve the best possible long-term outcome.

### What Is Post-Stroke Rehabilitation?

Rehabilitation helps stroke survivors relearn skills that are lost when part of the brain is damaged. For example, these skills can include coordinating leg movements in order to walk or carrying out the steps involved in any complex activity. Rehabilitation also teaches survivors new ways of performing tasks to circumvent or compensate for any residual disabilities. Patients may need to learn how to bathe and dress using only one hand, or how to communicate effectively when their ability to use language has been compromised. There is a strong consensus among rehabilitation experts that the most important element in any rehabilitation program is carefully directed, well-focused, repetitive practice—the same kind of practice used by all people when they learn a new skill, such as playing the piano or pitching a baseball.

Rehabilitative therapy begins in the acute-care hospital after the patient's medical condition has been stabilized, often within 24 to 48 hours after the stroke. The first steps involve promoting independent movement because many patients are paralyzed or seriously weakened. Patients are prompted to change positions frequently while lying in bed and to engage in passive or active range-of-motion exercises to strengthen their stroke-impaired limbs. (*Passive* range-of-motion exercises are those in which the therapist actively helps the patient move a limb repeatedly, whereas *active* exercises are performed by the patient with no physical assistance from the therapist.) Patients progress from sitting up and transferring between the bed and a chair to standing, bearing their own weight, and walking, with or without assistance. Rehabilitation nurses and therapists help patients perform progressively more complex and demanding tasks, such as bathing, dressing, and using a toilet, and they encourage patients to begin using their stroke-impaired limbs while engaging in those tasks. Beginning to reacquire the ability to carry out these basic activities of daily living represents the first stage in a stroke survivor's return to functional independence.

## What Disabilities Can Result from a Stroke?

The types and degrees of disability that follow a stroke depend upon which area of the brain is damaged. Generally, stroke can cause five types of disabilities: paralysis or problems controlling movement; sensory disturbances including pain; problems using or understanding language; problems with thinking and memory; and emotional disturbances.

### Paralysis or Problems Controlling Movement (Motor Control)

Paralysis is one of the most common disabilities resulting from stroke. The paralysis is usually on the side of the body opposite the side of the brain damaged by stroke, and may affect the face, an arm, a leg, or the entire side of the body. This one-sided paralysis is called hemiplegia (one-sided weakness is called hemiparesis). Stroke patients with hemiparesis or hemiplegia may have difficulty with everyday activities such as walking or grasping objects. Some stroke patients have problems with swallowing, called dysphagia, due to damage to the part of the brain that controls the muscles for swallowing. Damage to a lower part of the brain, the cerebellum, can affect the body's ability to coordinate movement, a disability called ataxia, leading to problems with body posture, walking, and balance.

### Sensory Disturbances Including Pain

Stroke patients may lose the ability to feel touch, pain, temperature, or position. Sensory deficits may also hinder the ability to recognize objects that patients are holding and can even be severe enough to cause loss of recognition of one's own limb. Some stroke patients experience pain, numbness, or odd sensations of tingling or prickling in paralyzed or weakened limbs, a condition known as paresthesia.

Stroke survivors frequently have a variety of chronic pain syndromes resulting from stroke-induced damage to the nervous system (neuropathic pain). Patients who have a seriously weakened or paralyzed arm commonly experience moderate to severe pain that radiates outward from the shoulder. Most often, the pain results from a joint becoming immobilized due to lack of movement and the tendons and ligaments around the joint become fixed in one position. This is commonly called a frozen joint; passive movement at the joint in a paralyzed limb is essential to prevent painful freezing and to allow easy movement if and when voluntary motor strength returns. In some stroke patients, pathways for sensation in the brain are damaged, causing the transmission of false signals that result in the sensation of pain in a limb or side of the body that has the sensory deficit. The most common of these pain syndromes is called *thalamic pain syndrome*, which can be difficult to treat even with medications.

The loss of urinary continence is fairly common immediately after a stroke and often results from a combination of sensory and motor deficits. Stroke survivors may lose the ability to sense the need to urinate or the ability to control muscles of the bladder. Some may lack enough mobility to reach a toilet in time. Loss of bowel control or constipation may also occur. Permanent incontinence after a stroke is uncommon. But even a temporary loss of bowel or bladder control can be emotionally difficult for stroke survivors.

## Problems Using or Understanding Language (Aphasia)

At least one-fourth of all stroke survivors experience language impairments, involving the ability to speak, write, and understand spoken and written language. A stroke-induced injury to any of the brain's language-control centers can severely impair verbal communication. Damage to a language center located on the dominant side of the brain, known as Broca's area, causes expressive aphasia. People with this type of aphasia have difficulty conveying their thoughts through words or writing. They lose the ability to speak the words they are thinking and to put words together in coherent, grammatically correct sentences. In contrast, damage to a language center located in a rear portion of the brain, called Wernicke's area, results in receptive aphasia. People with this condition have difficulty understanding spoken or written language and often have incoherent speech.

Although they can form grammatically correct sentences, their utterances are often devoid of meaning. The most severe form of aphasia, global aphasia, is caused by extensive damage to several areas involved in language function. People with global aphasia lose nearly all their linguistic abilities; they can neither understand language nor use it to convey thought. A less severe form of aphasia, called anomic or amnesic aphasia, occurs when there is only a minimal amount of brain damage; its effects are often quite subtle. People with anomic aphasia may simply selectively forget interrelated groups of words, such as the names of people or particular kinds of objects.

*Problems with Thinking and Memory*

Stroke can cause damage to parts of the brain responsible for memory, learning, and awareness. Stroke survivors may have dramatically shortened attention spans or may experience deficits in short-term memory. Individuals also may lose their ability to make plans, comprehend meaning, learn new tasks, or engage in other complex mental activities. Two fairly common deficits resulting from stroke are *anosognosia*, an inability to acknowledge the reality of the physical impairments resulting from stroke, and *neglect*, the loss of the ability to respond to objects or sensory stimuli located on one side of the body, usually the stroke-impaired side. Stroke survivors who develop *apraxia* lose their ability to plan the steps involved in a complex task and to carry the steps out in the proper sequence. Stroke survivors with apraxia may also have problems following a set of instructions. Apraxia appears to be caused by a disruption of the subtle connections that exist between thought and action.

*Emotional Disturbances*

Many people who survive a stroke feel fear, anxiety, frustration, anger, sadness, and a sense of grief for their physical and mental losses. These feelings are a natural response to the psychological trauma of stroke. Some emotional disturbances and personality changes are caused by the physical effects of brain damage. Clinical depression, which is a sense of hopelessness that disrupts an individual's ability to function, appears to be the emotional disorder most commonly experienced by stroke survivors. Signs of clinical depression include sleep disturbances, a radical change in eating patterns that may lead to sudden weight loss or gain, lethargy, social withdrawal, irritability, fatigue, self-loathing, and suicidal thoughts.

Post-stroke depression can be treated with antidepressant medications and psychological counseling.

## What Medical Professionals Specialize in Post-Stroke Rehabilitation?

Post-stroke rehabilitation involves physicians; rehabilitation nurses; physical, occupational, speech-language, and vocational therapists; and mental health professionals.

### Physicians

Physicians have the primary responsibility for managing and coordinating the long-term care of stroke survivors, including recommending which rehabilitation programs will best address individual needs. Physicians are also responsible for caring for the stroke survivor's general health and providing guidance aimed at preventing a second stroke, such as controlling high blood pressure or diabetes and eliminating risk factors such as cigarette smoking, excessive weight, a high-cholesterol diet, and high alcohol consumption.

Neurologists usually lead acute-care stroke teams and direct patient care during hospitalization. They sometimes remain in charge of long-term rehabilitation. However, physicians trained in other specialties often assume responsibility after the acute stage has passed, including physiatrists, who specialize in physical medicine and rehabilitation.

### Rehabilitation Nurses

Nurses specializing in rehabilitation help survivors relearn how to carry out the basic activities of daily living. They also educate survivors about routine health care, such as how to follow a medication schedule, how to care for the skin, how to manage transfers between a bed and a wheelchair, and special needs for people with diabetes. Rehabilitation nurses also work with survivors to reduce risk factors that may lead to a second stroke, and provide training for caregivers.

Nurses are closely involved in helping stroke survivors manage personal care issues, such as bathing and controlling incontinence. Most stroke survivors regain their ability to maintain continence, often with the help of strategies learned during rehabilitation. These strategies include strengthening pelvic muscles through special exercises and following a timed voiding schedule. If problems with incontinence continue, nurses can help caregivers learn to insert and manage catheters and to take special hygienic measures to prevent other incontinence-related health problems from developing.

*Physical Therapists*

Physical therapists specialize in treating disabilities related to motor and sensory impairments. They are trained in all aspects of anatomy and physiology related to normal function, with an emphasis on movement. They assess the stroke survivor's strength, endurance, range of motion, gait abnormalities, and sensory deficits to design individualized rehabilitation programs aimed at regaining control over motor functions.

Physical therapists help survivors regain the use of stroke-impaired limbs, teach compensatory strategies to reduce the effect of remaining deficits, and establish ongoing exercise programs to help people retain their newly learned skills. Disabled people tend to avoid using impaired limbs, a behavior called learned non-use. However, the repetitive use of impaired limbs encourages brain plasticity and helps reduce disabilities. (Plasticity is the ability of the brain to adapt and change.)

Strategies used by physical therapists to encourage the use of impaired limbs include selective sensory stimulation such as tapping or stroking, active and passive range-of-motion exercises, and temporary restraint of healthy limbs while practicing motor tasks. Some physical therapists may use a new technology, *transcutaneous electrical nerve stimulation* (TENS), that encourages brain reorganization and recovery of function. TENS involves using a small probe that generates an electrical current to stimulate nerve activity in stroke-impaired limbs.

In general, physical therapy emphasizes practicing isolated movements, repeatedly changing from one kind of movement to another, and rehearsing complex movements that require a great deal of coordination and balance, such as walking up or down stairs or moving safely between obstacles. People too weak to bear their own weight can still practice repetitive movements during hydrotherapy (in which water provides sensory stimulation as well as weight support) or while being partially supported by a harness. A recent trend in physical therapy emphasizes the effectiveness of engaging in goal-directed activities, such as playing games, to promote coordination. Physical therapists frequently employ selective sensory stimulation to encourage use of impaired limbs and to help survivors with neglect regain awareness of stimuli on the neglected side of the body.

*Occupational Therapists*

Like physical therapists, occupational therapists are concerned with improving motor abilities. They help survivors relearn motor skills needed for performing self-directed activities—occupations—such as housecleaning, gardening, and practicing arts and crafts. Therapists can teach some survivors how to adapt to driving and provide on-road training. They often teach people to divide a complex activity into its component parts, practice each part, and then perform the whole sequence of actions. This strategy can improve coordination and may help people with apraxia relearn how to carry out planned actions.

Occupational therapists also teach people how to develop compensatory strategies and how to change elements of their environment that limit goal-directed activities. For example, people with the use of only one hand can substitute Velcro closures for buttons on clothing. Occupational therapists also help stroke survivors learn how to use assistive devices, such as canes, walkers, or wheelchairs. Finally, many occupational therapists teach people how to make changes in their homes to increase safety, remove barriers, and facilitate physical functioning, such as installing grab bars in bathrooms.

*Speech-Language Pathologists*

Speech-language pathologists help stroke survivors with aphasia relearn how to use language or develop alternative means of communication. They also help people improve their ability to swallow.

Many specialized therapeutic techniques have been developed to assist people with aphasia. Some forms of short-term therapy can improve comprehension rapidly. Intensive exercises such as repeating the therapist's words, practicing following directions, and doing reading or writing exercises form the cornerstone of language rehabilitation. Conversational coaching and rehearsal, as well as the development of prompts or cues to help people remember specific words, are sometimes beneficial. Speech-language pathologists also help stroke survivors develop strategies for circumventing language disabilities. These strategies can include the use of symbol boards or sign language. Recent advances in computer technology have spurred the development of new types of equipment to enhance communication.

Speech-language pathologists use noninvasive imaging techniques to study swallowing patterns of stroke survivors and identify the exact source of their impairment. Difficulties with swallowing have many possible causes, including a delayed swallowing reflex, an inability to manipulate food with the tongue, or an inability to detect food remaining lodged in the cheeks after swallowing. When the cause has been pinpointed, speech-language pathologists work with the individual to devise strategies to overcome or minimize the deficit. Sometimes, simply changing body position and improving posture during eating can bring about improvement. The texture of foods can be modified to make swallowing easier; for example, thin liquids, which often cause choking, can be thickened. Changing eating habits by taking small bites and chewing slowly can also help alleviate dysphagia.

*Vocational Therapists*

Approximately one-fourth of all strokes occur in people between the ages of 45 and 65. For most people in this age group, returning to work is a major concern. Vocational therapists perform many of the same functions that ordinary career counselors do. They can help people with residual disabilities identify vocational strengths and develop resumés that highlight those strengths. They also can help identify potential employers, assist in specific job searches, and provide referrals to stroke vocational rehabilitation agencies.

Most important, vocational therapists educate disabled individuals about their rights and protections as defined by the Americans with Disabilities Act of 1990. This law requires employers to make reasonable accommodations for disabled employees. Vocational therapists frequently act as mediators between employers and employees to negotiate the provision of reasonable accommodations in the workplace.

## Where Can a Stroke Patient Get Rehabilitation?

Rehabilitation should begin as soon as a stroke patient is stable, often within 24 to 48 hours after a stroke. This first stage of rehabilitation usually occurs within an acute-care hospital. At the time of discharge from the hospital, the stroke patient and family coordinate with hospital social workers to locate a suitable living arrangement. Many stroke survivors return home, but some move into some type of medical facility.

*Inpatient Rehabilitation Units*

Inpatient facilities may be freestanding or part of larger hospital complexes. Patients stay in the facility, usually for 2 to 3 weeks, and engage in a coordinated, intensive program of rehabilitation. Such programs often involve at least 3 hours of active therapy a day, 5 or 6 days a week. Inpatient facilities offer a comprehensive range of medical services, including full-time physician supervision and access to the full range of therapists specializing in post-stroke rehabilitation.

*Outpatient Units*

Outpatient facilities are often part of a larger hospital complex and provide access to physicians and the full range of therapists specializing in stroke rehabilitation. Patients typically spend several hours, often 3 days each week, at the facility taking part in coordinated therapy sessions and return home at night. Comprehensive outpatient facilities frequently offer treatment programs as intense as those of inpatient facilities, but they also can offer less demanding regimens, depending on the patient's physical capacity.

*Nursing Facilities*

Rehabilitative services available at nursing facilities are more variable than are those at inpatient and outpatient units. Skilled nursing facilities usually place a greater emphasis on rehabilitation, whereas traditional nursing homes emphasize residential care. In addition, fewer hours of therapy are offered compared to outpatient and inpatient rehabilitation units.

*Home-Based Rehabilitation Programs*

Home rehabilitation allows for great flexibility so that patients can tailor their program of rehabilitation and follow individual schedules. Stroke survivors may participate in an intensive level of therapy several hours per week or follow a less demanding regimen. These arrangements are often best suited for people who lack transportation or require treatment by only one type of rehabilitation therapist. Patients dependent on Medicare coverage for their rehabilitation must meet Medicare's homebound requirements to qualify for such services; at this time lack of transportation is not a valid reason for home therapy. The major disadvantage of home-based rehabilitation programs is the lack of specialized equipment. However, undergoing treatment at home gives people the advantage of practicing skills and developing compensatory strategies in the context of their own living environment.

## What Research Is Being Done?

The National Institute of Neurological Disorders and Stroke (NINDS), a component of the Federal Government's National Institutes of Health (NIH), has primary responsibility for sponsoring research on disorders of the brain and nervous system, including the acute phase of stroke and the restoration of function after stroke. The NINDS also supports research on ways to enhance repair and regeneration of the central nervous system. Scientists funded by the NINDS are studying how the brain responds to experience or adapts to injury by reorganizing its functions (plasticity) by using noninvasive imaging technologies to map patterns of biological activity inside the brain. Other NINDS-sponsored scientists are looking at brain reorganization after stroke and determining whether specific rehabilitative techniques, such as constraint-induced movement therapy and transcranial magnetic stimulation, can stimulate brain plasticity, thereby improving motor function and decreasing disability. Other scientists are experimenting with implantation of neural stem cells, to see if these cells may be able to replace the cells that died as a result of a stroke.

## Additional Information

### BRAIN
P.O. Box 5801
Bethesda, MD 20824
Toll-Free: 800-352-9424
Tel: 301-496-5751; Fax: 301-402-2186
Website: http://ninds.nih.gov

### American Heart Association/American Stroke Association
7272 Greenville Avenue
Dallas, TX 75231-4596
Toll-Free AHA: 800-242-8721; ASA: 888-478-7653
Website: www.americanheart.org

### National Stroke Association
9707 East Easter Lane
Englewood, CO 80112-3747
Toll-Free: 800-STROKES (787-6537)
Tel: 303-649-9299; Fax: 303-649-1328
Website: www.stroke.org
E-mail: info@stroke.org

**Stroke Clubs International**
805 12ᵗʰ Street
Galveston, TX 77550
Tel: 409-762-1022
E-mail: strokeclub@aol.com

**National Easter Seal Society**
230 W, Monroe St., Suite 1800
Chicago, IL 60606-4802
Toll-Free: 800-221-6827
Tel: 312-726-6200
TTY: 312-726-4258
Fax: 312-726-1494
Website: www.easter-seals.org

**National Aphasia Association**
29 John Street, Suite 1103
New York, NY 10038
Tel: 212-267-2814
Fax: 212-267-2812
Website: www.aphasia.org
E-mail: naa@aphasia.org

**American Speech-Language-Hearing Association**
10801 Rockville Pike
Rockville, MD 20852-3279
Toll-Free: 800-638-8255
Tel: 301-897-5700
Website: www.asha.org
E-mail: actioncenter@asha.org

**Agency for Healthcare Research and Quality**
P.O. Box 8547
Silver Spring, MD 20907-8547
Toll-Free: 800-358-9295
TDD: 888-586-6340
Website: www.ahrq.gov
E-mail: info@ahrq.gov

**National Rehabilitation Information Center**
4200 Forbes Blvd., Suite 202
Lanham, MD 20706

## National Rehabilitation Information Center, continued
Toll-Free: 800-346-2742
Tel: 301-459-5900
Website: www.naric.com
E-mail: naricinfo@heitechservices.com

## Caregiving Information

### Eldercare Locator
National Association of Area Agencies on Aging
927 15th Street N.W., 6th Floor
Washington, DC 20005
Toll-Free: 800-677-1116
Website: www.eldercare.gov
E-mail: eldercare_locator@aoa.gov

### Family Caregiver Alliance
690 Market St., Suite 600
San Francisco, CA 94104
Toll-Free: 800-445-8106 (in California)
Tel: 415-434-3388
Fax: 415-434-3508
Website: www.caregiver.org
E-mail: info@caregiver.org

### National Family Caregivers Association
10400 Connecticut Ave., Suite 500
Kensington, MD 20895-3944
Toll-Free: 800-896-3650
Tel: 301-942-6430
Fax: 301-942-2302
Website: www.nfcacares.org
E-mail: info@nfcacares.org

### Well Spouse Foundation
63 W. Main St., Suite H
Freehold, NJ 07728
Toll-Free: 800-838-0879
Tel: 631-661-0421
Website: www.wellspouse.org
E-mail: wellspouse@aol.com

Chapter 30

# Physical Therapy Helps Stroke Patients Recover Skills

## Conditions That PM&R Physicians Treat: Stroke

Stroke is the third most common cause of death in the United States and is the most frequent cause of severe disability. There are 500,000 new stroke cases each year, even with the incidence declining over the past 20-30 years due to better control of risk factors like hypertension, high cholesterol, less smoking, and more exercise.

Working as part of a team, the physiatrist assists the patient in improving functional independence including personal care, mobility, and community skills. New equipment and new techniques are helping to achieve this.

### *Stroke Stats*

• There are 4.4 million stroke survivors alive today—up to half of them are totally or partially dependent on others to help them with daily activities.

This chapter includes "Conditions That PM&R Physicians Treat: Stroke," © 2000 American Academy of Physical Medicine and Rehabilitation, reprinted with permission; and "Rehabilitation Helps Stroke Patients Recover Skills," © 2000, American Academy of Physical Medicine and Rehabilitation, reprinted with permission. Also, a section is reprinted from *Fitness: A Way of Life*, with permission of the American Physical Therapy Association © 1987, reviewed October 2002 by David A. Cooke, MD, Diplomate, American Board of Internal Medicine; and a section is reprinted from *What You Need to Know about Balance and Falls*, with permission of the American Physical Therapy Association © 1998, reviewed October 2002 by David A. Cooke, MD, Diplomate, American Board of Internal Medicine.

- More than 60% of those who have experienced stroke, serious injury, or a disabling disease have never received rehabilitation.

- Only 40% of stroke patients reach the hospital within 24 hours— too late for some of today's most effective stroke treatments.

## Rehabilitation Helps Stroke Patients Recover Skills

### Therapy Helps in Regaining Coordination, Full Speech, and Other Abilities

Each year in the United States, approximately 730,000 people are affected by strokes, and that number is expected to surpass the 1 million mark by 2050. Today, the amount of stroke rehabilitation a patient receives can be severely limited by health plan restrictions, yet doctors and other medical professionals agree that a comprehensive rehabilitative therapy program provides the best chance for the recovery.

Of the 72 million Americans who have experienced serious injury, stroke, or other disabling disease, more than 60 percent never received proper rehabilitation. Yet the earlier rehabilitation begins, the more likely a patient is to regain the ability to function and return to a productive and satisfying life.

Treatment for a stroke begins immediately in the hospital with acute care, helping the patient to survive and avoid another stroke or similar attack. The next step, spontaneous recovery, happens naturally to most patients as they gradually regain some of their lost sensory and motor skill abilities. This usually happens during the first few weeks of recovery, but steady progress can take place over a longer period of time.

Rehabilitation programs are critical in helping patients regain lost skills, relearn tasks and work to be independent again. While many healthcare professionals are involved in administering a rehabilitation program, treatment is often managed by a doctor of physical medicine and rehabilitation (PM&R). This medical specialist will evaluate the patient's condition and develop a customized program of rehabilitation services designed to restore lost function.

Care may be provided by physical and occupational therapists, speech language pathologists, psychologists, rehabilitative nurses, social workers, geriatricians, neurologists, and other specialists as part of a treatment and rehabilitation team. The PM&R physician will manage the team, making sure that all components of the rehabilitation program are working together for the benefit of the patient. In addition to treating symptoms, the PM&R physician's role is to coordinate all aspects of the continuing treatment of a patient with stroke. It's important to have a coordinated effort, because it provides the best possible rehabilitative care for the patient. By directing the efforts of other professionals and gathering and analyzing information from their treatment sessions, the PM&R physician helps to ensure that continuity in care is covered and no aspects of treatment are unnecessarily duplicated.

This personalized rehabilitative care is designed to help the patient regain the ability to function as independently as possible at home, work, and in the community. It involves learning to perform the daily activities of living in order to achieve the best possible quality of life.

PM&R physicians help stroke survivors achieve this goal. There are nearly 4 million stroke survivors in the United States. The key word is survivor, because although a stroke may be debilitating, it's not the end of the road. There's life beyond a stroke. However, it is important to remember that stroke rehabilitation takes time. Patients and their families will need to take one day at a time. Each advance in a patient's skills and condition is a victory and over time, a number of small victories can add up dramatically.

## What You Need to Know about Balance and Falls

Anyone who has ever slipped on a patch of ice knows how unnerving it can be to lose your balance—for a moment your world is literally turned upside down. Yet balance—the ability to control and maintain your body's position as it moves through space—is such an integral, ever-present part of daily life that most people rarely give it conscious thought. There are conditions, however, that may impair your sense of balance and contribute to falls. The effects of aging are the most common causes of balance problems; injury and disease can also trigger problems. Because falling is such a common and potentially serious problem—1 in 4 people over the age of 65 (who live at home) will fall during the next year—it's important to find out what you can do to decrease your risk and improve your general health and mobility.

In this section we will discuss:

• How your body maintains its balance;

• Common problems with balance seen in older adults; and

• Advice and exercises for improving balance and preventing falls.

## *Drugs, Alcohol, and Balance*

Certain drugs (including tranquilizers, heart medicines, blood pressure medicines, and mood-altering drugs) and alcohol are major culprits when it comes to increased risk of falling because drowsiness, dizziness, and slowed reflexes are common side effects. Be especially aware of potentially dangerous drug interactions when taking multiple drugs (including over-the-counter medications and/or alcohol).

## *How Balance Works*

Your brain, muscles, and bones work together to maintain your body's balance and to keep you from falling, whether you're walking, rising from a chair, or climbing stairs. They also let you navigate sloping or uneven surfaces.

Balance relies on three types of sensory information. The first of these is visual: your eyes tell you about your environment and your place within it. They help you sense obstacles and potential dangers, and form motor memories that prevent falls. The second type of sensory information comes from your body's internal sense of spatial orientation, independent of vision. This allows you, for example, to close your eyes and then wiggle your foot in any direction, while still knowing which way your foot is pointed. The third type of sensory information is provided by your inner ears, which contain fluid-filled semicircular canals. These canals provide your brain and eyes with crucial information on the position of your head and its movement in space with respect to gravity. (Common problems related to the workings of the inner ear include dizziness on escalators and sea-sickness.) When your sense of balance is in good working order, the three elements of balance work together automatically with your musculoskeletal system to keep you mobile and to prevent falls.

There are various reasons why your sense of balance can become impaired. In older adults, poor posture—particularly if you tend to slouch forward and have rounded upper shoulders—can sometimes cause unsteadiness. Furthermore, your base of support is important in keeping you balanced: if you have a wide pyramid-type stance, you're less likely to lose your balance or fall than if your feet are close together in a pencil stance. Disease can also rob you of a strong sense of balance. People with diabetes, for example, may suffer from numbness in the lower extremities and feet—a problem that makes detecting obstacles or dangers more difficult. People with arthritis, or who have had surgery on their hips, knees, or feet, may lack the flexibility and range of motion necessary to avoid falling.

Strength, flexibility, and endurance are crucial to maintaining balance and preventing falls. Even if your basic perception of balance is good—you have normal vision and no inner ear problems—you can still be at risk for falls if your muscles are weakened or stiff, or if you tire easily. Older adults—particularly those with osteoporosis (the disease that causes brittle bones)—have very legitimate concerns about falling and often restrict their physical activities to prevent such a mishap. Ironically, lack of exercise only makes it more likely that a fall will occur—and a vicious cycle has been put into motion.

Fortunately, physical therapy can help you learn to cultivate and maintain higher levels of strength, flexibility, and endurance in a way that still feels safe and secure. Research indicates that the risk of falling in older adults can be reduced dramatically when specific exercises, activities, and interventions are prescribed by physical therapists. There are instances, however, in which physical therapy alone may not be appropriate. If you have an inner ear disorder, for example, you will need to consult a physician.

## Making Your Home Safer

Preventing falls is easier than treating them. Your physical therapist can help you evaluate your home environment with the goal of minimizing clutter, loose rugs, slippery conditions, uneven surfaces, and unsecured cords and wires—in short, anything that could cause a fall. Good lighting and well thought out placement of furniture can also help prevent mishaps.

## How Physical Therapy Can Help

If you consult a physical therapist about falls and balance, he or she will likely review your medical history and determine your general physical condition, as well as conduct an inventory of tests specifically designed to measure balance and gait (your individual style of walking). If you have fallen before, your physical therapist will ask you to describe the accident in some detail to find out what caused the fall. (Just as important as actual falls are near-falls—instances in which you were on your way down but managed to hang on.)

After your physical therapist has determined what is impairing your balance, he or she will design a program of exercises and activities just for you, with an emphasis on strength, flexibility, and proper gait. All exercises would be planned for maximum safety and security. Your physical therapist may also perform specific interventions to increase your range of motion and musculoskeletal flexibility. These may include electrical stimulation, massage, hydrotherapy, heat, cold, and ultrasound. If you have balance problems related to the inner ear, your physical therapist may also try interventions known as vestibular rehabilitation. Vestibular rehabilitation includes techniques that help the inner ear respond to a change in position. Conditions that may require vestibular rehabilitation include vertigo, dizziness, or nausea.

If necessary, your physical therapist may also prescribe assistive devices for walking (such as canes, crutches, or walkers). Make sure the tips on canes and crutches are large (and spiked, if necessary, for icy conditions) and that canes are high enough (they should come up to your hip).

Appropriate footwear is another major consideration. Wearing a good pair of lace-up walking shoes will help support your foot and provide necessary cushioning for your joints; this will make walking safer and more comfortable. Avoid high heels, slippers, and open-toed sandals, which can cause you to trip.

## Balance Is a Skill You Can Keep—or Recapture

The good news is that balance is a skill that almost all of us can keep throughout our lives. Much of the deterioration in balance associated with age is simply due to not using this skill. Sometimes this happens because of change in lifestyle—most of us become more sedentary as we grow older—or it can happen due to fear of falling.

Working with a physical therapist can produce exceptional results in many cases. Even if some of your innate sense of balance has been diminished over time, physical therapists are experts at retraining your body to make the most of its capabilities.

## Exercises to Improve Balance

### Eye Exercise for Balance

1.  Focus your eyes on a target 10-20 feet away while you change from sitting to standing and back again with your eyes open. Make sure that you land softly when you sit!

2.  Repeat with your eyes closed.

3. Feel the position of your body as you move. Be sure that you keep your weight forward on the front of your feet knees apart, chest forward and spine erect.

### *"All Fours" Balance Exercise*

1. Get on all fours, with your knees and also your hands 12-18 inches apart—like a table.

2. Pull your stomach muscles in tight. Keep your shoulders pinched back and your back flat.

3. Keep your chin in and your head straight.

4. Now lift each arm by itself and hold for 3-10 seconds.

5. Return arms to floor. Now lift each leg by itself, no more than 6" off the floor. Hold for 3-10 seconds.

6. Finally, lift the opposite arm and leg together no more than 1" and hold for 3-10 seconds. Reach out only if you feel ready. Repeat on opposite sides.

### *Toe, Heel, and Leg Rises*

1. Stand straight and tall, with your knees slightly bent and your toes pointed straight ahead. Line your knees up over the point of your shoes.

2. Look straight ahead. Keep your chin tucked and your shoulder blades pinched straight back. Tighten your stomach muscles.

3. Rise up on your toes. Lower yourself back down and repeat.

4. Keep your posture the same. This time, however, raise the front part of your foot, lower, and repeat. Remember to keep your stomach muscles tight.

5. Keep standing straight and tall, as before. Shift your weight forward to the front half of your feet. Lift one leg, keeping your standing leg in proper alignment. Hold 10-30 seconds. Lower and repeat with the other side.

6. Slowly and carefully repeat each exercise 3-5 times.

*Half-Circle Sway*

If you have experienced falls or problems with balance, get your physical therapist's permission before doing this exercise.

1. Stand with your feet shoulder-distance apart. Hold onto the kitchen sink counter for safety. Breathe deeply and relax.

2. Lean forward slowly from the ankles, without bending at the hips. Feel how about 70% of your body weight is now on the balls of your feet.

3. Return to the neutral starting position. Now lean slowly to the left. Feel how about 70% of your body weight is on the left sides of your feet.

4. Return to the upright position. This time lean slowly to the right, feeling the shift in your weight.

5. Now put it all together. Practice making graceful half-circle sways from left to center to right and back again. Begin with small half-circles, and gradually increase to see how far you can move your body without taking a step.

## Fitness: A Way of Life

### What Is Being Fit?

We would all like to be physically fit, but how many of us know what fit really means? Does playing softball twice a week make us fit? Or swimming at the neighborhood pool? Or walking to and from work? What amount of activity is enough to keep us fit? Do we all need to follow the same fitness program or are we all different?

Physical therapists answer these kinds of questions all the time. Realizing that each individual is unique, physical therapists have developed specific methods to determine how fit you are, and what types of activities your optimum level of fitness.

While each individual is unique, physical therapists support the Surgeon General's statement that everyone may substantially improve their health and quality of life by doing moderate-intensity physical exercise for at least 30 minutes every day. Physical therapists encourage people of all ages to begin a program of daily regular exercise to help prevent cardiovascular disease and musculoskeletal disorders.

Physical therapists are uniquely qualified to develop personalized conditioning programs that, if followed properly, will help prevent injury and promote fitness. Physical therapists would be the first to say they would rather see you before you embark on a fitness program, than after you have sustained a painful injury.

This section is designed to increase your understanding of fitness from a total body perspective—the approach used by physical therapists. Total fitness is achieved by matching your body and lifestyle to a fitness program that you will enjoy, a fitness program that can become a way of life.

## Six Elements of Fitness

### Fitness Is

Fitness as defined by physical therapists is an ongoing state of health whereby all systems of the body are conditioned to withstand physical stress and are able to perform at an optimum level without injury. A person who is physically fit has a properly aligned body structure; flexible and strong muscles; an efficient heart and healthy lungs; a good ratio of body fat to lean body mass; and good balance.

Note that the above definition does not say, "A person who is fit can run X amount of miles in X minutes." Being fit is just that—a state of being. What activities you choose to perform to achieve and maintain a state of fitness are really up to you!

And, as an added bonus, physical fitness also contributes to mental fitness. There's nothing like being in tip-top shape to give you a positive outlook on life.

The American Physical Therapy Association wants you to understand the total body approach to fitness by looking at the six elements of fitness:

1. Aerobic Capacity
2. Body Structure
3. Body Composition
4. Body Balance
5. Muscular Flexibility
6. Muscular Strength

We'll now look at each of these elements from the physical therapist's perspective, see how a therapist evaluates your body in

299

terms of these elements, and find out how that evaluation can help you achieve overall fitness.

### Aerobic Capacity

Aerobic capacity is an index of your cardiovascular system's ability to transport oxygen to working muscles, where the oxygen is used as fuel to produce energy for movement.

You can improve your aerobic capacity by achieving what is called an aerobic response. Although the level necessary to achieve an aerobic response varies with each individual, it is usually reached by exercising at 60 to 80 percent of your maximum heart rate. This ideal rate for exercise (60-80 percent of maximum) is called your target heart rate. Exercising at your target heart rate should be maintained for 20 to 30 minutes and occur at least three times a week for you to attain aerobic fitness.

There are many different types of activities that can generate an aerobic response. Walking can be an excellent activity that is a particularly good aerobic exercise. Some other aerobic activities include jumping rope, swimming, running, cross-country skiing, hiking, aerobic dancing, and bicycling.

### Target Heart Rate

To estimate your target heart rate, you must first determine your maximum heart rate. This is done by subtracting your age from 220. If a check-up by your physician indicates no problems, your target heart rate is 60 to 80 percent of your maximum rate. For example: If you are 20 years old, your maximum heart rate is 200. Your target heart rate is 60 to 80 percent of 200, or 120 to 160 beats per minute.

You can monitor your target heart rate by finding your pulse—either lay your fingertips on the palm side of your wrist or lightly against the side of your voice box—and count the pulse for 15 seconds; then multiply this number by four to get your pulse rate in beats per minute.

As you continue to exercise regularly, you will find that it takes more effort to reach your target heart rate. This is a good sign and means that your heart and lungs are getting stronger and that your aerobic capacity is improving.

### Resting Heart Rate

Another clear indicator of improved aerobic fitness is your resting heart rate. Take your pulse first thing in the morning, while you are still lying in bed. As your aerobic fitness level improves, your resting heart rate should decrease. This occurs because as your heart becomes a better pump, it can pump more blood with each beat, supplying your muscles with more of the oxygen they need. (Resting heart rates rarely go below 50 beats per minute and are usually between 60 to 100 beats per minute.)

## Body Structure

A physical therapist evaluates your body structure by looking for structural misalignments in upper and lower extremities (arms and legs), the head, neck, and trunk. The therapist will check your overall posture by looking at your head, neck, shoulders, spine, pelvis, knees, and feet, from front, side, and back views.

Even a small imbalance in the way you stand—too much weight on one foot, your shoulders slouched forward—may lead to pain and injury when you start exercising. If any problems are identified in the evaluation, the physical therapist may give you some exercises to strengthen weak muscles or improve the flexibility of tight muscles, teach you to become more aware of your posture while standing and walking, or recommend specific footwear.

## Body Composition

Body composition is the ratio of body fat to lean body mass (bones and muscles). You cannot determine your body composition simply by weighing yourself on a standard scale. In fact, body composition measurements tend to be a much better indicator of your current fitness level than your body weight. Some people who weigh a lot are not fat; they just may be muscular and muscles weigh more than fat. Conversely, a person who maintains a seemingly ideal weight may actually be carrying too much fat.

Your physical therapist can determine your body composition by taking fat measurements at various places on your body. Although ideal body fat levels vary with each individual, it is generally accepted that the ideal range of body fat is approximately 10 to 15 percent of total body mass for males and 15 to 22 percent for females; seasoned athletes often have much less. It is at the ideal fat-to-lean ratio that your body is its most efficient. An excessive fat-to-lean body composition puts unnecessary weight on your skeletal structure during exercise without helping you perform your task. Muscles at least work for you; fat just weights you down. (On the other hand, insufficient body fat isn't good for your health either and is common among some athletes and adolescents.)

And don't be discouraged if you gain a few pounds when you begin your fitness program—the extra weight means you're building up your muscles as you lose the fat.

### Body Balance

A physical therapist will check your balance by having you stand, with your eyes closed, on one leg for a brief period of time, then on the other. Although this seems a simple test, it may indicate if you have a neurological (nervous system) problem. Neurological testing evaluates the balance controlled by your brain.

Even a minor balance problem may place you at risk for possible injury. If a problem is identified, your therapist may give you some exercise tips that will help to improve your balance.

### Muscular Flexibility

Your muscles should be flexible to allow for the full range of motion required by life's many activities, such as stretching, lifting, reaching, and bending. Muscles should be able to lengthen without too much effort, allowing your body and limbs to move efficiently in many different ways.

Just as muscles can be stretched, due to their elastic nature, they can also become shortened when adapting to long periods of inactivity. A shortened or inflexible muscle may be more susceptible to stress and injury.

A physical therapist can determine your flexibility by measuring how far you can move your arms, legs, and torso. The therapist will notice if you have any specific areas of tightness and will suggest some gentle exercises to increase flexibility.

### Muscular Strength

In addition to being flexible, your muscles should be able to exert force and control movement. For example, flexible muscles will help you bend over to pick up a box, but it's your muscular strength that enables you to lift it.

The physical therapist will determine the strength of your major muscle groups by having you perform weight-resistance exercises and tests.

If your muscles need strengthening, you may embark on a strength-training program designed by your therapist. Usually these exercises do not require heavy lifting or strenuous exercise. You may only need to work with hand weights to strengthen one arm, or do strengthening exercises to bring muscles on one side of your body in balance with the other.

Strengthening exercises should condition those muscles that will be used to perform the activity of your choice. If you want to be a long-distance runner, you should condition your leg muscles to withstand stress for long periods of time.

## Additional Factors that Affect Fitness

It is important to be aware of, and tell your physical therapist about, any aspects of your lifestyle that may be considered risk factors to your fitness.

Do you:

• Smoke cigarettes?

• Eat junk food regularly?

• Take stimulants (drugs, caffeine, even vitamins)?

• Drink alcohol excessively?

• Have a stressful job?

• Feel depressed, lack motivation?

• Have a family health history that includes heart disease, diabetes, or high blood pressure?

Although some of these factors may seem unrelated to your fitness, they may have an effect on your general state of well-being, and may pose risks that should be considered when developing your fitness program.

## Fitness for People with Disabilities

There are many ways in which a physical therapist can tailor-make a fitness program for people with disabilities. The goal of anyone involved in a fitness program is to be at a level appropriate for his or her unique capacity. Your physical therapist is eager to help you meet your challenge and benefit from a fitness program that will keep you fit for life.

303

## *Starting Your Fitness Way of Life*

1. Decide what sports and activities you most enjoy. Do you play tennis? Swim? Jog? Do you enjoy walking? Make a list of your favorite activities, then list next to these activities a time when you feel you could perform them during an average week.

2. Consult a physical therapist who specializes in sports and orthopaedic physical therapy. To find an appropriate physical therapist near you, look in the yellow pages of your phone book, ask your physician or local hospital, or contact the local chapter of the American Physical Therapy Association. You'll be surprised how many physical therapists are ready to serve you right in your own area.

3. Ask your physical therapist to give you a fitness evaluation. This will determine your present level of fitness, based on the six elements of fitness as described in this chapter. The therapist will check your aerobic capacity, body structure, body composition, body balance, muscular flexibility, and muscular strength. The therapist will tell you what you need to do to improve your present condition.

4. Share the list you developed in Step 1 with your physical therapist. Together, you can choose activities for a balanced fitness program. Your choices should be based on your favorite activities and lifestyle, and on how much time during each week you want to commit to being fit.

5. Begin your fitness program, monitoring your progress based on the suggestions in this chapter, and the advice of your physical therapist. If you suffer an injury, no matter how minor you think it is, tell your physical therapist. it may be helpful in deciding what activities are best for you.

6. Although you may emphasize one area of conditioning as you develop your individualized fitness program, remember that total fitness requires a total body approach. Balance your program with activities that concentrate on the six elements of fitness: aerobic capacity, body structure, body composition, body balance, muscular flexibility, and muscular strength.

Achieving and maintaining fitness is a lifelong commitment. Perhaps you are currently active in sports; but what will you be doing

20 years from now? Your state of fitness need not lessen with age. Just because you may become less active as you grow older, you needn't resign yourself to being less fit.

As you become comfortable with your fitness program—enjoy yourself! Notice how much better you move, breathe, and feel. You were meant to be fit! It's just a matter of knowing where to start, and how to get to where you want to be. Remember—fitness is a way of life.

## About APTA

The American Physical Therapy Association (APTA) is a national professional organization representing physical therapists, physical therapist assistants, and students throughout the United States.

Physical therapists are vital members of the multidisciplinary health care team. They provide treatment and can refer clients to other health care specialists. APTA serves its members and the public by promoting understanding of the physical therapist's increasing role in the health care system. APTA also promotes excellence in the field with advancements in physical therapy practice, research, and education.

"Fitness: A Way of Life" Acknowledgments: Perry Esterson, MS, ATC, PT; Robert Finke, ATC, PT; Vanessa Mirabelli, PT; and Barbara Sanders, MS, PT

## Additional Information

### American Academy of Physical Medicine and Rehabilitation (AAPM&R)
One IBM Plaza, Suite 2500
Chicago, IL 60611-3604
Tel: 312-464-9700
Fax: 312-464-0227
Website: www.aapmr.org
E-mail: info@aapmr.org

### American Physical Therapy Association (APTA)
1111 North Fairfax Street
Alexandria, VA 22314-1488
Toll-Free: 800-999-APTA (2782)
Tel: 703-684-APTA (2782)
TDD: 703-683-6748
Fax: 703-684-7343
Website: www.apta.org

Chapter 31

# Occupational Therapy Is Important for Stroke Recovery

## Never Say Never by E.G. Richmond

At the age of 55, a severe stroke left this vibrant TV anchorman curled up in a wheelchair, unable to speak, his nose six inches from his knees. Fifteen years later, an occupational therapist got him talking, writing, and back on his feet.

It all started as I was scanning the local newspaper and a word in an ad caught my eye. Medical and Complex combined into one word—Mediplex. Reading on, I saw that the Mediplex Rehabilitation Hospital in Bowling Green, Ky., was going to host an open house, giving the public an opportunity to inspect its facilities and meet its personnel.

I showed the ad to my wife Rusty of 45 years who attended and returned, enthusiastically describing what she had seen. The next day Rusty called and made an appointment for me to be examined and interviewed. I should point out that I had never become reconciled to a wheelchair lifestyle. As a TV anchorman I had led a very active life prior to my stroke.

"Never Say Never," by E.G. Richmond © 2002 American Occupational Therapy Association, Inc. Reprinted with permission; "Occupational Therapy Is Important When You Are Recovering from Stroke," © 2002 American Occupational Therapy Association, Inc. Reprinted with permission; and "Finding an Occupational Therapist," © 2002 American Occupational Therapy Association, Inc. Reprinted with permission.

## I Can Breathe Again

My rehabilitation took a positive turn when I began to receive occupational therapy. Occupational therapist Marilyn McLaughlin explained the technique she was using as neurodevelopmental treatment. She said it is a technique used very effectively on brain-damaged stroke patients such as myself. It works on the principle that there are millions of pathways in the brain, many of which are never used. It is believed these pathways can take over for other pathways damaged by strokes or head injuries.

My trunk was curled in a "C" shape, affording me an excellent view of the floor and my shoes. Marilyn also determined she could improve this posture.

A first step was a new wheelchair that helped me sit in a better position. It took a bit of getting used to, but it did improve my posture and I felt better. And, I could breathe better, which meant I could also talk better.

## One Small Step

Marilyn told me that to get my brain to wake up and send messages to hold my torso straighter, she had to stand me up. So, with assistance from Marilyn, my wife, and a PT, I stood in a rolling walker and cautiously—very cautiously—moved my right leg a bit. My wife later told me that the OT and the PT looked at each other with an expression that silently asked, "Do you suppose he could take steps?"

The next time, I did take a step, then three steps. I felt like Astronaut Neal Armstrong, "One small step for a man . . . " After just those three steps I was worn out. Endurance was and continues to be my big problem. When I started therapy I could only tolerate 30 minutes at a time. Now I'm up to 90 minutes.

But, tired as I was, I could not and would not conceal my excitement—15 years after my devastating stroke I was walking!

According to OT Marilyn McLaughlin, Richmond wrote this article to let people know there is always hope. When it was written, Richmond was walking up to 100 feet with a rolling walker and was attending occupational therapy twice a week to improve sitting balance, trunk control, and hand function activities. He is able to look around and to use his right hand for typing and simple activities of daily living. He uses a computer up to five hours per day for writing and other communications.

Adapted from an article printed in the December 11, 1997 *OT Week*®

## *Occupational Therapy Is Important When You Are Recovering from Stroke*

This year, more than 500,000 Americans will have strokes. In spite of the problems that result from stroke, many of these people will return to their homes and live independent, productive lives with the skilled help of occupational therapy practitioners.

Problems resulting from a stroke may include:

• temporary or permanent weakness of one side of the body

• problems with vision and reading

• difficulties with memory or speech

These problems may interfere with your ability to:

• care for personal needs, like bathing and dressing

• prepare meals and care for your home

• move about in the community, drive a car, or use public transportation

• participate in work, educational, and leisure activities

While you are recovering, occupational therapy can help you:

• learn new ways to manage daily tasks, such as eating, dressing, and bathing

• obtain special assistive equipment to help you function more independently

• discover ways to increase your physical strength, endurance, and mobility

• compensate for losses of sensation and vision

• develop the skills necessary to return to work, household tasks, and community activities

To increase your independence, the occupational therapist may:

• recommend altering your home to eliminate hazards to walking or using a wheelchair

- recommend special devices or aids that help you to perform home and work tasks

- recommend methods of dressing and bathing

- recommend techniques and resources for improving your mobility in the home and community

**Occupational therapy practitioners** are important members of the health care team working with people recovering from stroke. They teach individuals who have had strokes to cope with disability and to become as independent as possible so they can continue their work and personal lives, manage stress and fatigue, and participate fully in family and community life.

**The occupational therapist is a health care professional** who has a bachelor's or master's degree and has completed a clinical internship. The occupational therapy assistant holds an associate degree and has also completed a clinical internship. Both occupational therapists and occupational therapy assistants must pass a national certification examination. Many states also regulate the practice of occupational therapy.

**The goal of occupational therapy** is to help individuals to become as independent as possible in daily life. Many people who have experienced strokes are meeting this goal with the help of occupational therapy.

**Occupational therapy services** are available in many hospitals, rehabilitation centers, and home health programs. To find occupational therapy professionals in your community, contact the occupational therapy department at your local hospital.

## Stroke Survivors Make an Important Contribution to Their Recovery by Being Informed and Active Participants in the Rehabilitation Process

They should ask for time to consider decisions being made about their care. If the stroke has made it difficult for an individual to speak, seek the assistance of a speech pathologist or enlist family members to aid in communication.

Family members help the stroke survivor by participating in education offered for survivors and family members. They can attend some rehabilitation sessions and encourage and help the person to practice skills. They can assist staff in choosing activities meeting the person's interests and needs.

To contact an occupational therapist in your community, check with your primary care physician, the occupational therapy department in your community hospital, or a home health agency.

## Finding an Occupational Therapist

Search the AOTA Specialist Directory. You may also wish to consult the Yellow Pages for the names of individuals in private practice. Further assistance may be available through State Occupational Therapy Associations located in all 50 of the United States, the District of Columbia, and Puerto Rico.

### The Facts about Occupational Therapy (OT)

Occupational therapy is skilled treatment that helps individuals achieve independence in all facets of their lives. Occupational therapy gives people the skills for the job of living they need to live satisfying lives. Services typically include:

- Customized treatment programs aimed at improving abilities to carry out the activities of daily living.

- Comprehensive evaluation of home and job environments and recommendations on necessary adaptation.

- Assessments and treatment for performance skills.

- Recommendations and training in the use of adaptive equipment to replace lost function.

- Guidance to family members and attendants in safe and effective methods of caring for individuals.

Occupational therapy practitioners are skilled professionals whose education includes the study of human growth and development with specific emphasis on the social, emotional, and physiological effects of illness and injury. The occupational therapist enters the field with a bachelor's, master's, or doctoral degree. The occupational therapy assistant generally earns an associate's degree. Practitioners must complete supervised clinical internships in a variety of health care settings, and pass a national examination. Most states also regulate occupational therapy practice.

## Who Benefits from Occupational Therapy?

A wide variety of people can benefit from occupational therapy, including those with:

- work related injuries such as low back problems or repetitive stress injuries
- limitations following a stroke or heart attack
- arthritis, multiple sclerosis, or other serious chronic conditions
- birth injuries, learning problems, or developmental disabilities
- mental health or behavioral problems including Alzheimer's, schizophrenia, and post-traumatic stress
- substance abuse problems or eating disorders
- burns, spinal cord injuries, or amputations
- broken bones or other injuries from falls, sports injuries, or accidents
- vision or cognitive problems that threaten their ability to drive

### How OT Works

Every day, countless people of all ages experience problems that significantly affect their ability to manage their daily lives. With the help of occupational therapy, many of these individuals can achieve or regain a high level of independence. From the infant with a birth defect or injury to the person affected by aging, occupational therapy helps people make the most of their abilities. When skill and strength cannot be developed or improved, occupational therapy offers creative solutions and resources for carrying out the person's daily activities.

### Stroke

Helen Richards is a publishing executive, respected for her business skills and admired for her perfect grooming. Three months ago Helen had a stroke. During her recovery she had to relearn many things, but her first goal was to face the world with her hair and makeup in place. Helen's occupational therapist understood. Together they found the right combination of tools and techniques so Helen could handle her personal grooming. They also worked on the other tasks she would need to manage in her home and upon return to work.

From makeup to management, occupational therapy helped Helen recover the skills she needed.

## Links to Consumer Organizations

### ASPIIRE Partnership
Website: www.ideapractices.org

The IDEA Practices website is a resource-rich and highly interactive website that gives parents, schools, service providers, and local administrators information and support for IDEA-related concerns, issues, and strategies that work.

### Consortium for Citizens with Disabilities
Website: www.c-c-d.org

The Consortium for Citizens with Disabilities is a coalition of approximately 100 national disability organizations working together to advocate for national public policy that ensures the self determination, independence, empowerment, integration, and inclusion of children and adults with disabilities in all aspects of society.

### National AMBUCS, Inc.
Website: www.aota.org/featured/area6/links/LINK09.asp

AMBUCS (formerly known as the American Business Clubs) is a national service organization composed of a diverse group of men and women dedicated to creating independence and opportunities for people with disabilities. They do this by performing community service, by providing AmTrykes, the therapeutic tricycle, to children with disabilities, and by providing scholarships for therapists through the AMBUCS Scholars program.

### VSA arts
Website: www.vsarts.org

VSA arts is an international organization that creates learning opportunities through the arts for people with disabilities. The organization offers arts based programs in creative writing, dance, drama, music, and the visual arts implemented primarily through their affiliate network in 41 states and the District of Columbia and 86 international affiliates in 83 countries. VSA arts' programs now serve 4.3 million Americans and 1.3 million people in other parts of the world.

# Additional Resources

## *Administration on Aging*
1 Massachusetts Ave., NW
Washington, DC 20201
Toll-Free: 800-677-1116
Tel: 202-619-0724
Website: www.aoa.gov
E-mail: aoainfo@aoa.gov

Call for list of community services for older Americans in your area.

## *AHA Stroke Connection*
American Heart Association
7272 Greenville
Dallas, TX 75231
Toll-Free: 800-4-STROKE
Website: www.strokeassociation.org
E-mail: strokeconnection@heart.org

## *National Stroke Association*
8480 East Orchard Rd., Suite 1000
Englewood, CO 80111
Toll-Free: 800-787-6537
Tel: 303-649-9299
Fax: 303-649-1328
Website: www.stroke.org

Serves as information referral clearinghouse on stroke.

## *The American Occupational Therapy Association, Inc.*
4720 Montgomery Lane
P.O. Box 31220
Bethesda, MD 20824-1220
Tel: 301-652-2682
TDD: 800-377-8555
Fax: 301-652-7711

Chapter 32

# Aphasia and Dysarthria—
# Speech Difficulties Following
# Stroke

The use of speech to communicate is unique to humans. When
speech is impaired or absent, the impact on the person and his family is profound. One of the most heartbreaking and devastating disabilities is aphasia. Most people have not heard about aphasia, nor
do they know the term until someone in their family or a friend ac-
quires aphasia.

## What Is Aphasia?

Aphasia is an impairment of language, affecting the production or
comprehension of speech and the ability to read or write. Aphasia is
always due to injury to the brain—most commonly from a stroke, particularly in older individuals. But brain injuries resulting in aphasia
may also arise from head trauma, brain tumors, or infections.

Aphasia can be so severe as to make communication with the patient almost impossible, or it can be very mild. It may affect mainly a
single aspect of language use, such as the ability to retrieve the names
of objects, or the ability to put words together into sentences, or the
ability to read. More commonly, however, multiple aspects of communication are impaired, while some channels remain accessible for a

This chapter includes "Aphasia Fact Sheet," 1988, revised June 22, 1999,
© NAA, reprinted with permission of the National Aphasia Association (NAA),
and "Communicating with People Who Have Aphasia," © NAA, reprinted with
permission of the National Aphasia Association (NAA); also "Adult Aphasia:
Recent Research," National Institute on Deafness and Other Communication
Disorders (NIDCD), NIH Pub. No. 01-4257, June 2001.

315

limited exchange of information. It is the job of the professional to determine the amount of function available in each of the channels for the comprehension of language, and to assess the possibility that treatment might enhance the use of the channels that are available.

## Varieties and Special Features of Aphasia

Over a century of experience with the study of aphasia has taught us that particular components of language may be particularly damaged in some individuals. We have also learned to recognize different types or patterns of aphasia that correspond to the location of the brain injury in the individual case. Some of the common varieties of aphasia are:

**Global aphasia**—This is the most severe form of aphasia, and is applied to patients who can produce few recognizable words and understand little or no spoken language. Global aphasics can neither read nor write. Global aphasia may often be seen immediately after the patient has suffered a stroke and it may rapidly improve if the damage has not been too extensive. However, with greater brain damage, severe and lasting disability may result.

**Broca's aphasia**—This is a form of aphasia in which speech output is severely reduced and is limited mainly to short utterances, of less than four words. Vocabulary access is limited in persons with Broca's aphasia, and their formation of sounds is often laborious and clumsy. The person may understand speech relatively well and be able to read, but be limited in writing. Broca's aphasia is often referred to as a non-fluent aphasia because of the halting and effortful quality of speech.

**Mixed non-fluent aphasia**—This term is applied to patients who have sparse and effortful speech, resembling severe Broca's aphasia. However, unlike persons with Broca's aphasia, they remain limited in their comprehension of speech and do not read or write beyond an elementary level.

**Wernicke's aphasia**—In this form of aphasia the ability to grasp the meaning of spoken words is chiefly impaired, while the ease of producing connected speech is not much affected. Therefore Wernicke's aphasia is referred to as a fluent aphasia. However, speech is far from normal. Sentences do not hang together and irrelevant words intrude—

sometimes to the point of jargon, in severe cases. Reading and writing are often severely impaired.

**Anomic aphasia**—This term is applied to persons who are left with a persistent inability to supply the words for the very things they want to talk about—particularly the significant nouns and verbs. As a result their speech, while fluent in grammatical form and output, is full of vague circumlocutions and expressions of frustration. They understand speech well, and in most cases, read adequately. Difficulty finding words is as evident in writing as in speech.

**Other varieties of aphasia**—In addition to the foregoing syndromes that are seen repeatedly by speech clinicians, there are many other possible combinations of deficits that do not exactly fit into these categories. Some of the components of a complex aphasia syndrome may also occur in isolation. This may be the case for disorders of reading (alexia) or disorders affecting both reading and writing (alexia and agraphia), following a stroke. Severe impairments of calculation often accompany aphasia, yet in some instances patients retain excellent calculation in spite of the loss of language.

## Disorders That May Accompany or Be Confused with Aphasia

There are a variety of disorders of communication that may be due to paralysis, weakness, or incoordination of the speech musculature or to cognitive impairment. Such impairment may accompany aphasia or occur independently and be confused with aphasia. It is important to distinguish these disorders from aphasia because the treatment(s) and prognosis of each disorder are different.

**Apraxia** is a collective term used to describe impairment in carrying out purposeful movements. People with severe aphasia are usually extremely limited in explaining themselves by pantomime or gesture, except for expressions of emotion. Commonly they will show you something in their wallet, or lead you to show you something, but this is the extent of their non-verbal communication. Specific examination usually shows that they are unable to perform common expressive gestures on request, such as waving good-bye, beckoning, or saluting, or to pantomime drinking, brushing teeth, etc. (limb apraxia). Apraxia may also primarily affect oral, non-speech movements, like pretending to cough or blow out a candle (facial apraxia). This disorder may even extend to the inability to manipulate real objects. More often, however, apraxia is not very apparent unless one asks the patient to perform or imitate a pretended action. For this reason it is almost never presented as a complaint by the patient or the family. Nevertheless it may underlie the very limited ability of people with aphasia to compensate for the speech impairment by using informative gestures.

**Apraxia of speech.** This term is frequently used by speech pathologists to designate an impairment in the voluntary production of articulation and prosody (the rhythm and timing) of speech. It is characterized by highly inconsistent errors.

**Dysarthria** refers to a group of speech disorders resulting from weakness, slowness, or incoordination of the speech mechanism due to damage to any of a variety of points in the nervous system. Dysarthria may involve disorders to some or all of the basic speech processes: respiration phonation, resonance, articulation, and prosody. Dysarthria is a disorder of speech production not language (e.g., use of vocabulary and/or grammar). Unlike apraxia of speech, the speech errors that occur in dysarthria are highly consistent from one occasion to the next.

**Dementia** is a condition of impairment of memory, intellect, personality, and insight resulting from brain injury or disease. Some forms of dementia are progressive, such as Alzheimer's disease, Picks disease, or some forms of Parkinson's disease. Language impairments are more or less prominent in different forms of dementia, but these are usually overshadowed by more widespread intellectual loss. Since dementia is so often a progressive disorder, the prognosis is quite different from aphasia.

## How Many People Have Aphasia?

It has been estimated that about one million people in the United States have acquired aphasia. The majority have it as the result of stroke. About one-third of severely head-injured persons have aphasia.

## Who Can Have Aphasia?

Aphasia may occur in persons of any age, sex, race, or nationality. Vocation and education are not determining factors.

## Can Aphasia Be Temporary?

Yes. Temporary aphasia, called transient aphasia, refers to a communication problem that lasts only a few hours or days. More than half of those who initially show symptoms of aphasia recover completely within the first few days.

## Can Aphasia Be Prevented?

There are no definitive steps that can be taken to prevent the onset of aphasia in the event of a stroke or head trauma. The condition is determined by the location and size of the area of damage in the brain.

## Can Aphasia Be Cured?

No medicine or drugs have been known to cure aphasia, as yet. Surgery is successful in those occasions where pressure from a brain tumor or a hematoma impacts a critical speech center. Surgery is not useful in cases of aphasia following stroke, which represent the vast majority of instances. Speech therapy is often provided to persons with aphasia, but does not guarantee a cure. The purpose of speech therapy is to help the patient to fully utilize remaining skills and to learn compensatory means of communication.

## Communicating with People Who Have Aphasia

Aphasia is a communication impairment usually acquired as a result of a stroke or other brain injury. It affects both the ability to express oneself through speech, gesture, and writing, and to understand the speech, gesture, and writing of others. Aphasia thus changes the way in which we communicate with those people most important to us: family, friends, and co-workers.

The impact of aphasia on relationships may be profound, or only slight. No two people with aphasia are alike with respect to severity, former speech and language skills, or personality. But in all cases it is essential for the person to communicate as successfully as possible from the very beginning of the recovery process.

## How to Communicate with a Person Who Has Aphasia

- Talk to the person with aphasia as an adult and not as a child. Avoid talking down to the person.

- During conversation, minimize or eliminate background noise (i.e., television, radio, other people) whenever possible.

- Make sure you have the person's attention before communicating.

- Praise all attempts to speak; make speaking a pleasant experience and provide stimulating conversation. Encourage and use all modes of communication (speech, writing, drawing, yes/no responses, choices, gestures, eye contact, facial expressions).

- Give them time to talk and permit a reasonable amount of time to respond.

- Accept all communication attempts (speech, gesture, writing, drawing) rather than demanding speech. Downplay errors and avoid frequent criticisms/corrections. Avoid insisting that each word be produced perfectly.

- Keep your own communication simple, but adult. Simplify sentence structure and reduce your own rate of speech. Keep your voice at a normal volume level and emphasize key words.

- Augment speech with gesture and visual aids whenever possible. Repeat a statement when necessary.

- Encourage people with aphasia to be as independent as possible. Avoid being overprotective or speaking for the person except when absolutely necessary. Ask permission to do so.

- Whenever possible continue normal home activities (i.e., dinner with family, company, going out). Do not shield people with aphasia from family or friends or ignore them in a group conversation. Rather, try to involve them in family decision-making as much as possible keeping them informed of events but not burdening them with day to day details.

These guidelines are intended to enhance communication with persons who have aphasia. However, they cannot guarantee that communication will be immediate or on a par with former skills.

## Adult Aphasia: Recent Research

### Aphasia Treatment

In general, treatment strives to improve a person's ability to communicate. The most effective treatment begins early in the recovery process and is maintained consistently over time. Major factors that influence the amount of improvement include the cause of the brain damage, the area of the brain that was damaged, the extent of the injury, and the person's general health.

Usually a speech-language pathologist works with other rehabilitation and medical professionals, such as physicians, nurses, neuropsychologists, occupational therapists, physical therapists, and social workers, as well as families, to provide a comprehensive evaluation and treatment plan for the person with aphasia.

## Aphasia Research at NIDCD

The National Institute on Deafness and Other Communication Disorders (NIDCD) is one of the Institutes of the National Institutes of Health. The NIDCD supports and conducts biomedical and behavioral research and research training on normal and disordered processes of hearing, balance, smell, taste, voice, speech, and language. Currently supported aphasia research focuses on evaluating, characterizing, and treating the disorder, as well as on improving the understanding of the relationship between the language disorder and the brain.

## New Approaches to Evaluation

Scientists are attempting to reveal the underlying problems that cause specific aphasia symptoms. The goal is to understand how injury to a particular brain structure impairs specific portions of a person's language process. The results could be useful in treating many types of aphasia, since the underlying cause can vary.

Other research is attempting to develop a model of sentence comprehension and production that can help provide a functional explanation for aphasia symptoms. These studies look at how difficulties in word representations and processes contribute to problems with sentence production and comprehension so specific symptoms can be traced back to identifiable processing deficits. This would help focus treatment on the responsible word processes or representations.

## New Approaches to Characterization

Since the same types of aphasia look different from one language to another, some scientists are attempting to distinguish between universal symptoms of the disorder and those that are language specific. Others are examining how people with aphasia maintain their knowledge of a language, but seem to have difficulty accessing that knowledge. Scientists are also comparing aspects of language that are at risk or are protected within and across language types and assessing the effect of stress on language expression in people without aphasia. These studies may help with the development of tests tailored to specific characteristics of individual languages and in clinical services to bilingual communities.

## New Therapeutic Approaches

Pharmacotherapy is a new, experimental approach to treating aphasia. Some studies are testing how drugs can be used in combination with speech therapy to improve recovery of various language functions by increasing the task-related flow of activation in the left hemisphere of the brain. These studies indicate that drugs may help improve aphasia in acute stroke and as an adjuvant to language therapy in post-acute and chronic aphasia.

Other treatment approaches use computers to improve the language abilities of people with aphasia. Studies have shown that computer-assisted therapy can help people with aphasia retrieve and produce verbs. People who have auditory problems perceiving the difference between phonemes can benefit from computers, which can be used for speech-therapeutic auditory discrimination exercises.

Researchers are also looking at how treatment of other cognitive deficits involving attention and memory can improve communication deficits.

## A Closer Look at the Brain

To understand recovery processes in the brain, some researchers are attempting to use functional MRI (magnetic resonance imaging) to uncover the anatomical organization of the human brain regions involved in comprehending words and sentences. This type of research may improve understanding of how these areas reorganize after focal brain injury. The results could have implications for both the basic understanding of brain function and the diagnosis and treatment of neurological diseases.

## About the Recent Research Series

This series is intended to inform health professionals, patients, and the public about progress in understanding the normal and disordered processes of human communication through recent advances made by NIDCD-supported scientists in each of the Institute's seven program areas: hearing, balance, smell, taste, voice, speech, and language.

## Additional Information

***National Institute on Deafness and Other Communication Disorders (NIDCD) Clearinghouse***
1 Communication Avenue
Bethesda, MD 20892-3456
Toll-Free: 800-241-1044 Toll-Free TTY: 800-241-1055
Website: www.nidcd.nih.gov
E-mail: nidcdinfo@nidcd.nih.gov

***Academy of Neurologic Communicative Disorders and Sciences***
P.O. Box 26532
Minneapolis, MN 55426
Tel: 952-920-0484; Fax: 952-920-6098
Website: www.duq.edu/ancds
E-mail: ancds@incnet.com

***American Speech-Language-Hearing Association***
10801 Rockville Pike
Rockville, MD 20852
Toll-Free: 800-638-8255
Tel: 301-897-5700
Website: www.asha.org
E-mail: actioncenter@asha.org

***Aphasia Hope Foundation***
2436 West 137th Street
Leawood, KS 66224
Toll-Free: 866-449-5804
Tel: 913-402-8306; Fax: 913-402-8315
Website: www.aphasiahope.org

***National Aphasia Association***
29 John Street, Suite 1103
New York, NY 10038
Toll-Free: 800-922-4622
Fax: 212-267-2812
Website: www.aphasia.org
E-mail: naa@aphasia.org

Chapter 33

# Activities of Daily Living and Stroke Recovery

Editor's Note: Although initially written for individuals with Parkinson's disease, this information is also helpful for people who have experienced stroke.

Activities of daily living include tasks such as bathing, grooming, dressing, preparing food, eating, and caring for the home. Walking and general mobility—getting from place to place—are also important aspects of a person's life. Individuals with declining abilities may have difficulty caring for themselves. People with Parkinson's disease often have tremors, rigidity, and slowness of movement, all of which may interfere with their ability to care for themselves.

This chapter contains suggested techniques and useful aids which can help people to remain independent and assist with activities of daily living. The adaptive devices mentioned can be purchased at a surgical supply store or through the catalogues listed in the "Resources for Independent Living" section at the end of the chapter. There are many things that can be done to increase independence and safety in self-care and mobility. For further information, consult your physician, occupational therapist, or physical therapist.

The information in this chapter is reprinted from *Be Independent*, a booklet published by The American Parkinson Disease Association, 1250 Hylan Boulevard, Suite 4, Staten Island, NY 10305. © 1999 American Parkinson Disease Association. Reprinted with permission.

## The Bedroom

The bedroom should be kept free of clutter and be large enough to allow free access to the bed, bureau, closet, and hallway doors. Scatter rugs increase the risk of falling and should be avoided. If they are used, they must be taped or tacked to the floor even if they have nonskid rubber pads beneath them. Casters should be removed from furniture, since objects that roll provide unstable handholds. Shoes and other small objects should be kept off the floor, especially at night.

Special equipment and aids can be used in the bedroom to help maintain independence and safety while increasing comfort.

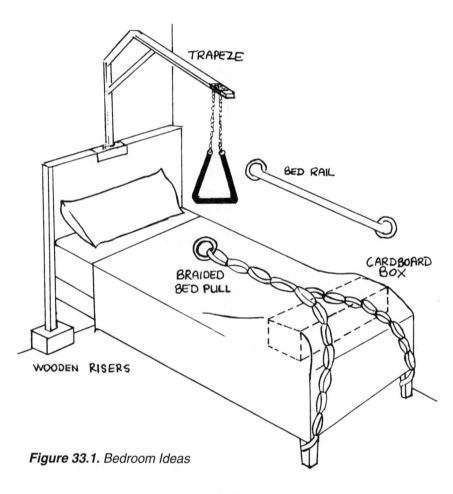

**Figure 33.1.** *Bedroom Ideas*

## *Bedroom Equipment*

1. Bed pulls can be attached to the frame at the end of the bed. They are useful to assist in rising to a seated position or turning in bed, and can be either purchased or made at home. To make: Braid three pieces of tightly woven fabric, such as sheeting, together in a length that reaches from the base of the bed to your hand when you are lying down. Sew a large wooden curtain ring to the end to serve as a grasp. Then sew a small binder clip near the ring so that the bed pull can be clamped to the bedding and remain within your reach. Bed pulls can also be attached to the sides of the bed to assist in turning.

2. A trapeze installed over the head of the bed can help individuals to change position. It may be purchased at a surgical supply store and can be mounted to most standard beds.

3. A sturdy cardboard box can be placed under the covers at the foot of the bed. This "bed cradle" keeps feet and lower legs free of the sheets while turning.

4. A urinal may be kept within reach on a bed table, or a commode may be placed at the bedside for nighttime use. The urinal or commode helps reduce walks to the bathroom.

5. Disposable incontinence garments are designed to address the problem of accidental urination and may be especially helpful at night.

6. A chair with armrests and a firm seat should be part of the bedroom furniture. Dressing can be accomplished while sitting in the chair, thus eliminating the risk of falling. Try to avoid sitting in a low chair. A firm pillow, secured to the chair, makes it easier to rise from a low surface.

7. The bed should be no lower than knee height for ease in getting in and out. If the bed is too high, a carpenter can cut two or three inches off the legs. If the bed is too low, use a thicker mattress or mattress padding.

8. A railing can be installed on a bedroom wall ten inches higher than the level of the bed, and the bed placed against the wall under the railing. The railing becomes an assist for rising from and turning in bed. Commercially made bed rails are

available and can be mounted on most beds. Satin sheets are smooth and can also facilitate turning.

9. For difficulty in sitting up in bed, place a foam wedge cushion under the mattress at the head of the bed, or place wooden risers under the legs at the head of the bed.

10. Nightlights should be installed in a wall socket near the bedroom door, in the hallway leading to the bathroom, and in the bathroom. They are indispensable in helping you avoid accidents.

11. A communication device such as a bell or intercom system may be needed to ensure safety at night, especially if you have decreased voice volume.

## The Bathroom

Safety is essential in the bathroom. It is the most dangerous room in your house. The tile floor is slippery and the surfaces of the shower or tub are extremely slick, especially when wet. The average bathroom is often small and furnished with porcelain fixtures that jut out from the walls and restrict walking space. A call for help may go unheard, especially if the water is running or the door is closed.

It is important that the bathroom be made as safe as possible. Adequate equipment and awareness of danger increases the ease and safety of bathing and grooming. Bathing is easier if you are organized and keep everything that you need arranged safely within or near the tub.

### Bathroom Safety

1. Non-skid decals or strips, attached to a tub or shower floor, or the use of a rubber mat, help to eliminate falls. Small bathroom rugs are easy to trip over, and should not be used. Use a large rug that covers most of the floor, wall-to-wall carpeting, or bare flooring. Do not wax the floor.

2. Grab bars or tub rails placed in strategic locations provide balance and support for getting in and out of the tub or shower. Never use towel racks or wall soap holders as grab bars. They are not designed for this and may break away under pressure.

3.  Tub seats or shower chairs make bathing easier and safer. A flexible shower hose or a hand-held shower massage allows for safer bathing while seated. A shower nozzle with a turn-off knob is more convenient than a free-flow nozzle.

4.  A raised toilet seat makes sitting on and rising from the toilet easier. Arm rails attached to the toilet, or a grab bar installed on the wall adjacent to the toilet, provide convenient hand holds.

5.  If you have difficulty holding objects, do not use glass tumblers. Paper or plastic cups are safer.

6.  A nightlight should always be installed in a bathroom wall socket.

7.  The hot water heater in your house should be turned down to prevent accidental scalding.

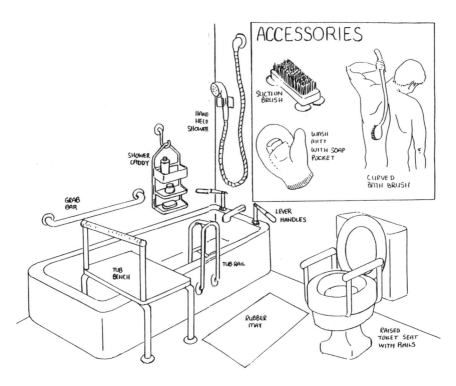

**Figure 33.2.** Bathroom Ideas

## *Grooming*

1. Soap on a rope keeps soap conveniently within reach while showering or taking a tub bath.

2. A suction nailbrush makes grooming easier and safer. It can be secured to the tub, reducing the risk of injury from falling.

3. A long-handled sponge reaches the lower legs, feet, and back. It helps eliminate bending and is necessary if you have a problem with balance. A curved bath sponge can be useful for washing your back.

4. Wash mitts are terry cloth gloves that eliminate the need for holding onto a washcloth.

5. An electric razor should be used for safety, particularly if you have hand tremor. A variety of electric razor holders, which make grasp easier, are commercially available.

6. Round-headed faucets require a twisting motion to operate. This is difficult for people with impaired strength or coordination. They can be replaced with a lever-type handle or a single arm control faucet. The round-headed faucet can be improved by adding tap-turner adaptations.

7. Adding a commercial built-up handle, a bicycle handle, or a wrist cuff makes your tooth brush, hairbrush, or comb handles larger and easier to grip. Extension handles may be helpful if your shoulder or arm movement is limited.

## *Dressing*

The fine hand coordination and strength needed for dressing is sometimes impaired. Pain and stiffness in the limbs can also complicate putting on and taking off clothing, particularly underwear, socks, and slacks. There are many simple and useful aids that can help people remain independent.

Try to choose clothing that is easy to manage. Loose fitting, stretchy clothes with simple fastenings are easier to put on and take off. For some people, pullover tops may be more convenient. They eliminate the need for buttoning. Front-closing garments are easier to manage than zipper and button-back garments.

Knee-length stockings can be worn instead of panty hose only if they have wide elasticized tops to prevent constriction of circulation.

**Never** wear stockings rolled down and secured with a rubber band or garter. This impairs circulation.

Clothing should be placed, in order of wear, on a chair near the individual. Take time and, if possible, do not allow anyone to rush the care recipient. Try to maintain their independence.

### *Dressing Devices*

1. Velcro closures are excellent substitutes for buttons and zippers. Sew tabs of velcro over the buttonhole and on the underside of the button. Press the velcro strips together to fasten your shirt.

2. A button hook or button aid slips through the buttonhole and pulls the button back through it. The handles of these tools are more easily grasped than a small button when fine hand coordination is impaired.

3. Large, easily grasped zipper pulls or rings make opening and closing trouser flys, jackets, and coats less difficult.

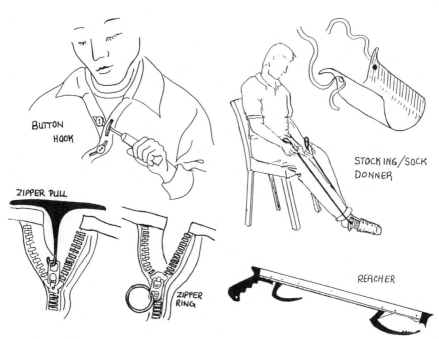

BUTTON HOOK

ZIPPER PULL

ZIPPER RING

STOCKING/SOCK DONNER

REACHER

**Figure 33.3.** Dressing Ideas

331

4.  Small cuff buttons can be difficult to manipulate. Use elastic thread to sew buttons onto cuffs. Keep them buttoned all the time and slide your hand through. You can also join the cuff with a velcro closure.

5.  A dressing stick or reacher is useful for pulling pants and undergarments up over your legs. It allows you to remain seated while dressing and reduces the risk of falling. Reachers are also useful for picking up objects that have dropped to the floor.

6.  Elastic shoelaces need to be tied only once, thus converting laced shoes to slip-on shoes. Standard tie shoes can be closed with Velcro strips. A shoemaker can stitch them on.

7.  A front-closing bra is easier to put on and take off. You can adapt a back-closing bra by sewing up the rear closure, cutting the front open, and attaching velcro strips.

8.  A long-handled shoehorn and a sock donner reduce bending and straining when putting on socks and shoes.

## The Kitchen

Decreased strength, range of motion, and coordination problems can limit your ability to perform kitchen activities such as: meal preparation, food storage, eating, cleaning, and clearing up after meals. Many ingenious aids have been devised to improve safety and efficiency in the kitchen.

The kitchen should be kept well organized with dishes, utensils, and foods stored near to where they are used and within easy reach. Coffee and tea for instance, should be stored as close as possible to the teakettle. Store utensils you rarely use behind those used everyday. If there is wall space, install a pegboard at an accessible height and hang utensils there.

Pace yourself during kitchen activities and plan before you start to avoid unnecessary energy-consuming steps. If you have impaired balance, slowness of movement, or decreased hand coordination, meal preparation is safer and easier if done while seated.

### Kitchen Equipment

1.  A Lazy Susan, placed in the center of the kitchen table or on a counter, holds numerous frequently used items and eliminates

the need to gather each one before meals. The Lazy Susan can also be used as a shelf organizer to reduce the need to reach for objects at the back of the shelf.

2. Reachers can be used in the kitchen to pick up light objects that fall to the floor. Heavy objects should be placed in counter-height cabinets.

3. A rubber pad or wet dishcloth can be placed under bowls and pans to stabilize them while you are preparing food.

4. Electric can openers are useful and convenient, especially if fine hand coordination is impaired.

5. A jar opener eases the problem of opening jars.

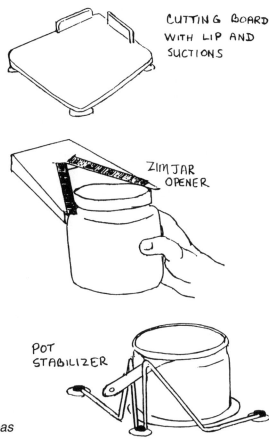

CUTTING BOARD WITH LIP AND SUCTIONS

ZIM JAR OPENER

POT STABILIZER

***Figure 33.4.*** *Kitchen Ideas*

6. A cutting board with a raised edge prevents diced vegetables and small pieces of meat from scattering off the board. A nail hammered into the board skewers food while dicing or cutting. The nail also helps when buttering bread or toast. Suction cups can be attached to the bottom of your cutting board to prevent it from sliding.

7. A microwave, used instead of a stove, reduces the risk of injury from burns.

8. A long-handled dustpan enables you to collect floor sweepings without bending to the floor. A sponge mop should be kept accessible as spills should be wiped up immediately to reduce the chance of falling.

9. Your strength and hand function should affect your choice of pots and pans. If you have limited strength, use aluminum pots and pans and lightweight dishes. Make sure that the shape and size of the handles are suited to your grasp strength. A long pot handle allows for two-handed lifting.

10. A pot stabilizer keeps the handle steady when you stir.

11. Kitchen scissors can help you to open plastic packages and boxes that are difficult to rip.

## *Mealtime*

There are many attractive and durable commercially available mealtime aids. They have been designed to enable people to continue to eat with as much independence as possible.

If a special or adapted piece of silverware is used at home, take it along when dining in a restaurant. If a person has difficulty cutting food, ask the waiter to have the food cut in the kitchen before it is presented. This prevents someone from having to reach across the table to assist. Take time while eating and try not to rush.

### *Mealtime Equipment*

1. Attachable plate guards provide a rim on one side of the plate. Food, especially small vegetables, can be pushed against the guard, where they fall onto the fork. Plate guards also prevent spills. Scoop dishes contoured with raised edges serve the same purpose.

2. Silverware with built up plastic handles is more easily grasped. Tubular foam padding can be attached to the utensil to widen the grip.

   Soup spoons can be used instead of forks when eating small pieces of food. Sporks are a combination spoon and fork. This one utensil can spear as well as hold food. A rocking knife may be used instead of a straight knife if you have problems with coordination. Weighted utensils may help to decrease hand tremors, thus allowing the utensil to reach your mouth more easily.

3. If you have a tremor, flexible plastic straws help you to drink.

4. A mug with a large handle for easy grasp should be used if your tremor is severe. An insulated mug with a lid reduces the risk of burns from spills when drinking hot liquids.

5. A rubber pad or a moist paper towel can be placed under plates, cups, and serving dishes to keep them from sliding.

## *Walking*

The ability to get from one place to another inside or outside the home is very important. There are a number of assistive devices that can help a person with decreased balance, coordination, or mobility to walk safely.

Canes can be used to compensate for minor balance problems. They come in a variety of shapes and sizes and increase an individual's base of support.

The standard J-Handle cane offers some stability as well as a sense of security. An ortho-cane or a quad cane may also be used. Each offers an increasing degree of support and balance.

If more assistance than a cane is needed, a walker can be prescribed. A walker that folds is good if you need to store or transport it in limited space—for example, in a car. Wheels can be added if you have difficulty coordinating the advancement of the walker or are unable to lift it off the floor. A braking mechanism which locks with downward pressure can be attached to the front or back wheels. It is important to note, however, that although the rolling walker is easier to advance, it can be unsafe on rugs and other uneven surfaces.

If you are unable to walk, or can walk only short distances in your home, a wheelchair provides more functional mobility.

In order to best suit your individual needs, a physical therapist should be consulted so that the appropriate ambulatory device or wheelchair is provided.

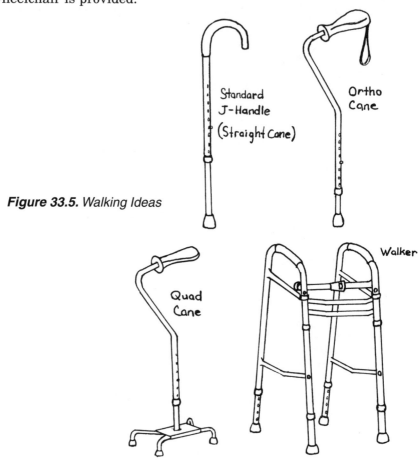

Standard
J-Handle
(Straight Cane)

Ortho
Cane

Quad
Cane

Walker

**Figure 33.5.** *Walking Ideas*

## Negotiating Stairs

Stairs often become a major barrier to a person who has limited strength, balance, and mobility. The following guidelines make stair climbing easier.

If there is a handrail available, use it as long as it is well secured. Hold onto the handrail with one hand and an assistive device, if needed, in the other hand. Both hands can also be placed on the handrail to sidestep up and down the stairs one at a time.

If you are unable to go up or down the stairs safely in a step-over-step manner, negotiate the stairs one step at a time. Place one foot on the step; place the second foot on that same step before you move on to the next.

If someone is assisting you, that person should stay by your side. The assisting person should stagger their feet so that their lead foot is one step down from yours. This maintains good balance.

If you cannot safely climb stairs, you can be carried up and down in a wheelchair. A lift may be installed, but it is expensive.

Specific instructions for walking up and down the stairs or being assisted in a wheelchair can best be given by a physical therapist.

## Getting In or Out of a Car

There are ways to make getting in or out of a car easier. First, the car must be parked far enough away from the curb so that you can step onto the level ground before you go into or get out of the car. To get into a car turn so that you back in for the last steps. Your buttocks should lead. Then sit down and swing your legs in.

To exit the car, swing both legs out together and stand up. Sit in the front or back seat, whichever gives you more room. Use pillows to make it easier to get up from a low car. Specific techniques should be taught by and practiced with a physical therapist or occupational therapist.

## Miscellaneous Tips

If you have a problem with shuffling, small steps, and stopping while walking, arrange the furniture so as to avoid congested areas. Keep hallways free of obstacles. Plan a route through the house so that there is always a safe handhold available in case you lose your balance.

Railings can be installed on the walls to provide support. Your family should consult with you before they rearrange the furniture so that you do not lose familiarity with your surroundings.

Avoid low couches and chairs as it is often extremely difficult to rise from them without help. A straight back chair with armrests and a firm seat is easier to get up from. A firm cushion can be used to acquire the height that is suitable for you. Pneumatic lifter seats can assist someone who has severe difficulty rising from a chair.

Handrails should be installed on all staircases, especially those outside.

Use a carpet sweeper instead of a vacuum. It is lighter and easier to manipulate.

The "Fone Holder" is a long, flexible shaft that attaches to most tables and can be positioned to hold the telephone receiver so a person can use the handset without having to move or even touch it. Another device adapts huge push buttons to the small touch-tone buttons of a standard phone to make dialing easier.

Handwriting can be a serious problem for persons with Parkinson's disease. Various pens, pencils, and writing devices are available to stabilize your grip. A weighted pen may help reduce tremors and improve writing.

A door knob turner fits over the door handle and converts the round knob into a lever. This makes it easier to open.

## A Word to the Family

In order to preserve independence in activities of daily living, people should do all that they can for themselves. Because of tremor, rigidity, and slowness of movement, each activity may take more time than it used to.

It is tempting to do or to complete tasks for people. It saves time and, perhaps, frustration. However, this may lead to dependence, because it decreases people's motivation to help themselves.

The physical ability of persons with Parkinson's disease varies throughout the day in response to anti-Parkinson's medication. Tremor, rigidity, and slowness of movement may be more pronounced in the morning than in the afternoon. People's ability to dress or to eat may be impaired at one time and not another.

To decrease misunderstanding and further frustration, families should be aware that their relatives are not malingering but that it is the variability of the disease that causes fluctuation in independence. People may require help some of the time, but not all of the time.

It is vitally important for the families of people with Parkinson's disease to help them remain as independent as possible.

## Resources for Independent Living

*Adaptability*
75 Mill Street
Colchester, CT 06415
Toll-Free: 800-937-3482
Website: www.adaptability.com

*After Therapy Catalog*
North Coast Medical
18305 Sutter Blvd.
Morgan Hill, CA 95037-2845
Toll-Free: 800-821-9319
Tel: 408-776-5000

338

*Verizon Center for Customers with Disabilities*
280 Locke Drive, 4th Floor
Marlboro, MA 01752
Toll-Free: 800-974-6006
Fax: 508-624-7645
Website: www22.verizon.com

*Bruce Medical Supply*
411 Waverly Oaks Rd., Suite 154
P.O. Box 9166
Waltham, MA 02452
Toll-Free: 800-225-8446
Fax: 781-894-9519
Website: www.brucemedical.com
E-mail: sales@brucemedical.com

*Comfort House*
189 Frelinghuysen Avenue
Newark, NJ 07114-1595
Toll-Free: 800-359-7701
Tel: 973-242-8080
Fax: 973-242-0131
Website: www.comforthouse.com
E-mail:
customerservice@comforthouse.com

*Dr. Leonard's Health Care Catalog*
P.O. Box 7821
Edison, NJ 08818
Toll-Free: 800-785-0880
Fax: 732-572-2118
Website: www.drleonards.com
E-mail:
custserv@drleonards.com

*Dressing Tips and Clothing Res. for Making Life Easier*
The Best 25 Catalogues Resources for Making Life Easier
9042 Aspen Grove Lane
Madison, WI 53717
Tel: 608-824-0402
Fax: 608-824-0403
Website:
www.meetinglifechallenges.com
E-mail:
help@meetinglifechallenges.com

*Metro Medical Equipment*
12985 Wayne Road
Livonia, MI 48150
Toll-Free: 800-877-7285
Fax: 734-522-9380

*Durable Medical Equipment (over 3500) Plate Guards, Aids for Daily Living*
Yes I Can
35-325 Date Palm Drive
Suite 131
Cathedral City, CA 92234
Toll-Free: 888-366-4226
Tel: 760-321-1717
Fax: 760-321-7780
Website: http://yesican.com
E-mail: info@yesican.com

*Sammons Preston and Enrichments*
4 Sammons Court
Bolingbrook, IL 60440
Toll-Free: 800-323-5547
Fax: 800-547-4333
Website:
www.sammonspreston.com
E-mail:
ap@sammonspreston.com

## Fashion Ease
1541 60ᵗʰ Street
Brooklyn, NY 11219
Toll-Free: 800-221-8929
Tel: 718-871-8188 (NY State)
Fax: 718-436-2067
Website: www.fashionease.com
E-mail: info@fashionease.com

## Independent Living Aids Inc.
200 Robbins Lane
Jericho, NY 11753
Toll-Free: 800-537-2118
Tel: 516-937-1848
Fax: 516-937-3906
Website:
www.independentliving.com
E-mail:
can-do@independentliving.com

## J C Penny's Easy Dressing Catalog
P.O. Box 2021
Milwaukee, WI 53201
Toll-Free: 800-222-6161
Website: www.jcpenney.com

## Patients Transfer Systems
Beatrice M. Brantman, Inc.
207 E. Westminster
Lake Forest, IL 60045
Toll-Free: 800-232-7987
Fax: 847-615-8894
E-mail: beasyets@aol.com

## Personal Pager
The Greatest of Ease Company
2443 Fillmore Street, #345
San Francisco, CA 94115
Tel: 415-441-6649
Fax: 415-441-4319
Website: http://
personalpagers.tripod.com/go
E-mail: greatestofease@aol.com

## Sears Health Care Catalog
Sears Roebuck and Company
P.O. Box 804203
Chicago, IL 60680-4203
Toll-Free: 800-326-1750

## The Speedo Aquatic Exercise System
7911 Haskell Avenue
Van Nuys, CA 91409
Toll-Free: 800-547-8770
Website: www.speedo.com

## The Do Able Renewable Home
Consumer Affairs Program Dept.
American Association of Retired Persons (AARP)
P.O. Box 2240
Long Beach, CA 90801
Toll-Free: 800-424-3410

*Voice Amplifiers*

*Rand Voice Amplifier*
Park Surgical Company, Inc.
5001 New Utrecht Avenue
Brooklyn, NY 11219
Toll-Free: 800-633-7878
Tel: 718-436-9200
Fax: 718-854-2431
Website: www.parksurgical.com

*Luminaud Inc.*
8688 Tyler Blvd.
Mentor, OH 44060-4348
Toll-Free: 800-255-3408
Fax: 440-255-2250
Website: www.luminaud.com
E-mail: info@luminaud.com

*Anchor Audio, Inc.*
3415 Lomita Blvd.
Torrance, CA 90505
Toll-Free: 800-262-4671
Tel: 310-784-2300
Fax: 310-784-0066
Website: www.anchoraudio.com
E-mail: sales@anchoraudio.com

*Walkers*

*Noble Motion Inc.*
P.O. Box 5366
6741 Reynolds Street
Pittsburgh, PA 15206
Toll-Free: 800-234-9255
Fax: 412-363-7189
Website:
www.wheels4walking.com
E-mail: info@noblemotion.com

Chapter 34

# *Understanding Paralysis and Spasticity after Stroke*

## *Mobility Issues Facing Stroke Survivors and Their Families*

Moving around safely and easily is not something you may think about, unless you have had a stroke. Each year more than 750,000 Americans suffer strokes. In some instances paralysis and/or balance problems may result. One out of every three Americans age 65 and older falls. Ten percent of those individuals fracture a bone, dislocate a joint, or experience other serious injuries due to their balance and/ or paralysis problems. This chapter provides helpful information about home adaptations and lifestyle changes that may increase your safety and ability to move more easily.

## *Understanding Paralysis and Spasticity*

Paralysis is the inability of a muscle or group of muscles to move voluntarily. When messages from the brain to the muscles don't work properly due to a stroke, a limb becomes paralyzed or develops a condition called spasticity.

Spasticity is tight, stiff muscles that make movement, especially of the arms or legs, difficult or uncontrollable. Characteristics of the condition can include any of the following: a tight fist, bent elbow, arm pressed against the chest, stiff knee and/or pointed foot that can in-

"Spasticity after Stroke," © 2002 National Stroke Association, reprinted with permission.

terfere with walking. These long periods of forceful contractions in major muscle groups can cause painful muscle spasms. The spasms produce a pain similar to athletic cramping.

## What Are the Symptoms or Effects of Spasticity?

* Stiffness in the arms, fingers, or legs

* Painful muscle spasms

* A series of involuntary rhythmic contractions and relaxation in a muscle or group of muscles that lead to uncontrollable movement or jerking, called clonus

* Increased muscle tone

* Abnormal posture

* Hyperexcitable reflexes

## Treatment Options

Treatment for spasticity is often a combination of many therapies and medications. This approach is used to achieve the best function possible. It's important to remember that all therapies and drugs may have potential side effects that should be weighed against their benefits. Patients need to discuss appropriate options with their healthcare provider.

### Stretching and Temporary Strategies

Spasticity treatment often includes full range-of-motion exercises at least three times a day; gentle stretching of tighter muscles; frequent repositioning of body parts, and splinting or casting.

### Oral Medications

Oral medications are available to treat the general effects of spasticity by acting on multiple muscle groups in the body. Side effects may range from drowsiness and confusion to depression and liver abnormalities, among other things.

### Injections

Injections using Botulinum Toxin Type A (Botox®) or Phenol relax stiff muscles by blocking the chemicals that make them tight. While oral medications affect multiple muscle groups in the body, these injections target only specific limbs or muscle groups affected by spasticity. A single injection can relax affected muscles for three to six months and improve some activities of daily living. Since the medication is targeted to affected muscles, side effects are minimized. Side effects may include mild soreness at injection site and temporary fatigue.

*Intrathecal Medication*

ITB (Intrathecal Baclofen) Therapy delivers Lioresal Intrathecal, a liquid form of the drug Baclofen, directly into the spinal fluid. A programmable pump is surgically placed just below the skin near the abdomen where it continuously delivers small doses of medication. Since the drug is delivered to affected areas and does not circulate throughout the body, side effects are minimized. Possible side effects include drowsiness, nausea, and headache.

*Surgery*

Neurosurgery and orthopedic surgery are generally used as last resorts for spasticity treatment. Surgery may help block pain and restore movement to limited degrees.

Healthcare providers should try to customize spasticity treatment, taking into consideration the extent of the problems, individual symptoms, and personal lifestyle goals.

## Safety at Home

Stroke survivors and caregivers may be apprehensive about being on their own at home. With some simple modifications and education, fears can be overcome and recovery enhanced.

*Assistive Devices*

Modifying home environments with assistive devices, such as grab bars and ramps, may provide additional safety and easier movement around the home.

Other useful devices:

• Raised toilet seat
• Tub bench
• Hand-held shower head

- Plastic adhesive strips on the bottom of the tub
- Long handled brushes, washing mitts with pockets for soap
- Electric toothbrushes and razors

Many areas of the home can be made safer if throw rugs and furniture are removed or securely fastened to the floor.

### Movement Aids

Braces, canes, walkers, and wheelchairs may also help stroke survivors gain strength and move about more freely. It is important to use the braces or other devices exactly as a therapist recommends.

Foot drop is a common problem during stroke recovery. The condition is caused by a person's foot or ankle dropping down when lifting a leg to take a step. It may cause a person to trip and fall if the foot and ankle are not supported by a brace at all times.

The most common brace for this long-term problem is an ankle-foot orthosis (AFO). The AFO starts below the knee and encompasses and controls the ankle and foot. Certain types of these braces or adjustments to these braces can also influence knee movement. Other variations and adjustments can be made to braces to fit individual needs.

A physical therapist or orthotist can recommend the appropriate device. Training in safety procedure and proper use of orthotics, including proper fit and maintenance, is essential.

### Lifestyle Can Affect Safe Movement

Lifestyle modifications in relation to diet and exercise should be individualized to meet a person's specific environment and needs. Weak leg muscles, poor vision, dizziness, and medications that may compromise balance may put people at risk for falls. Your health care provider should be aware of the symptoms and help provide guidance regarding dosage and side effects.

You can also prevent falls by:

- Remaining active

- Strengthening leg muscles and balance through weight training and/or Tai chi classes

- Wearing flat, wide-toed shoes

- Eating calcium-rich foods and taking calcium supplements, if necessary, to increase bone strength

- Following your therapists' recommendations regarding limitations and walking needs

- Not relying on furniture for support while walking. Use the assistive device prescribed by your therapist

- Recognizing that certain medications may make you drowsy, and taking precautions

- Limiting walking when distracted

- Never walking without prescribed assistive aids such as braces

Be on the safe side and don't take chances. Listen to the advice of healthcare professionals and experienced caregivers. Regaining independence requires patience.

Chapter 35

# Nutrition for Stroke Victims

Stroke is the most common cause of neurological disabilities in western countries. Although vascular injury to the brain can occur as part of a number of relatively rare diseases, most cerebrovascular illnesses are related to arteriosclerosis, hypertension, or a combination of both.

There are several types of strokes:

- Cerebral Insufficiency—This stroke occurs because of a temporary disturbances of blood flow to blood vessel in the brain.

- Cerebral Infarction—This stroke occurs due to a blood clot in a blood vessel in the brain.

- Cerebral Hemorrhage—This stroke occurs due to a broken or leaking blood vessel in the brain.

- Cerebral arteriovenous malformation—This stroke may cause mass lesions, infarctions, or hemorrhages.

## General Recommendations

In order to help prevent strokes, you should treat the conditions that lead to strokes (i.e., high blood pressure and arteriosclerosis).

"Nutrition Review: Stroke, Cerebrovascular Accident, CVA, Brain Attack," by Mary Schmidt, RD, LD, © 2001 Agenet, Inc. Reprinted with the permission of Agenet Inc., providing a comprehensive offering of eldercare products, services, and information through its *Solutions for Better Aging* program, and at www.caregivers.com.

Strokes can vary in severity; they can result in either minor or major disabilities. People who suffer severe strokes may need to have the texture of their food modified. Food may need to be chopped, ground, or pureed. Liquids may need to be thickened. Consult with a speech therapist for advice on how to prevent the individual from experiencing swallowing or choking problems.

Adaptive equipment such as swivel spoons, rocking knives, plate guards, special cups, and glasses with straws can be of great help. An occupational therapist can assist in determining the most appropriate adaptive equipment; selection will depend upon the severity of the disease.

## Nutritional Considerations

### Fluid

Depending upon the type of stroke and other conditions, a stroke victim may need to either increase or decrease their fluid intake. Stroke victims who do not have to restrict their fluids can use the following formula to determine how much fluid to consume daily:

- Body weight in pounds
  divided by 17 =
  number of cups (8oz) of fluid per day.

The aforementioned formula does not apply to every stroke victim, however. For people judged by their physician to be dehydrated, a different formula is appropriate:

- Body weight in pounds
  divided by 13 =
  number of cups (8oz) of fluid per day.

If a stroke resulted in some paralysis, it may be difficult for a stroke victim to physically consume beverages. In some cases, mental, cognitive, or communicative problems may also interfere with the person's ability to recognize thirst or ask for beverages. Therefore, it is important that caregivers regularly offer water, juice, and other non-caffeinated beverages and encourage consumption. It may be necessary to provide straws, special water bottles, or adaptive drinking glasses to ensure adequate hydration. Dehydration can lead to urinary tract infections, confusion, skin ulcers, and constipation.

## *Fat*

Because strokes are often a result of atherosclerosis, nutrition therapy should be geared toward reducing foods that might contribute to atherosclerosis. Many people with high levels of triglycerides and cholesterol have an increased risk of developing atherosclerosis. Nutrition therapy emphasizes reducing and changing the type of fat in the diet.

**Table 35.1.** Fat in the Diet

| | |
|---|---|
| Total Fat | should comprise 30% or less of total daily calories |
| Cholesterol | should not exceed 300 mg per day. |
| Saturated Fat | should not exceed 7-8% of calories (bad fat) |
| Polyunsaturated Fat | should comprise up to 10% of calories (okay fat) |
| Monounsaturated Fat | should comprise up to 15% of calories (good fat) |

## *Protein*

Protein keeps the immune system functioning, increases resistance to infection, prevents skin breakdown, and promotes healing; therefore, it is important to consume protein. Protein can be found in meat, eggs, poultry, fish, cheese, nuts, nut butters, soybeans, legumes, and milk. A minimum of 6 ounces of meat or meat equivalent should be consumed each day. If intake is limited due to poor appetite, the meals can be supplemented with a high protein nutritional beverage such as an instant breakfast, Ensure, Boost, or Resource. If protein needs to be restricted due to other conditions, please consult your physician.

## *Sodium*

In many cases, people who have had a stroke have problems with edema (water retention) or related conditions. Therefore, your physician should be consulted about sodium restriction levels. As a general rule, stroke victims should limit their sodium intake to 3 to 4 grams of sodium per day.

## *Vitamins and Minerals*

The best way to obtain sufficient vitamins and minerals is to eat at least five servings of fruits and vegetables per day. Because a stroke often prevents regular exercise, constipation can be a problem.

Consuming five servings of fruits and vegetables a day can help to prevent it. Keep in mind that there are also some very powerful anti-oxidants that can be found in fruits and vegetables that cannot be duplicated in supplements.

If your intake does not include a variety of fruits and vegetables, a multivitamin or mineral supplement may be necessary. Be sure to choose a supplement that is balanced and contains 100% of the recommended daily value. Taking excessive amounts of vitamins or minerals can be toxic or result in a deficiency of other vitamins and minerals. Avoid vitamin supplements that contain vitamin K. If

**Table 35.2.** Specific Nutritional Recommendations

| | |
|---|---|
| Eggs | Eat only 3 egg yolks per week. Limit your intake of foods made with eggs, (custards, eggnog, etc) unless they are made with cholesterol free eggs. Cholesterol free eggs (like EggBeaters) may be used in place of regular eggs. |
| Meat, poultry, and fish | Limit meat, poultry, and fish to 6 oz per day. Cut visible fat off, and bake, broil, or roast; avoid breading and frying. Remove skin from poultry. Avoid lunchmeats such as bologna, salami, sausage, and frankfurters. Use peanut butter made from 100% peanuts. Avoid foods that contain hydrogenated fat. |
| Milk/Milk Products | Consume 2 to 3 servings of low fat dairy products per day. Choose dairy products made from skim, 1%, or 2% milk, including low fat milk, yogurt, and cheese. |
| Salt | Limit the amount of salt added to food. Read labels and limit foods containing 300 mg of sodium or more per serving. Avoid foods in brines, as well as foods that are salt-cured or smoked. Avoid seasonings labeled "salt," such as celery salt and seasoning salt. Celery powder, garlic powder, and other seasonings that do not contain salt may be used. Some seasonings, such as lemon pepper, may be deceptive, because they contain significantly more salt than their name would imply. Salt substitutes may be used if approved by your physician. Many salt substitutes contain potassium, so if potassium in the stroke victim is restricted because of renal disease, salt substitutes may need to be avoided. |

coumadin (anticoagulant) is taken, read the section on food/drug interactions.

## Fiber

Stroke victims often experience a decline in exercise due to paralysis. Such a decline can lead to constipation. Fiber is extremely important to a stroke victim because it helps to prevent constipation and reduce cholesterol in the blood. Approximately 25 to 35 grams of fiber should be consumed each day. Fiber should be increased gradually. It

**Table 35.2.** Specific Nutritional Recommendations, continued

| | |
|---|---|
| Breads/ Cereals | Eat 6 or more servings of breads and cereals per day. Try to include whole grain bread and cereals with bran to increase fiber in the diet. Avoid highly processed foods since much of the fiber, vitamins, and minerals in these foods have been removed or destroyed. Avoid foods that are made with hydrogenated fat. Limit breads that are high in total fat, such as croissants, biscuits, and pastries. |
| Fruits/ Vegetables | Eat at least 5 servings of fruits and vegetables per day. Dark green or orange fruits and vegetables (greens, spinach, squash, cantaloupe, carrots, etc.) contain vitamin A and beta-carotene. The latter is a powerful antioxidant. Vitamin C, which is found in citrus fruits, juices, strawberries, and broccoli, is another excellent antioxidant. Fruits and vegetables also contribute a significant amount of fiber to the diet. However, when taking Coumadin, be sure to keep vitamin K foods to a minimum. (See food/drug interaction section). |
| Fats/Oils | Consume less than 6 to 8 tablespoons per day. Monounsaturated fats appear to have the best effect on blood cholesterol. Monounsaturated fats include olive oil, peanut oil, canola oil, and grapeseed oil. Limit the amount of saturated fats such as coconut oil, palm kernel oil, butter, lard, and shortening. Avoid margarine and fats that contain hydrogenated fat or trans-fatty acids. Always read labels for ingredients. |

is extremely important to include plenty of fluids in the diet when fiber is increased.

### Food/Drug Interactions

Many people who have had a stroke take an anticoagulant called Coumadin. Coumadin helps to prevent blood clots from forming. People who take Coumadin will have their blood tested every couple of weeks to be sure it is at the proper anticoagulant level. Coumadin may be adjusted according to results of the test. It is important not to change the diet drastically, especially when it comes to foods that affect blood clotting.

- Vitamin K, which is found in deep green leafy vegetables, decreases the anticoagulant effects of coumadin. Try to remain consistent with your consumption of green leafy vegetables; if more vitamin K foods are eaten, the anticoagulant effect of Coumadin will be reduced.

- Herbs that decrease the anticoagulant affect of Coumadin include ginseng and alfalfa. Herbs that increase the anticoagulant effects are bromelain, cinchona, cayenne, feverfew, garlic, danshen, ginkgo biloba, quinine, and ginger.

- Vitamin E will increase the anticoagulant effects of Coumadin.

- Alcohol increases or decreases the anticoagulant effects if consumption is suddenly increased or decreased. Increased amounts will intensify the anticoagulant effect, and decreased amounts will weaken the anticoagulant effect.

## Additional Information

### AgeNet, Inc.
17 Applegate Ct., Suite 200
Madison, WI 53713
Toll-Free: 888-405-4242
Fax: 608-256-3944
Website: http://agenet.com
E-mail: support@betteraging.com

Chapter 36

# Life at Home for Stroke Survivors and Family

## How Stroke Affects People

### Effects on the Body, Mind, and Feelings

Each stroke is different depending on the part of the brain injured, how bad the injury is, and the person's general health. Some of the effects of stroke are:

**Weakness (hemiparesis: hem-ee-par-EE-sis) or paralysis (hemiplegia: hem-ee-PLEE-ja) on one side of the body.** This may affect the whole side or just the arm or the leg. The weakness or paralysis is on the side of the body opposite the side of the brain injured by the stroke. For example, if the stroke injured the left side of the brain, the weakness or paralysis will be on the right side of the body.

This chapter includes an excerpt from "Recovering after a Stroke: A Patient and Family Guide," AHCPR publication No. 95-0664, May 1995, Agency for Healthcare Research and Quality, reviewed October 2002 by Dr. David A. Cooke, MD, Diplomate, American Board of Internal Medicine; and "Life at Home: Survivors and Family," © 2002 National Stroke Association, reprinted with permission. Also, reprinted with permission of the University of Maryland Medical System are three News Releases from the *University of Maryland Medical News*: "University of Maryland Study Finds Certain Coping Strategies Impact Recovery from Stroke," February 7, 2002; "Personality Influences Psychological Adjustment," February 14, 2001; and "Job Demands Sway Speed of Return to Work after Stroke," February 15, 2001.

**Problems with balance or coordination.** These can make it hard for the person to sit, stand, or walk, even if muscles are strong enough.

**Problems using language (aphasia and dysarthria).** A person with aphasia (a-FAY-zha) may have trouble understanding speech or writing. Or, the person may understand but may not be able to think of the words to speak or write. A person with dysarthria (dis-AR-three-a) knows the right words but has trouble saying them clearly.

**Being unaware of or ignoring things on one side of the body (bodily neglect or inattention).** Often, the person will not turn to look toward the weaker side or even eat food from the half of the plate on that side.

**Pain, numbness, or odd sensations.** These can make it hard for the person to relax and feel comfortable.

**Problems with memory, thinking, attention, or learning (cognitive problems).** A person may have trouble with many mental activities or just a few. For example, the person may have trouble following directions, may get confused if something in a room is moved, or may not be able to keep track of the date or time.

**Being unaware of the effects of the stroke.** The person may show poor judgment by trying to do things that are unsafe as a result of the stroke.

**Trouble swallowing (dysphagia: dis-FAY-ja).** This can make it hard for the person to get enough food. Also, care must sometimes be taken to prevent the person from breathing in food (aspiration: as-per-AY-shun) while trying to swallow it.

**Problems with bowel or bladder control.** These problems can be helped with the use of portable urinals, bedpans, and other toileting devices.

**Getting tired very quickly.** Becoming tired very quickly may limit the person's participation and performance in a rehabilitation program.

**Sudden bursts of emotion, such as laughing, crying, or anger.** These emotions may indicate that the person needs help, understanding, and support in adjusting to the effects of the stroke.

**Depression.** This is common in people who have had strokes. It can begin soon after the stroke or many weeks later, and family members often notice it first.

## *Depression after Stroke*

It is normal for a stroke survivor to feel sad over the problems caused by stroke. However, some people experience a major depressive disorder, which should be diagnosed and treated as soon as possible. A person with a major depressive disorder has a number of symptoms nearly every day, all day, for at least 2 weeks. These always include at least one of the following:

• Feeling sad, blue, or down in the dumps.

• Loss of interest in things that the person used to enjoy.

A person may also have other physical or psychological symptoms, including:

• Feeling slowed down or restless and unable to sit still.

• Feeling worthless or guilty.

• Increase or decrease in appetite or weight.

• Problems concentrating, thinking, remembering, or making decisions.

• Trouble sleeping or sleeping too much.

• Loss of energy or feeling tired all of the time.

• Headaches.

• Other aches and pains.

• Digestive problems.

• Sexual problems.

• Feeling pessimistic or hopeless.

• Being anxious or worried.

• Thoughts of death or suicide.

If a stroke survivor has symptoms of depression, especially thoughts of death or suicide, professional help is needed right away. Once the depression is properly treated, these thoughts will go away.

357

Depression can be treated with medication, psychotherapy, or both. If it is not treated, it can cause needless suffering and also makes it harder to recover from the stroke.

### Disabilities after Stroke

A disability is difficulty doing something that is a normal part of daily life. People who have had a stroke may have trouble with many activities that were easy before, such as walking, talking, and taking care of activities of daily living (ADLs). These include basic tasks such as bathing, dressing, eating, and using the toilet, as well as more complex tasks called instrumental activities of daily living (IADLs), such as housekeeping, using the telephone, driving, and writing checks.

Some disabilities are obvious right after the stroke. Others may not be noticed until the person is back home and is trying to do something for the first time since the stroke.

## Life at Home: Survivors and Family

After a stroke, both the stroke survivor and the family often are apprehensive about being on their own at home. Among the common concerns are fear:

• that a stroke might happen again

• that the stroke survivor may be unable to accept the disabilities

• that the survivor might be placed in a nursing home

• that the caregiver may not be prepared to face the responsibility of caring for the stroke survivor

• that friends and family will abandon them

### Behavior

The confused cautious stroke survivor needs an ordered environment. The stroke survivor with poor judgment must be guided when making important decisions. The apathetic stroke survivor, on the other hand, should not live in a world so quiet and simple that there is little to react to. The caregiver needs to be aware of the reasons for the stroke survivor's behavior, without overlooking the fact that he or she may also be depressed.

### Depression

Depression is nearly universal among people who have had a stroke. It can be overwhelming, affecting the spirit and confidence of everyone involved. A depressed person may refuse or neglect to take medications, may not be motivated to perform exercises which will improve mobility or may be irritable with others. The stroke survivor's depression may dampen the family's enthusiasm for helping with recovery or drive away others who want to help. This deprives the stroke survivor of the social contacts which could help dispel depression, and creates a vicious cycle.

It is possible that as time goes by and a stroke survivor's deficits improve, the depression may lift by itself. Family can help by trying to stimulate interest in other people, encouraging leisure activities, and providing opportunities to participate in spiritual activities. If necessary, chronic depression can be treated with individual counseling, group therapy, or antidepressant drugs.

### Emotional Lability

Sudden laughing or crying for no apparent reason and difficulty controlling emotional responses, known as emotional lability, affects many stroke survivors. There may be no happiness or sadness involved, and the emotional display will end as quickly as it started.

### Neglect

Some stroke survivors neglect the side of their world corresponding to the side of their brain which was injured by the stroke. Those with left-sided neglect do not perceive what is on their left side. For example, the stroke survivor with left-sided neglect may ignore the left side of the face when washing or not eat food on the left side of the plate. If the stroke survivor's head is moved to the left, neglected objects may become apparent. If the plate is turned around, he or she will finish eating the meal.

### Memory Loss

Some changes in behavior, such as memory loss, can be so subtle the family may not notice them at first. A stroke survivor may be anxious and cautious, needing a reminder to finish a sentence or know what to do next. Some stroke survivors have difficulty with numbers and calculating. Their family will need to learn to keep things in the same place, do things in the same sequence, tell the stroke survivor in advance what is going to happen, and possibly take over some responsibilities.

## Communication Problems

If a stroke causes damage to the language center in the brain, there will be language difficulties. Some stroke survivors are unable to understand or speak at all. Others do not make sense when they speak. Some can no longer read or write. Many have difficulty pronouncing words. Communication problems are among the most frightening after-effects of stroke for both the survivor and the family, often requiring professional help.

## Daily Task Difficulties

Stroke survivors will find that completing simple tasks around the house which they took for granted before the stroke are now extremely difficult or impossible. Many adaptive devices and techniques have been designed especially for stroke survivors to help them retain their independence and function safely and easily. The home usually can be modified so that narrow doorways, stairs, and bathtubs do not interfere with the stroke survivor's ability to care for personal needs.

Helpful bathroom devices include grab bars, a raised toilet seat, a tub bench, a hand-held shower head, no-slip pads, a long-handled brush, a washing mitt with pockets for soap, soap-on-a-rope, an electric toothbrush, and an electric razor.

There are many small electric appliances and kitchen modifications which also make it possible for the stroke survivor to participate in meal preparation.

## Dressing and Grooming

Dressing oneself is a basic form of independence. The added value of being neatly and attractively dressed enhances a stroke survivor's self-image. There are many ways to eliminate the difficulties in getting dressed. Stroke survivors should avoid tight-fitting sleeves, armholes, pant legs and waistlines; as well as clothes that must be put on over the head. Clothes should fasten in front. Velcro fasteners should replace buttons, zippers, and shoelaces. Devices which can aid in dressing and grooming include a mirror which hangs around the neck, a long-handled shoehorn, and a device to help pull on stockings.

## Diet, Nutrition, and Eating

A low-salt, low-fat, low-cholesterol diet can help prevent a recurrent stroke. People with high blood pressure should limit the amount of salt they eat. Those with high cholesterol or hardening of the arteries should avoid foods containing high levels of saturated fats (i.e., animal fats). People with diabetes need to follow their doctor's advice on diet. These diet controls can enhance the benefits of the drugs which may have been prescribed for control of a specific condition.

Weight control is also important. Inactive people can easily become overweight from eating more than a sedentary lifestyle requires. Obesity can also make it difficult for someone with a stroke-related disability to move around and exercise.

Some stroke survivors may have a reduced appetite. Ill-fitting dentures or a reduced sense of taste or smell can make food unappealing. The stroke survivor who lives alone might even skip meals because of the effort involved in buying groceries and preparing food. Soft foods and foods with stronger flavors may tempt stroke survivors who are not eating enough. Nutrition programs, such as Meals on Wheels, or hot lunches offered through community centers have been established to serve the elderly and the chronically ill.

Special utensils can help people with physically-impaired arms and hands at the table. These include flatware with built-up handles which are easier to grasp, rocker knives for cutting food with one hand, and attachable rings which keep food from being pushed off the plate accidentally.

Stroke survivors who have trouble swallowing need to be observed while eating so that they do not choke on their food. The same is true of those with memory loss who may forget to chew or to swallow. Tougher foods should be cut into small pieces.

## Skin Care

Decubitus ulcers (sometimes called bed sores) can be a serious problem for stroke survivors who spend a good deal of time in bed or who use a wheelchair. The sores usually appear on the elbows, buttocks, or heels.

To prevent bed sores, caregivers should make sure the stroke survivor does not sit or lie in the same position for long periods of time. Pillows should be used to support the impaired arm or leg. The feet can hang over the end of the mattress so that the heels don't rest on the sheet, or pillows can be put under the knees to prop them so that the soles of the feet rest flat on the bed. Sometimes, a piece of sheep-skin placed under the elbows, buttocks, or heels can be helpful. Special mattresses or cushions reduce pressure and help prevent decubitus ulcers.

## Pain

A stroke survivor may suffer pain for many reasons. The weight of a paralyzed arm can cause pain in the shoulder. Improperly-fitted braces, slings, or special shoes can cause discomfort. Often the source of pain can be traced to nerve damage, bed sores, or an immobilized joint. Lying or sitting in one position too long causes the body and joints to stiffen and ache.

## Sexuality

The quality of a couple's sexual relationship following a stroke differs from couple to couple. Most couples do find that their sexual relationship has changed, but not all find this to be a problem. The closeness that a couple shares before a stroke is the best indicator of how their relationship will evolve after the stroke. It is important to remember that sexual satisfaction, both giving and receiving, can be accomplished in many ways. Whatever is comfortable and acceptable between partners is normal sexual activity.

# University of Maryland Study Results

## University of Maryland Study Finds Certain Coping Strategies Impact Recovery from Stroke

Following a stroke, almost two-thirds of people turn to religion on a regular basis and about 12 percent frequently use humor to cope with the stress that results from having a stroke. That's according to researchers at the University of Maryland School of Medicine in Baltimore, who also found that about two-thirds of stroke patients use acceptance as a way to move forward and deal with their new challenges.

Results of the study, which showed that certain coping strategies enable people to adjust better to life after a stroke, were presented at the American Heart Association's 27th International Stroke Conference in San Antonio, Texas, on February 7, 2002.

The study evaluated the coping style and psychological adjustment of 56 stroke survivors treated at the University of Maryland Medical Center (34 women and 22 men) one year after their stroke. The most common strategies among the patients were turning to religion, acceptance, and positive reinterpretation and growth, which means that they tried to find something positive from their experience, shifted their priorities, and gained new appreciation for their family and friends. Almost half of the patients studied used positive reinterpretation and growth on a daily basis.

While many patients use a variety of coping strategies, the researchers looked at the most dominant ones used on a regular basis by patients in the study.

"Individuals who used humor and positive reinterpretation were more outgoing, active, and positive a year after their stroke," says the study's lead author, Lynn Grattan, Ph.D., an associate professor of neurology at the University of Maryland School of Medicine and a neuropsychologist at the University of Maryland Medical Center.

"Turning to religion can also help patients cope effectively following a stroke, especially if they are using it to seek strength to deal with the challenges they face," says Dr. Grattan.

The researchers also found that stroke patients who avoided addressing the issues related to their stroke had higher levels of depression one year after the stroke. These individuals used behavioral disengagement as a coping strategy, acting as though their stroke didn't happen and diverting their attention away from activities that would help them with rehabilitation and recovery. For example, they may have skipped follow-up doctor or physical therapy appointments or ignored recommendations on diet, exercise, and other lifestyle changes to prevent a future stroke. Behavioral disengagement was used frequently by seven percent of patients in the study.

A stroke can lead to feelings of frustration, anxiety, anger, apathy, or depression. By avoiding the emotional and behavioral aspects of what they went through, Dr. Grattan says patients who disengage are not dealing with natural feelings of loss and are not allowing themselves to take steps that could improve their condition.

"We believe these findings are important to keep in mind as we work with patients early in the recovery process," according to Dr. Grattan.

"Two people with the same stroke-related disabilities can have very different outcomes. One person may return to work and social activities, while the other may end up on permanent disability. We believe pre-stroke personality and coping strategies play a major role in how well patients recover," she adds.

Dr. Grattan says health care providers should first assess the patient's dominant coping style and tailor therapy to that individual.

"Through counseling, stroke support groups, and other methods, we can encourage patients to use the most effective coping strategies, especially during the year following a stroke, to maximize their adjustment and recovery," she says.

In a related study, Dr. Grattan and her colleagues found that patients who had adjusted most successfully one year after their stroke had received support from family and friends. The most useful types of support included driving them to doctor appointments, picking up prescriptions, and empathic listening, which means listening with sensitivity to the person's needs and point of view without being judgmental.

Stroke is the leading cause of serious disability among adults. About 600,000 people suffer from a stroke each year in the U.S.

The following University of Maryland School of Medicine researchers collaborated with Dr. Grattan on the study: Natasha Kabitski, Marjan Ghahramanlou, Christopher Vaughan, Marcella Wozniak, Steven Kittner, and Thomas Price.

## *Personality Influences Psychological Adjustment*

Pre-stroke personality has a greater influence on stroke recovery than the brain injury itself, according to research presented on February 14, 2001 at the American Stroke Association's 26th International Stroke Conference. The American Stroke Association is a division of the American Heart Association.

Some stroke survivors are highly susceptible to emotional changes from the brain injury and psychological reactions to that injury. How they cope with the changes—and how well they recover—is based on the individual's unique pre-stroke persona, according to new research.

"In some cases, two people with the exact same stroke-related deficits can have very different results," says Lynn M. Grattan, Ph.D., lead author and associate professor of neurology at the University of Maryland School of Medicine in Baltimore. "One person might return to work and social and leisure activities, while the other may end up on permanent disability. Our research is the first to demonstrate that in many cases, personality has a greater influence than the brain injury itself."

Grattan says healthcare providers should act promptly to identify an individual's pre-existing personality features including previous methods of coping, problem-solving, and emotional styles and sensitivities.

"By harnessing and mobilizing their strengths early on, you can help reduce the disappointment, confusion, and pain brought on by the stroke and engage them immediately in the rehabilitation process," says Grattan.

She suggests that this can easily be done with a brief neuropsychological examination of the patient within the first few days of a stroke.

The psychological reaction to having a stroke can cause feelings of frustration, anxiety, apathy, anger, or depression. Depression can seriously hinder an individual's willingness and ability to participate in rehabilitation, as well as their ability to avoid another stroke.

In this study, researchers hoped to identify which elements of an individual's baseline personality changed and determine which personality types are vulnerable to depression after a stroke. Investigators studied the personalities of 35 stroke survivors—20 female, 15 male with an average age of 57. They administered standard psychological tests to the close relatives (spouse, child, or sibling) of the individuals who had a stroke. They were asked questions about the patients' interpersonal style, degree of extroversion or introversion, openness to new experiences, and how they coped with stress. The test was given a few days after the stroke and again one year later.

Researchers found that people whose families described them as highly self-conscious or as deep thinkers were most vulnerable to post-stroke depression.

"After the stroke, these people became more self-conscious, moody, withdrawn, and socially isolated," says Grattan. "Their subsequent depression made it very difficult for them to participate in and benefit from rehabilitation as they lacked the energy or interest to succeed."

In contrast, people described as more energetic, outgoing, flexible, and self-confident before a stroke can often successfully dedicate themselves to a rigorous post-stroke rehabilitation routine and get themselves back to a higher level of recovery, she says.

Much of stroke care has focused on medically stabilizing patients and sending them home, she says. "While this is clearly crucial for recovery, more attention should be placed on working with patients and their families soon after hospital admission to understand the changes a stroke can cause so that they can all better deal with the stroke-related deficits and subsequent disability."

"Pre-existing personality is exceedingly important to how an individual faces the painful aspects of stroke recovery, how they approach the challenge of rehabilitation, and maximize recovery," she says.

Ultimately, the researchers hope to develop counseling and medical regimes that will optimize psychosocial outcomes following stroke.

Grattan's research was supported by a grant from the National Institutes of Health/National Institute of Neurological Disorders and Stroke.

## Job Demands Sway Speed of Return to Work after Stroke

Job characteristics may be a key determinant in how soon an individual returns to work after having a stroke, according to research presented on February 15, 2001 at the American Stroke Association's 26th International Stroke Conference. The American Stroke Association is a division of the American Heart Association.

It was the first study to examine job characteristics and compare them with the time stroke survivors take to return to work or whether they return at all.

"The type and characteristics of the job are very important in determining who will return to work," says lead researcher Marcella A. Wozniak, M.D., Ph.D., an associate professor of neurology at the University of Maryland School of Medicine in Baltimore.

"By understanding why some individuals do not return to work, we can develop programs to help more people get back to their jobs. Similarly, we can learn to identify those who will have great difficulty resuming work."

Researchers found that both the physical and mental demands of the job were important in predicting patients' return. Individuals who were back to work within 12 months had significantly less physically and psychologically demanding jobs. They felt their jobs were very secure, felt more job satisfaction, and believed they had more authority to make decisions on the job.

"Survivors who felt their job was secure returned to work significantly sooner than those who felt they were at risk of losing their job," says Wozniak. "Those with authority to make decisions about their job and with supportive co-workers and employers also tended to return to work sooner."

The results are important in light of the aging of America's workforce. Wozniak notes that the risk of stroke increases dramatically with age, that the average age of workers is increasing, and that the Social Security Administration recently has changed its policies.

"They've increased the minimum retirement age to 67 for people born after 1959," says Wozniak. "For people born between 1934 and 1959, a sliding scale to determine retirement age is in place. Therefore, more people will be working at the time of stroke and, as more effective treatments are developed, more survivors will be facing the possibility of re-employment."

The study, conducted at the University of Maryland Medical Center, recruited patients who had their first ischemic stroke (a stroke due to blood-vessel blockage) between the ages of 24 and 64 and were employed full-time outside of the home. Of 150 patients, 64 percent were male and 48 percent were black. They were all able to go home or to a rehabilitation center immediately after their stroke.

Six weeks later, study participants completed standardized questionnaires that measured their perceptions of their jobs. These questionnaires have been used in other studies examining the association of heart disease and other illnesses with employment. Patients were asked to rate their agreement or disagreement with statements about their job such as: "My job is very hectic;" "I have a lot to say about what happens on my job;" "My prospects for career development and promotions are good;" and "I can take it easy and still get my work done."

Patients were phoned at six and 12 months after the stroke to determine when they returned to work.

"Our prior analysis and work by others had found that white-collar, more educated, and wealthier patients were more likely to return to work," says Wozniak. "On one level, this seems obvious because blue-collar jobs are more likely to be physically demanding. On other levels, white-collar jobs would have more cognitive demands, and educated patients with higher-paying jobs would be more likely to have disability insurance and other financial resources to retire early. These factors should make it less likely for white-collar workers to return."

Other factors that may help employees make the decision to return to work could include their perceived ability to change or modify their job environment, their assessment of how easily they could be replaced at work, how likely they feel they are to lose the job, and their social support network at work.

"How the other factors play into what is clearly a complex relationship is mostly speculation right now," says Wozniak. "It is interesting that even in people who regain their independence in daily activities, only about 60 percent return to work."

Chapter 37

# Stroke Caregivers: What to Do and How to Do It?

## Caring for Someone Who Has a Stroke, Recommendations from the American Heart Association

### *What Should a Caregiver Do?*

No one job description explains what caregivers do. Each person's responsibilities vary according to the unique needs of the stroke survivor, and each person must determine what type and amount of care he or she is able to provide. This may require several adjustments, role changes, and learning new skills. Common responsibilities of caregiving include:

- Physical help with day-to-day activities

- Managing financial, legal, and business affairs

---

This chapter includes "Caring for Someone Who Has a Stroke," Reprinted with permission from the American Heart Association World Wide Web Site, www.americanheart.org © 2002, Copyright American Heart Association. Additional information in this chapter is excerpted with permission from *Stroke Caregivers Handbook* by Joyce W. Dreslin, © 2001 Joyce Dreslin. To view the complete text of the handbook and find additional information about stroke, please visit the Website of S.A.F.E., Stroke Awareness For Everyone, Inc., at www.strokesafe.org.

- Monitoring behavior to ensure safety and well-being
- Coordinating medical and rehabilitative care
- Providing emotional support for the stroke survivor and his or her family members

### Is There Help for Caregivers?

Don't make the mistake of not asking for help when you need it. Ask relatives, friends, clergy, or social workers for suggestions about people who might be able to help you. There are lots of places to seek help, including:

- Adult day care
- Adult foster homes
- Meal programs such as Meals on Wheels
- Home healthcare services
- Homemaker assistance
- Public health nursing services
- Respite care
- Transportation services

You can get information on the availability and cost of these services from your doctor or other healthcare professional, your state and community service department, and stroke support groups such as the American Stroke Association's Stroke Family Support Network. Just dial 1-888-7-STROKE to reach someone who really understands what you're going through. They also have a list of other stroke information pages on the Internet.

### Stay Informed and Stay in Touch

The more you learn about stroke and its aftermath, the better equipped you'll be as a caregiver. The American Stroke Association has many materials that can help you understand what the stroke survivor is feeling and experiencing. Call the Stroke Family Support Network at 1-888-4-STROKE to get information sent to you. Or visit the pages American Stroke Association for help in understanding stroke and its affects.

## Keeping Hope Alive for the Challenges Ahead

Editor's Note: The following information is excerpted from *Stroke Caregiver's Handbook*, by Joyce W. Dreslin

One thing all stroke victims have in common is that life will be forever changed in some way. In addition, everyone close to the victim will experience a life-altering adjustment. No family member or good friend escapes the reach of this paralyzing agent. And the degree of recovery can be in direct proportion to the amount of support put forth by the family-and-friend network.

Once you've been assured that the stroke's threat to life has waned, be wary of statements from people (often medical professionals) who say there is no recovery after "x" amount of time. For many, recovery continues for years, and sometimes a lifetime. Recovery usually comes more quickly during that first year, but seldom ceases. The brain continues to form new pathways as it heals, and there'll be times when recovery is great and times when it slows.

If you are facing a situation where your loved one has been felled by stroke, it is very important to understand that, in most cases, nobody (not even the most experienced medical professionals) can really predict how much the strokee will or will not recover. No matter what you are told, stroke recovery is very unpredictable and varies with each individual. Try to take each day one at a time. Take joy in each moment of progress, and know that there is always room for hope. Sometimes neurologists and other doctors, even though knowing their territory very well, will communicate through statistics, and their talent in understanding the complexities of the brain does not necessarily extend to understanding the emotional needs of a new strokee and their family. We're complex too. And we don't need to be frightened by someone rattling off the statistics of average recovery or possibility of recurring stroke. As we said, every stroke is different. And we certainly don't want to be thrown into the heap called average.

## Stroke Caregiver: An Unwelcome Job Opportunity

It's not a job you apply for. Chances are, if already employed, you don't need or want another job, much less this one. Usually you have no prior experience, you don't know the language, you don't have the proper tools to do it, the pay isn't compensatory to the task, it may come at a time in your life when you don't have the energy required to do the job well, you may be expected to do it without giving up all the other jobs you may have, but there IS job security—as it may last forever.

It's like you're on your way to the restroom at the theater on opening night, and someone says, "You!" The star is sick, the conductor hasn't shown up, the stagehands have gone on strike, and you've been tapped to step in and make sure the show goes on for 20 years. If you don't, someone dies (or so you're led to believe). Caregiving isn't like parenthood where you have had nine months to prepare. You were once a kid, and you've seen millions of parents in the act of doing their job prior to having to do it yourself. And it's not a decision you can just say no to, like when you were threatened with not having your kid in Scouts unless you became the scout leader. So? The kid can play soccer and not be a Scout. This is a bigger deal. Stroke offers few options.

Suddenly you're front and center stage in the wrong outfit and totally clueless. Quick, someone give that person a manual.

## Intensive Care—Be Faithful

### Checklist

- Take care of yourself first.
- Take mountains of notes.
- Keep *all* records in a safe and easy-to-find location.
- Contact victim's employer to determine benefits.
- Don't pay any bills yet, other than meeting required deductibles.

Chances are that during this stage, friends and family will come to your aid. There are cards, flowers, concern, attention, food, visitors, and offers of help. Take it all. Especially the offers of help. Line up people to be with the patient, in shifts, to take notes when doctors appear, to remind nurses and aides that if they had read the chart, they'd know this patient can't move one side, etc. Do not try to do it all yourself. This is going to be a long haul. You'll need to conserve your energy and get plenty of sleep (ask your doctor about drugs to assist in sleep, if necessary, to insure this happens). Don't allow someone to get rid of their guilt and sense of duty by just dropping off one lasagna. The answer to "Is there anything I can do?" is always yes. (Freeze the lasagna for use later. You may get ten the first week, but chances are you won't see another one for the next ten years.) Don't forget to thank profusely as you come up with another small task to be done. "Pick up stamps at the post office, take in dry cleaning, etc. Please!"

Keep a notebook. Better, keep two notebooks. Label them appropriately. Caregiving 101 will be the toughest course you'll ever study. Invest in a three-hole punch if you don't have one, a couple of very fat three-ring binders, and some index tab separators. Save every scrap of paper and document. Use one notebook for notes (with names, dates, and times) from every encounter with any and all medical personnel. You may also want to utilize a tape recorder (ask permission to use it— "Can I record this? I always get things mixed up.") to have a more accurate record of doctors' orders or answers to questions you ask. It can also save a lot of grief when coming home with a survivor who "remembers exactly" what the doctor said.

Use the other notebook for all medical records and correspondence, insurance receipts, and medical bills. You are entitled to copies of all test results and medical records. Sign a release, and keep them in the notebook. Always keep an up-to-date list of all medications, dosages, and prescription filling histories handy. It will be needed every time you see a doctor, therapist, or have to have the stroke victim hospitalized. It might help to create this list on a computer, so it's easy to update and print. Likewise, a scanner can be used to scan and print out copies of medical bills to send to the insurance company. Saves making copies, and keeping a backup on a floppy disk gives one extra place to look for receipts that are lost.

And, if all this organization is simply too much for you at this very stressful time—see if someone can help with this task, or else, find yourself a big box, and put every scrap of paper and every record into that box, then deal with it when your head is clearer. Store the box in an easy-to-find place. There will come a time when you will be glad you took five minutes to do this.

Do not pay any bills before the insurance company goes through their entire approval process—which may be months in the making. If the insurance company disallows any payment, it is your right to appeal that judgment. One major insurance provider admitted that 98% of all judgments are reversed when appealed. Once you pay $1 of a bill, you are claiming full responsibility for that bill, and once you pay a doctor or hospital yourself, you will spend years trying to get that money back from the insurance company, if at all.

## Hospitalization—Be Vigilant

### Checklist

- Ask questions—make sure they're answered clearly to your satisfaction.

- Arrange for a swallow assessment.

- Physical therapies begin now—be proactive.

- Health Care Proxy, Powers of Attorney, Do Not Resuscitate (DNR) Orders should be negotiated, as appropriate.

- Maintain a positive attitude, but be realistic.

- Don't allow negative comments in front of the patient. They may not be able to speak, but can hear. They may also understand.

- Make hospital environs cheery with appropriate comforts of home.

This is no time to be shy and demure. There are times in life when it's smart to pretend to know what you don't. Not now. In the schematic of a stroke time line, you're the equivalent of a two-year-old—so act like one. Ask "Why?" "How come?" and "What for?" a hundred times a day. Throw a tantrum if things don't go the way you think they should. Be a tattletale and go to authority figures if those beneath them misbehave. (Also give thank you's in the form of hugs and complimentary notes to those in charge, telling them who was especially good.) If you can't transform yourself into an aggressive, in-your-face, don't-give-me-any-guff type of personality, call in a big brother to help fight your battles. But don't be a whiner. Nobody likes a whiner at any age. You are fighting for the life of someone you love, and you deserve respect from everyone.

Stroke may be hard for you to swallow emotionally, but, physically speaking, swallowing may be the survivor's first problem. Muscles on one side may not be working properly, and the opposite of what you think is true: the thinner the consistency, the harder it is to go down. Water and thin liquids come back up, or worse, aspirate into the lungs. Foods may need to be puréed until a swallow test can be done. It's sort of like a moving x-ray where therapists watch as dyed liquids are ingested to see where they go—successfully down the esophagus, or unsuccessfully elsewhere. Only after they pass the test should a stroke victim be allowed real food. If they flunk, don't despair. That doesn't mean they'll never eat again. The swallow muscles can often be therapeutically rehabilitated just as the bigger ones can.

Physical, occupational, and speech therapies should begin in the hospital, as soon as the patient is medically stable enough to tolerate them. To reduce their descriptions to the lowest possible terms, physical therapy takes care of legs, occupational therapy takes care of the hands and arms and personal care skills, and speech takes care of verbal communications.

Occupational therapy may be the hardest concept to figure out because at this stage it has nothing to do with one's occupation. It doesn't matter if the patient is a doctor, lawyer, or Indian chief. After a stroke, their main job is to learn how to dress, brush teeth, and learn life's basic skills, coping with the disabilities the stroke has handed them. That's the job of the occupational therapist.

It's important that all non-working parts be put through the motions they would do if they were working normally. These are called range-of-motion (ROM) exercises. Impress the therapists by asking them to teach you how to administer these. They can also give you instructional sheets to keep in your notebook. This will be your first hands-on job since you're the one with two working hands. Jump in and keep the patient's limbs loose. Besides being valuable physically, it will send a strong message of love and commitment that will be missed by no one. If and when the brain recovers enough to tell those limbs to move again, they must be ready to respond. "I forgot" is seldom a good excuse in any situation, so move on in and don't allow muscles to forget their moves.

Riddle: What is life's greatest luxury that you will have more of while the stroke victim is in the hospital, but you won't realize it until the patient is home and then you'll have none of it. Answer: Time.

Take advantage of that little lifesaver on the hospital nightstand called the telephone and get your lives in order before time runs out. Here's who should be called to hear your call for help:

*The Hospital Social Worker*

Do you have a Durable Power of Attorney in your loved one's will? You will need both a regular (financial) Durable Power of Attorney and a Medical Power of Attorney. Get the social worker to access the hospital's Notary Public (this should be free) and have these two forms signed. Do not leave an ending date for the term of the contract. This may legally be left open. Have the hospital put this in the file and ask them to make it part of the permanent medical file. Even if you have these forms at home or in your safety deposit box, do this anyway and save time. If things go bad, you will not have time for attorneys to review forms. Be prepared.

*The Employer of the Stroke Survivor*

Speak to the immediate supervisor and to the Human Resources person-in-charge. Get names and phone numbers. Discuss long-term disability, sick leave, and Social Security Disability with them. (The social worker above may be helpful in this regard as well.) Find out how much they can do for you, and let them do it. Remember the answer to the question, "Can I do something for you?" is always a resounding "Yes."

*Social Security Office*

Look in the phone book for the local phone number, or you can find Social Security online at http://www.ssa.gov. Find out what benefits are available and how to go about applying for them. This process takes months. The paperwork is monumental, but once the application is approved, the benefits pay back to the date of the beginning of the disability. Get it going while you're sitting bedside.

*Insurance Company*

Get the name and direct phone number of a caseworker you can call regularly. They may become your best friend. They may cringe every time they hear your name, but recognition is better than starting anew every time you have to call.

## Life at the Rehab Facility

### Checklist

- Continually reevaluate your decision of selecting this facility.

- Get to know therapy and therapists.

- Establish yourself as the advocate in charge and liaison between patient and staff.

- Realize recovery isn't fast; celebrate the small steps.

- Be a constant source of positive encouragement.

- Make surroundings pleasant, but getting out of there often is more pleasant.

You've selected the facility you feel is a good match to your strokee, and they move in. One thing to keep in the back of your mind is that this is not an irreversible decision. If things don't work out the way you thought they would, remember that the door that you walked in through also has the capability to let you back out.

At the beginning, it's very important for the caregiver to be there to make sure the patient settles in well and has some understanding of the routine. Meet every person that has a role in your loved one's care. Introduce yourself to each therapist and sit in on the sessions. Have the therapists explain exactly what they're doing and why, and then ask how you can help and what activities you can do during "off-therapy" time, weekends, or during visitation. It's important to establish your position as someone who wants the best possible care for your patient and one who is willing to help get it.

Depending on your loved one's condition, it may be difficult for them to verbally communicate needs and pain to the therapist. For the first few sessions it may be up to you to devise a communication method between therapist and patient to signify what hurts and the degree of pain or displeasure. This may be a hand, finger, nod, or an eyebrow signal. The method of communication doesn't matter as long as there is a dialogue that is understood. You know the patient best; in your role as advocate, it's to everyone's advantage to make sure the therapists get to know them, their physical discomforts and emotional needs as well.

## Evaluating the Competency of Therapists

Carry that symbol of authority, the clipboard, and take notes.

1:00    Individual PT scheduled.

1:05    Inquired as to whereabouts of therapist. No explanation can be given.

1:10    Supervisor makes calls. "Therapist is on the way."

1:22    Therapist appears, looks around for equipment.

1:30    Area is finally ready for therapy. Patient asked to do 12 leg lifts. Can patient count to 12? Can patient do leg lifts? Does patient even know what a leg lift is? Therapist leaves before finding answers.

1:40   Therapist returns, wakes up patient, asks if 12 leg lifts have been done. "Yes" is the reply. "No" should have been the reply.

If these are the sort of notes you're taking, and the therapist is acting in that manner while you're obviously taking notes on a clipboard, imagine what happens when you're not there. That's why you're there. As soon as you realize what you are documenting is a negative trend, do something about it.

Determine if the problem is with one therapist or aide and request a change from the supervisor. Sometimes there is a personality conflict between patient and therapist. While you may not be qualified to judge a therapist's technical expertise, you certainly can tell if they're condescending, impatient, belittling, apathetic, cruel, negligent, heavy-handed, harsh, or just plain gives up on the patient. You should be aware that many therapists are necessarily "tough" because they must be, to motivate an otherwise unmotivated patient—and do try observe enough to sort this out first. And, often, a patient will express a great dislike for a therapist that drives them hard, and challenges them. But, the match-up between patient and therapist has to be a productive one. This isn't a marriage—it's more important than that. A life is at stake. Some patients do better with male therapists rather than female (men patients who have an abundance of women running their lives especially may need a male presence). Always have good documentation to back up your request for a change in personnel.

If your documentation shows that the whole place is operating at substandard efficiency, run to the nearest phone and demand an audience with the Executive Director of the facility. Remind them and yourself again how the door to the facility works both in and out. If there's no other alternative facility to threaten with, threaten to go to the one with the big bucks: the insurance provider. Insist on a breakdown of billings for all services rendered. Make sure you have a log to back up disputes: show that the one hour billed was, in fact, 20 minutes. It can turn into an unpleasant job, but you'll need to dig your heels in and fight for what you know to be right.

Your loved one deserves an opportunity to regain as much as their developmental functions as they can. Good therapy will help maintain and retrain a stroke victim's body, spirit, and mind, including muscle tone, flexibility, coordination, motor skills, cognition, and speech. A good rehabilitation facility should be committed to make this happen. You may have to remind its administration of these basic rights and that you intend to do whatever is necessary to obtain them. Your right to do so is granted by virtue of the fact that you love the person who can't fight for himself. A good rehab facility has a staff that will listen to the caregiver and ask your opinions. You are the only one there who knows who and what the patient was before the stroke.

## In the Best of Times, in the Best of Rehabs

One thing to keep in mind is that even if you found the finest rehab facility with the very best therapists in the world, progress in stroke recovery is usually measured in very small increments. This is not a fast process. Walking, talking, moving the affected arm do not come overnight even if the therapy is timely, and the therapist works every minute of their allotted time. Individual results often vary. Two strokes are seldom the same. Unfortunately, there is no published timetable available to determine the degree of recovery and when it's going to come. Recovery doesn't end at three weeks, or three years. It continues for a lifetime. And if you think it's slow now, guess what? It's going to get slower with time, so rehab is the time to utilize the staff and the doctors and to "make hay while the sun shines." Use this time wisely and to the best advantage of the patient. Make sure everyone around your loved one thinks and acts in a positive manner. There isn't a place for negativity in this scenario. Try very hard not to make comparisons to others in therapy. Make others (friends, relatives) aware as well—that every brain recovers at a different rate and to a different degree, no matter how motivated the patient, how much therapy is provided or by whom. Don't ever allow the word never to be uttered.

If your patient is receiving pain or muscle-relaxing medication, make sure that it's given at a time when it will most benefit therapy. It certainly is easier to do physical tasks when one is pain-free, so be sure that those medications aren't just dispensed at a X o'clock without regard for when the therapy will take place. No, the doctors and nurses don't always think of that.

Because progress is so slow, it's very important to continually encourage the patient to work hard and not give up. Celebrate the improvements, no matter how dinky.

Get a big calendar like the ones used as desk blotters. Circle the date of the stroke and write in all milestones when they are achieved: first solid food, first step, etc. Make the patient aware of the date—

numbers and names of days and months are often lost—it helps them in their awareness and time frames. It's also helpful when they're discouraged: "Look two weeks ago you couldn't even do _____. Now you're an expert."

When something big happens (first step, first glimmer of movement, any recognizable accomplishment), have a party. Have balloons and approved "party food and drink" on hand for such an occasion. Impatience is a big part of stroke so it's important to not have to wait for a celebration. Just show the patient how very proud you are of them right then and there, and don't forget to write it down on the calendar, surrounded by stars. Take pictures or videos—because it is nearly guaranteed that the patient will be unlikely to see their own progress. They just remember how they were before the stroke, and are constantly aware that they're not that way any more.

Try hard to keep the strokee aware of their presence in the real world. Watch the news and discuss it, if language isn't a barrier. Watch comedies. Listen to radio, listen to music. Talk about what you are seeing, doing, and hearing. Talk about family and friends, about all things you would normally have talked to them about in the same voice you used to use. Yes, they have suffered a stroke, but they need to know that the outside world is still there and waiting for their return.

Just as you did during acute care hospitalization, decorate the patient's room. Put up pictures of friends and family. This helps the strokee remember who they are and gives the staff another dimension of the fallen soul lying there: this was an active person with a family, loved ones. Looking through photos with the patient is mentally stimulating, but go easy. The brain at this stage needs to heal, it can quickly overload and result in exhaustion. Ask if there is anything from home they'd like in the room, any magazine from the newsstand, if they are able to read.

If possible, take the patient for walks/rides throughout the facility. Explore every nook and cranny, inside and out. Take advantage of outings they may have—make sure your patient gets signed up, even if you have to sign on too as a chaperone for the group. Try to get the strokee out of their room as much as possible. The room is for sleeping and resting, not a place to hide or escape from the world. As soon as it is allowed, take the patient out on a pass away from the facility. This may require some testing by the staff to be sure that you can transfer the patient and attend to whatever needs may arise. Go get a noninstitutional type meal. Just be careful not to overload the senses. After being in a controlled environment, Saturday afternoon at a mall at Christmastime probably isn't a good idea.

# Can We Go Home Now?

Your idea, and the insurance company's idea, of when the time is right for Home Sweet Home are not likely to coincide. Twenty years ago, a patient might have convalesced in a rehab facility many months until they could go home and live independently, but no more. Some inpatient rehab stays are as short as a few weeks. The main criterion for leaving the rehab facility may be as basic as being able to transfer to and from a wheelchair with assistance. It may also be that the patient is not recovering sufficiently (in the "Great Eyes" of the insurance case worker) to continue to benefit from a continual program of inpatient rehab.

So, no matter how you cut it, the burden is placed squarely on your shoulders as the caregiver. (And, this is the instant when you will begin to treasure that time when your loved one was out of medical danger, but temporarily under care and feeding of someone else.)

You'll generally face one of two scenarios at this point. Sadly, neither heralds the end of this long road. The most positive one: the patient has recovered enough to go home (often with lots of daily assistance), and can continue with outpatient therapy, sometimes at the same inpatient facility. In the second scenario: recovery has been limited, and the patient pretty much requires full-time care. Typically, therapy is no longer covered by insurance, and it becomes a decision whether the patient can be cared for at home or requires continued stay in a nursing facility.

# Part Five

# Stroke Prevention

Chapter 38

# Stroke Prevention Guidelines

1. Know your blood pressure. Have it checked at least annually. If it is elevated, work with your doctor to keep it under control.

   • High blood pressure (hypertension) is a leading cause of stroke.

   • Have your blood pressure checked at least once a year—more often if you have a history of high blood pressure.

   • If the higher number (your systolic blood pressure) is consistently above 130, or if the lower number (your diastolic blood pressure) is consistently over 85, consult your doctor.

   • If your doctor confirms that you have high blood pressure, s/he may recommend changes in your diet, regular exercise, and possibly medication.

2. Find out if you have Atrial Fibrillation (also called AF). If you have AF, work with your doctor to manage it.

   • Atrial fibrillation (AF) can cause blood to collect in the chambers of your heart. This blood can form clots and cause a stroke.

This chapter includes "Stroke Prevention Guidelines," © Research Center for Stroke and Heart Disease, available at www.strokeheart.org, reprinted with permission; and an excerpt from "WHI HRT Update—2002," National Heart, Lung, and Blood Institute (NHLBI).

385

- Your doctor can diagnose AF by carefully checking your pulse. AF can be confirmed with an ECG (Electrocardiogram).

- If you have AF, your doctor may choose to lower your risk for stroke by prescribing medications such as Coumadin® or Aspirin.

3. If you smoke, stop.

- Smoking doubles the risk for stroke.

- If you stop smoking today, your risk for stroke will immediately begin to drop.

- Within five years, your stroke risk may be the same as that of a non-smoker.

4. If you drink alcohol, do so in moderation.

- Drinking up to two glasses of wine or the alcohol equivalent, each day may actually lower your risk for stroke (*provided that there is no other medical reason that you should avoid alcohol*).

- Heavy drinking increases your risk for stroke.

- Remember that alcohol is a drug. It can interact with other drugs you are taking, and alcohol is harmful in large doses.

5. Know your cholesterol number. If it is high, work with your doctor to control it.

- Lowering your cholesterol may reduce your risk for stroke. Having high cholesterol can indirectly increase stroke risk by putting you at greater risk of heart disease which is another important stroke risk factor.

- Some cholesterol lowering medications have been shown to reduce the risk of stroke in some high risk individuals.

- High cholesterol can be controlled in many individuals with diet and exercise; some may need medication.

- Recent studies show that some individuals with normal cholesterol may lower their risk for stroke by taking specific medications for cholesterol.

6. If you are diabetic, follow your doctor's recommendations carefully to control your diabetes.

   • Having diabetes puts you at increased risk for stroke.

   • Often, diabetes may be controlled through careful attention to what you eat.

   • Your doctor can prescribe a nutrition program, lifestyle changes, and medicines that can help control your diabetes.

7. Include exercise in the activities you enjoy in your daily routine.

   • A brisk walk or other activity for as little as 30 minutes a day can improve your health in many ways, and may reduce your risk for stroke.

   • Try walking with a friend, this will make it more likely that you'll make it a habit.

   • If you don't enjoy walking, choose another exercise activity that suits your lifestyle; bicycling, golfing, swimming, dancing, playing tennis, or aerobics.

8. Enjoy a lower sodium (salt), lower fat diet.

   • By cutting down on sodium and fat in your diet, you may be able to lower your blood pressure, and most importantly, lower your risk for stroke.

9. Ask your doctor if you have circulation problems which increase your risk for stroke. If so, work with your doctor to control them.

   • Fatty deposits caused by atherosclerosis or other diseases can block the arteries which carry blood from your heart to your brain. This kind of blockage, if left untreated, can cause stroke.

   • You can be tested for atherosclerosis by your doctor.

   • If you have blood problems such as sickle cell disease, or severe anemia, work with your doctor to manage these problems. Left untreated, these problems can cause stroke.

   • Circulation problems can usually be treated with medications.

   • Occasionally surgery is necessary to remove a blockage.

## *Postmenopausal Hormone Therapy*

### *What Were the Main Findings in the Women's Health Initiative Study on Estrogen Plus Progestin?*

The main findings show that compared to women taking placebo pills:

- The number of women who developed breast cancer was higher in women taking estrogen plus progestin.

- The numbers of women who developed heart attacks, strokes, or blood clots in the lungs and legs were higher in women taking estrogen plus progestin.

- The numbers of women who had hip and other fractures or colorectal cancer were lower in women taking estrogen plus progestin.

- There were no differences in the number of women who had endometrial cancer (cancer of the lining of the uterus) or in the number of deaths.

### *What Are the Increased Risks for Women Taking Estrogen Plus Progestin?*

For every 10,000 women taking estrogen plus progestin pills:

- 38 developed breast cancer each year compared to 30 breast cancers for every 10,000 women taking placebo pills each year.

- 37 had a heart attack compared to 30 out of every 10,000 women taking placebo pills.

- 29 had a stroke each year, compared to 21 out of every 10,000 women taking placebo pills.

- 34 had blood clots in the lungs or legs, compared to 16 women out of every 10,000 women taking placebo pills.

### *What Are the Reduced Risks for Women Taking Estrogen Plus Progestin?*

For every 10,000 women taking estrogen plus progestin pills:

- 10 had a hip fracture each year, compared to 15 out of every 10,000 women taking placebo pills each year.

- 10 developed colon cancer each year, compared to 16 out of every 10,000 women taking placebo pills.

## What Are the Conclusions from These Findings?

The main conclusions are:

- The estrogen plus progestin combination studied in WHI does not prevent heart disease.

- For women taking this estrogen plus progestin combination, the risks (increased breast cancer, heart attacks, strokes, and blood clots in the lungs and legs) outweigh the benefits (fewer hip fractures and colon cancers).

## Additional Information

### National Institute of Neurological Disorders and Stroke
Information Office
P.O. Box 5801
Bethesda, MD 20824
Toll-Free: 800-352-9424
Tel: 301-496-5751
TTY: 301-468-5981
Website: www.ninds.nih.gov

### National High Blood Pressure Education Program
NHLBI Information Center
P.O. Box 30105
Bethesda, MD 20824-0105
Toll-Free: 800-757-WELL (9355)
Tel: 301-592-8573
Fax: 301-592-8563
Website: www.nhlbi.nih.gov/about/nhbpep
E-mail: NHLBIInfo@rover.nhlbi.nih.gov

### The National Stroke Association
9707 East Easter Lane
Englewood, CO 80712-3747
Toll-Free: 800-STROKES (787-6537)
Tel: 303-649-9299
Fax: 303-649-1328
Website: www.stroke.org

## American Stroke Association
A Division of the American Heart Association
7272 Greenville Ave
Dallas, TX 75231-4596
Toll-Free: 888-4-STROKE (478-7653)
Website: www.strokeassociation.org
E-mail: strokeconnection@heart.org

## National Institute on Aging (NIA)
Building 31, Room 5C27
31 Center Drive, MSC 2292
Bethesda, MD 20892
Tel: 301-496-1752
Website: www.nia.nih.gov

## Office on Women's Health
8550 Arlington Blvd., Suite 300
Fairfax, VA 22031
Toll-Free: 800-994-9662
TTD: 888-220-5446
Website: www.4women.gov

Chapter 39

# Carotid Endarterectomy for Stroke Prevention

## What Is a Carotid Endarterectomy?

A carotid endarterectomy is a surgical procedure in which a doctor removes fatty deposits blocking one of the two carotid arteries, the main supply of blood for the brain. Carotid artery problems become more common as people age. The disease process that causes the buildup of fat and other material inside the artery walls is called atherosclerosis, popularly known as "hardening of the arteries." The fatty deposit is called plaque; the narrowing of the artery is called stenosis. The degree of stenosis is usually expressed as a percentage of the normal diameter of the opening.

## Why Is Surgery Performed?

Carotid endarterectomy is performed to prevent stroke. Two large clinical trials supported by the National Institute of Neurological Disorders and Stroke (NINDS) have identified specific individuals for whom the surgery is beneficial when performed by surgeons and in institutions that can match the standards set in those studies. The surgery has been found highly beneficial for persons who have already had a stroke or experienced the symptoms of a stroke and have a severe stenosis of 70 to 99 percent. In this group, surgery reduces the

"Questions and Answers about Carotid Endarterectomy," Office of Scientific and Health Reports, National Institute of Neurological Disorders and Stroke (NINDS), January 1998, reviewed July 1, 2001.

estimated 2-year risk of stroke or death by more than 80 percent, from greater than 1 in 4 to less than 1 in 10.

For patients who have already had transient or mild stroke symptoms due to moderate carotid stenosis (50 to 69 percent), surgery reduces the 5-year risk of stroke or death by 6.5 percent. The failure rate for ipsilateral stroke or death for the medical group is 22.2 percent, and for the surgery group is 15.7 percent from greater than 1 in 4 to less than 1 in 7. Individuals who have already had stroke symptoms, and who have carotid stenosis greater than 50 percent, may wish to consider surgery to prevent future stroke. With the completion of the NASCET trial, patients with moderate (50 to 69 percent) stenosis will be better able to make more informed decisions.

In another trial, the procedure has also been found highly beneficial for persons who are symptom-free but have a carotid stenosis of 60 to 99 percent. In this group, the surgery reduces the estimated 5-year risk of stroke by more than one-half, from about 1 in 10 to less than 1 in 20.

## What Is a Stroke?

A stroke occurs when blood flow is cut off from part of the brain. In the same way that a person suffering a loss of blood to the heart can be said to be having a heart attack, a person with a loss of blood to the brain can be said to be having a brain attack. There are two kinds of stroke, hemorrhagic and ischemic. Hemorrhagic strokes are caused by bleeding within the brain. Ischemic strokes, which are far more common, are caused by a blockage of blood flow in an artery in the head or neck leading to the brain. Some ischemic strokes are due to stenosis, or narrowing of arteries due to the build up of plaque, fatty deposits, and blood clots along the artery wall. A vascular disease that can cause stenosis is atherosclerosis, in which deposits of plaque build-up along the inner wall of large and medium-sized arteries, decreasing blood flow. Atherosclerosis in the carotid arteries, two large arteries in the neck that carry blood to the brain, is a major risk factor for ischemic stroke.

## What Are the Symptoms of a Stroke?

Symptoms of stroke include:

• Sudden numbness, weakness, or paralysis of face, arm, or leg, especially on one side of the body.

- Sudden confusion, trouble talking, or understanding speech.

- Sudden trouble seeing in one or both eyes.

- Sudden trouble walking, loss of balance, or coordination.

- Sudden severe headache with no known cause (often described as the worst headache in a person's life).

Symptoms may last a few moments and then disappear. When they disappear within 24 hours or less, they are called a transient ischemic attacks (TIA).

## How Important Is a Blockage as a Cause of Stroke?

A blockage of a blood vessel is the most frequent cause of stroke and is responsible for about 80 percent of the approximately 700,000 strokes in the United States each year. With nearly 150,000 stroke deaths each year, stroke ranks as the third leading killer in the United States after heart disease and cancer. Stroke is the leading cause of adult disability in the United States with 2 million of the 3 million Americans who have survived a stroke sustaining some permanent disability. The overall cost of stroke to the nation is $40 billion a year.

## How Many Carotid Endarterectomies Are Performed Each Year?

In 1995, statistics from the National Hospital Discharge Survey indicate there were about 132,000 carotid endarterectomies performed in the United States. The procedure was first described in the mid-1950s. It began to be used increasingly as a stroke prevention measure in the 1960s and 1970s. Its use peaked in the mid-1980s when more than 100,000 operations were performed each year. At that time, several authorities began to question the trend and the risk-benefit ratio for some groups, and the use of the procedure dropped precipitously. The NINDS-supported North American Symptomatic Carotid Endarterectomy Trial (NASCET) and the NINDS-supported Asymptomatic Carotid Atherosclerosis Study (ACAS) were launched in the mid-1980s to identify the specific groups of people with carotid artery disease who would clearly benefit from the procedure.

393

# What Are the Risk Factors and How Risky Is the Surgery?

Important risk factors in addition to the degree of stenosis include, gender, diabetes, the type of stroke symptoms, and blockage of the carotid artery on the opposite side. Without other complicating illnesses, age alone is not a worrisome risk factor. Risk factors can affect patients in two ways. They can, particularly in combination, greatly increase a person's risk of having a stroke. In addition, these risk factors can increase the likelihood of surgical complications.

## How Is Carotid Artery Disease Diagnosed?

In some cases, the disease can be detected during a normal checkup by a physician. In other cases further testing is needed. Some of the tests a physician can use or order include ultrasound imaging, arteriography, and magnetic resonance angiography (MRA). Frequently these procedures are carried out in a stepwise fashion: from a doctor's evaluation of signs and symptoms to ultrasound, MRA, and arteriography for increasingly difficult cases.

- **History and physical exam.** A doctor will ask about symptoms of a stroke such as numbness or muscle weakness, speech or vision difficulties, or lightheadedness. Using a stethoscope, a doctor may hear a rushing sound, called a bruit (pronounced "broo-ee"), in the carotid artery. Unfortunately, dangerous levels of disease sometimes fail to make a sound, and some blockages with a low risk can make the same sound.

- **Ultrasound imaging.** This is a painless, noninvasive test in which sound waves above the range of human hearing are sent into the neck. Echoes bounce off the moving blood and the tissue in the artery and can be formed into an image. Ultrasound is fast, risk-free, relatively inexpensive, and painless compared to MRA and arteriography.

- **Arteriography.** This can be used to confirm the findings of ultrasound imaging which can be uncertain in some cases. Arteriography is an x-ray of the carotid artery taken when a special dye is injected into the artery. A burning sensation may be felt when the dye is injected. An arteriogram is more expensive and carries its own small risk of causing a stroke.

394

- **Magnetic Resonance Angiography (MRA).** This is a new imaging technique that avoids most of the risks associated with arteriography. An MRA is a type of image that uses magnetism instead of x-rays to create an image of the carotid arteries.

## What Is "Best Medical Therapy" for Stroke Prevention?

The mainstay of stroke prevention is risk factor management: smoking cessation, treatment of high blood pressure, and control of blood sugar levels among persons with diabetes. Additionally, physicians may prescribe aspirin, warfarin, or ticlopidine for some individuals.

Chapter 40

# Cholesterol Control Reduces Stroke Risk

## Cholesterol Is the Jekyll and Hyde of the Body

Like the literary split personality, cholesterol has a good side because it is needed for certain important body functions. But for many Americans, cholesterol also has an evil side. When present in excessive amounts, it can injure blood vessels and cause heart attacks and stroke.

The body needs cholesterol for digesting dietary fats, making hormones, building cell walls, and other important processes. The bloodstream carries cholesterol in particles called lipoproteins that are like blood-borne cargo trucks delivering cholesterol to various body tissues to be used, stored, or excreted. But too much of this circulating cholesterol can injure arteries, especially the coronary ones that supply the heart. This leads to accumulation of cholesterol-laden plaque in vessel linings, a condition called atherosclerosis.

When blood flow to the heart is impeded, the heart muscle becomes starved for oxygen, causing chest pain (angina). If a blood clot completely obstructs a coronary artery affected by atherosclerosis, a heart attack (myocardial infarction) or death can occur.

"Keeping Cholesterol Under Control," by John Henkel, *FDA Consumer*, January-February 1999, U.S. Food and Drug Administration, updated in October 2002 by David A. Cooke, MD, Diplomate, American Board of Internal Medicine; and "Cholesterol Lowering in Elderly Reduces Heart Disease and Strokes," NIH News Release, August 8, 1999, National Heart, Lung, and Blood Institute (NHLBI).

Heart disease is the number one killer of both men and women in this country. More than 90 million American adults, or about 50 percent, have elevated blood cholesterol levels, one of the key risk factors for heart disease, according to the National Heart, Lung, and Blood Institute's National Cholesterol Education Program.

While the institute estimates that heart disease killed nearly half a million in 1996, the most recent year for which figures are available, a study published in the *New England Journal of Medicine* in September 1998 says heart disease deaths have declined steadily over the last 30 years. Indeed, between 1990 and 1994, heart disease deaths decreased by 10.3 percent, the study says. From this and other studies, it appears that this is due largely to improvements in medical care after heart attack, a reduction in the number of repeat heart attacks, and better prevention of heart disease development.

A key factor in this drop is that the public, patients, and doctors today are better informed about the risks associated with elevated cholesterol and the benefits of lifestyle changes and medical measures aimed at lowering blood cholesterol. "Public health initiatives such as the National Cholesterol Education Program have raised consumer awareness, promoted effective interventions, and have likely contributed to the reduction in heart disease deaths," says David Orloff, MD, of the Food and Drug Administration's division of metabolic and endocrine drug products.

Another factor in the drop may be a relatively new class of drugs called statins. These have provided doctors with an arsenal of therapies to lower elevated blood cholesterol levels, often dramatically. To date, FDA has approved six statin drugs.

## When Blood Cholesterol Becomes a Problem

Two types of lipoproteins and their quantity in the blood are main factors in heart disease risk:

- Low-density lipoprotein (LDL)—This bad cholesterol is the form in which cholesterol is carried into the blood and is the main cause of harmful fatty buildup in arteries. The higher the LDL cholesterol level in the blood, the greater the heart disease risk.

- High-density lipoprotein (HDL)—This good cholesterol carries blood cholesterol back to the liver, where it can be eliminated. HDL helps prevent a cholesterol buildup in blood vessels. Low HDL levels increase heart disease risk.

One of the primary ways LDL cholesterol levels can become too high in blood is through eating too much of two nutrients: saturated fat, which is found mostly in animal products, and cholesterol, found only in animal products. Saturated fat raises LDL levels more than anything else in the diet.

Several other factors also affect blood cholesterol levels:

- Heredity—High cholesterol often runs in families. Even though specific genetic causes have been identified in only a minority of cases, genes still play a role in influencing blood cholesterol levels.

- Weight—Excess weight tends to increase blood cholesterol levels. Losing weight may help lower levels.

- Exercise—Regular physical activity may not only lower LDL cholesterol, but it may increase levels of desirable HDL.

- Age and gender—Before menopause, women tend to have total cholesterol levels lower than men at the same age. Cholesterol levels naturally rise as men and women age. Menopause is often associated with increases in LDL cholesterol in women.

- Stress—Studies have not shown stress to be directly linked to cholesterol levels. But experts say that because people sometimes eat fatty foods to console themselves when under stress, this can cause higher blood cholesterol.

Though high total and LDL cholesterol levels, along with low HDL cholesterol, can increase heart disease risk, they are among several other risk factors. These include cigarette smoking, high blood pressure, diabetes, obesity, and physical inactivity. If any of these is present in addition to high blood cholesterol, the risk of heart disease is even greater.

The good news is that all these can be brought under control either by changes in lifestyle—such as diet, losing weight, or an exercise program—or quitting a tobacco habit. Drugs also may be necessary in some people. Sometimes one change can help bring several risk factors under control. For example, weight loss can reduce blood cholesterol levels, help control diabetes, and lower high blood pressure.

But some risk factors cannot be controlled. These include age (45 years or older for men and 55 years or older for women) and family history of early heart disease (father or brother stricken before age 55; mother or sister stricken before age 65).

## What Is High Blood Cholesterol?

Cholesterol levels are determined through chemical analysis of a blood sample taken from a finger prick or from a vein in the arm. Home cholesterol kits, first approved in 1993, test only for total cholesterol levels but are as accurate as tests done in a doctor's office, says Steven Gutman, M.D., director of FDA's division of clinical laboratory devices. "These tests can give a consumer very valuable information when screening for high cholesterol," he says. "But they shouldn't be considered substitutes for a test conducted in a doctor's office." He adds that if test results are elevated, consumers should see a doctor right away for a more refined blood analysis. The National Cholesterol Education Program considers cholesterol testing in a doctor's office to be the preferred way because the patient can get advice immediately about the meaning of the results and what to do.

Besides determining total cholesterol levels, doctors often order a lipoprotein profile that shows the amounts of LDL, HDL, and another type of blood fat called triglycerides. This information gives doctors a better idea of heart disease risk and helps guide any treatment.

Cholesterol levels are measured in milligrams per deciliter (mg/dL). The National Cholesterol Education Program developed the following classifications for people over age 20 who do not have heart disease:

- Desirable blood cholesterol—Total blood cholesterol is less than 200 mg/dL; LDL is lower than 130 mg/dL.

- Borderline high cholesterol—Total level is between 200 and 239 mg/dL or LDL is 130 to 159 mg/dL.

- High blood cholesterol—Total level is greater than 240 mg/dL or LDL is 160 mg/dL or higher. For patients with heart disease, LDL above 100 mg/dL is too high. In addition, an HDL level less than 40 mg/dL is considered low and increases the risk of heart disease.

The main goal of cholesterol treatment is to lower LDL in people without heart disease. If the LDL level is in the high category and fewer than two other risk factors for heart disease are present, the goal is an LDL level lower than 160 mg/dL. If two or more risk factors are present, the goal is less than 130 mg/dL. If a patient already has heart disease, or is diabetic, LDL levels should be 100 mg/dL or less. By reducing LDL, heart disease patients may prevent future heart attacks, prolong their lives, and slow down or even reverse cholesterol buildup in the arteries, according to the National Heart, Lung, and Blood Institute.

## Treating High Blood Cholesterol

When a patient without heart disease is first diagnosed with elevated blood cholesterol, doctors often prescribe a program of diet, exercise, and weight loss to bring levels down. National Cholesterol Education Program guidelines suggest at least a six-month program of reduced dietary saturated fat and cholesterol, together with physical activity and weight control, as the primary treatment before resorting to drug therapy. Typically, doctors prescribe the Step I / Step II diet to lower dietary fat, especially saturated fat. Many patients respond well to this diet and end up sufficiently reducing blood cholesterol levels. Study data reinforce these benefits. For example, a 1998 Columbia University study examined 103 male and female patients of diverse ages and ethnic backgrounds and found that reducing dietary saturated fat directly affected blood cholesterol. For every 1 percent drop in saturated fat, the study showed a 1 percent lowering of LDL in patients.

But sometimes diet and exercise alone are not enough to reduce cholesterol to goal levels. Perhaps a patient is genetically predisposed to high blood cholesterol. In these cases, doctors often prescribe drugs. The National Cholesterol Education Program estimates that as many as 9 million Americans take some form of cholesterol-lowering drug therapy. The most prominent cholesterol drugs are in the statin family, an array of powerful treatments that includes Mevacor (lovastatin), Lescol (fluvastatin), Pravachol (pravastatin), Zocor (simvastatin), and Lipitor (atorvastatin). Many doctors say statin drugs have revolutionized patient care.

"These drugs have had a fantastic impact on cholesterol treatment," says Redonda Miller, M.D., assistant professor of medicine at Johns Hopkins University School of Medicine. "They all lower cholesterol levels, but the side effects are minimal."

A study published in the medical journal *Circulation* in 1998 showed that statins dramatically lower the risk of dying from heart disease. Research found that for every 10 percentage points cholesterol was reduced, the risk of death from heart disease dropped by 15 percent.

So far, only three of the drugs—Mevacor, Zocor, and Pravachol—have been studied in long-term, controlled trials. "Based on existing evidence, [statin drugs] all have similar safety profiles and are effective at lowering cholesterol in appropriately selected patients," says FDA's Orloff. "The difference between drugs lies mainly in their absolute capacity to lower cholesterol—that is, at the highest approved daily doses."

One landmark study completed in 1994, the Scandinavian Simvastatin Survival Study, or 4S, showed a 42 percent reduction in deaths from heart disease and a 30 percent drop in death from all causes over five years in patients with coronary heart disease whose high LDL levels were lowered with Zocor. The West of Scotland study, reported in 1995, revealed similar benefits from lowering LDL levels with Pravachol in patients without heart disease. And the Cholesterol and Recurrent Events (CARE) study, reported in 1996, showed that lowering LDL levels with Pravachol reduced heart attacks and deaths in patients with a previous heart attack but with cholesterol levels relatively average for the general population. This study showed that Pravachol treatment not only reduced death from heart disease but also death from all causes in a group of heart disease patients with average cholesterol levels.

A 1997 study, the Air Force/Texas Coronary Atherosclerosis Prevention Study, showed that Mevacor helped prevent a first heart attack or unstable angina in men and women with average cholesterol levels but with below-average HDL.

Statins work by interfering with the cholesterol-producing mechanisms of the liver and by increasing the capacity of the liver to remove cholesterol from circulating blood. Statins can lower LDL cholesterol by as much as 60 percent, depending on the drug and dosage.

Heart patient Norbert Hoffmann, 65, of Northfield, Minn., saw what he calls "a dramatic drop" in cholesterol levels after taking Zocor for three months. For example, his total cholesterol went from 270 to 145 mg/dL and LDL from 182 to 82 mg/dL.

But patients can respond differently to drugs. Some patients may have fewer side effects with one drug than another. "I had problems such as stomach cramps with Zocor," says Oklahoma patient Linden Gilbert, 50. His doctor ultimately switched him to Lipitor, which he credits with lowering his total cholesterol from 230 to 150 mg/dL.

It is worth noting that studies of statins have shown that at-risk patients treated with them have lower rates of death from all causes, not just cardiovascular disease, than patients not treated with the drugs. This shows that for most patients, any negative effects of the drugs are more than outweighed by their benefits. However, while the majority of patients tolerate statins very well, they are not entirely free of side effects. Blood tests are recommended to be performed at regular intervals while patients are on statins due to the rare occurrence of liver inflammation. All statins are known to rarely cause muscle inflammation (myopathy), which may lead to symptoms of muscle soreness and weakness. Very rarely, this is severe, and can lead to kidney damage and/or failure and death. One statin, Baycol (cervistatin), was pulled off the market by the FDA after it was found to cause myopathy far more frequently and severely than other statins, especially when combined with another cholesterol-lowering drug called gemfibrozil.

## Other Drug Treatments

These include:

- Nicotinic acid (niacin)—This lowers total and LDL cholesterol and raises HDL cholesterol. It also can lower triglycerides. Because the dose needed for treatment is about 100 times more than the Recommended Daily Allowance for niacin and thus can potentially be toxic, the drug must be taken under a doctor's care.

- Resins—Doctors have been prescribing Questran (cholestyramine) and Colestid (colestipol) for about 20 years. These resins bind bile acids in the intestine and prevent their recycling through the liver. Because the liver needs cholesterol to make bile, it increases its uptake of cholesterol from the blood. A newer drug, Welchol (colesevelam) works in the same manner.

- Fibric acid derivatives—Used mainly to lower triglycerides, Lopid (gemfibrozil) and Tricor (fenofibrate) can also increase HDL levels.

- Aspirin—Because studies have shown that aspirin can have a protective effect against heart attacks in patients with clogged blood vessels, doctors often prescribe the drug to patients with heart disease.

The decision of which drug to prescribe is one the doctor makes based on factors such as degree of cholesterol lowering desired, side effects, and cost. "If a patient has only a modest cholesterol elevation, I might prescribe Mevacor," says Johns Hopkins' Miller. "But if a more drastic reduction is needed, especially of LDL, I'll prescribe Lipitor."

The potential for drug interaction is a crucial concern, says FDA's Orloff. "Some statin drugs are known to interact adversely with other drugs, and that information may guide a decision about which statin to use." In June 1998, FDA announced the withdrawal of the drug Posicor (mibefradil), used to treat high blood pressure and stable angina, because it caused adverse reactions in patients taking various other drugs, including Mevacor and Zocor. Similarly, the statin drug Baycol (cervistatin) was withdrawn in 2001 due to severe adverse reactions, most of which occurred when it was combined with a non-statin cholesterol drug, Lopid (Gemfibrozil).

Though it is impossible to know yet just how many lives cholesterol-lowering therapies have saved, public health experts say awareness efforts such as the National Cholesterol Education Program are getting the word out to Americans about heart disease, its prevention, and management. Reflecting on his own experience with elevated cholesterol, Hoffmann says, "Get informed [about cholesterol]. Read books, search the Internet, look at your risk factors, and most of all, don't wait to do something about it if you have a [cholesterol] problem."

## Food for Thought

One of the main ways blood cholesterol can reach undesirable levels is through a diet high in saturated fat and cholesterol. Fatty cholesterol deposits can collect in blood vessels, raising the risk of heart disease.

Drugs, exercise, and other therapies may be prescribed. But in many cases, cholesterol levels can be lowered by revising dietary habits and limiting the kinds of foods known to boost cholesterol, such as those high in saturated fat. This doesn't mean totally eliminating all your favorite foods, such as desserts, says the National Cholesterol Education Program (NCEP). It means taking a more prudent approach to the kinds and amounts of foods you eat.

When elevated cholesterol is first discovered in a person without heart disease, doctors often start patients on the Step I diet recommended by the American Heart Association and NCEP. On this program, patients should eat: 8 to 10 percent of the day's total calories from saturated fat, 30 percent or less of total calories from fat, less than 300 milligrams of dietary cholesterol a day, and just enough calories to achieve and maintain a healthy weight. A doctor or a registered dietitian can suggest a reasonable calorie level. Food labels also are very helpful in determining how much saturated fat, cholesterol, and calories are in various foods.

If the Step I diet doesn't result in desirable cholesterol levels, doctors may try the Step II diet, which changes the daily saturated fat limits to below 7 percent of daily calories and dietary cholesterol to below 200 milligrams. Step II also is the diet for people with heart disease.

In many patients, blood cholesterol levels should begin to drop a few weeks after starting on a cholesterol-lowering diet. Just how much of a drop depends on factors such as how high the cholesterol level is and how each person's body responds to changes made. With time, cholesterol levels may be reduced 10 to 50 milligrams per deciliter or more, a clinically significant amount.

## Cholesterol Lowering in Elderly Reduces Heart Disease and Strokes

Older Americans have the Nation's highest rate of coronary heart disease (CHD) and can benefit greatly from lowering elevated cholesterol, according to a new report from the National Cholesterol Education Program (NCEP). The report notes that cholesterol lowering also has been shown to reduce the risk of strokes. NCEP is coordinated by the National Heart, Lung, and Blood Institute (NHLBI), part of the National Institutes of Health.

The report, which appeared in the August 1999 issue of the *Archives of Internal Medicine*, makes clear the NCEP's stand on the controversial issue of cholesterol lowering in those age 65 and older. "Some investigators have questioned the value of testing cholesterol and treating high levels in the elderly," said NHLBI Director Dr. Claude Lenfant. "But an overview of the research shows that cholesterol lowering can improve both the quality and length of life for many older Americans."

"Because most older Americans have cholesterol buildup in their arteries, an elevated cholesterol causes more cases of CHD in the elderly than in any other age group," said Dr. Scott Grundy, Director of the Center for Human Nutrition at The University of Texas Southwestern Medical Center at Dallas and lead author of the NCEP report. "It is clear that cholesterol counts in the elderly."

Dr. James Cleeman, NCEP Coordinator and a co-author of the report said, "The new report reviews the evidence from epidemiological studies and clinical trials, and concludes that controlling cholesterol produces significant benefits in the elderly. For those with CHD, it can prolong life and dramatically reduce their risk of having a heart attack. For healthy seniors, it will reduce their high risk of developing CHD."

NCEP recommends that older Americans keep their cholesterol in check by following an eating pattern lower in saturated fat, total fat, and cholesterol, being physically active, and maintaining a healthy weight.

High cholesterol is a major risk factor for CHD. It leads to hardening of the arteries, or atherosclerosis, in which cholesterol deposits build up in vessel walls, including the coronary arteries that feed the heart. According to the new report, two-thirds to three-quarters of those over age 65 have either obvious CHD or "silent" atherosclerosis. In the latter form, the person has no symptoms but plaques have formed in arteries. As noted, older Americans have more CHD than any other age group and suffer more coronary events, such as heart attacks and angina. Most first CHD events strike after age 65, according to the report.

The report notes that, in the past decade, treatment of high cholesterol has expanded and includes a wider range of cholesterol-lowering drugs, especially the statins, which produce the largest reduction in cholesterol levels. The report adds that cholesterol-lowering treatment works for both women and men.

The report's recommendations include:

- Older Americans should have their total cholesterol tested once every 5 years, and if an accurate measurement is available, their high density lipoprotein (HDL, the good cholesterol)—the same recommendation as for all American adults. The test should be done in a medical setting, so the presence of other CHD risk factors can be checked.

- Those with high cholesterol should take steps to lower it, especially if they also have other CHD risk factors. These include cigarette smoking, high blood pressure, physical inactivity, overweight, and diabetes.

- For seniors without CHD who need to lower a high cholesterol, the first line of treatment should be the adoption of the healthy life habits noted—eating a diet lower in saturated fat, total fat, and cholesterol, being physically active, and maintaining a healthy weight.

- When life habit changes do not sufficiently lower cholesterol and seniors are at high risk for CHD, drug therapy may be advisable. However, physicians should evaluate a patient's overall health status in making that decision.

- For most seniors with CHD, life habit changes and medication should be used together from the start of treatment.

- Postmenopausal women who are judged to need drug treatment to reduce their risk for CHD should consider cholesterol-lowering drugs instead of hormone replacement therapy. A study of women with CHD found that a combination of estrogen and progesterone did not reduce the risk of CHD events. By contrast, studies have shown that postmenopausal women at high risk for CHD benefit greatly from treatment with statin drugs.

- "It is important for older Americans to pay attention to their cholesterol," said NCEP's Cleeman. "Even if you're 70 and feeling fine, you can develop CHD, so you should take action."

- "Whether you are old or young, cholesterol counts—you can improve your quality of life by caring about your cholesterol," he added.

## Additional Information

### National Cholesterol Education Program
NHLBI Information Center
P.O. Box 30105
Bethesda, MD 20824-0105
Toll-Free: 800-575-WELL (9355)
Tel: 301-592-8573
Fax: 301-592-8563
Website: www.nhlbi.nih.gov
E-mail: NHLBIinfo@rover.nhlbi.nih.gov

Chapter 41

# Take Your Pulse for Life™— 60 Seconds Once a Month Can Help Prevent a Stroke

Stroke is the third leading cause of death in America. But strokes can be prevented. One way to help prevent strokes is as easy as taking your pulse. A risk factor for stroke, responsible for over 80,000 strokes each year, is characterized by an irregular pulse—a pulse that is not constant, but beats in an unsteady way.

You should learn how to check your pulse. If you discover you have a pulse that is not steady and constant, you should check with your doctor. With appropriate medical treatment, you can potentially avoid a devastating stroke.

The medical information presented is meant for general educational purposes only. Persons should consult qualified physicians regarding specific medical concerns or treatment.

## How Was This Technique Developed?

The Take Your Pulse for Life™ technique was created and validated by the Research Center for Stroke and Heart Disease. Since most people with Atrial Fibrillation (AF) are unaware they have the condition, teaching people to check the rhythm of their pulse can potentially prevent many strokes, especially since current treatment reduces the risk of stroke by about 70%. An irregular heartbeat is a telltale sign of AF.

The information in this chapter is from "Take Your Pulse for Life™," © 2001 Research Center for Stroke & Heart Disease, www.strokeheart.org, reprinted with permission.

In 1997, to validate the idea that people might be able to detect an irregular heartbeat, the Research Center for Stroke and Heart Disease, in partnership with the National Stroke Association, conducted a clinical research trial based out of five hospitals in the United States. The results of the trial proved that over 91% of individuals could determine whether a pulse was regular or irregular.

The self-screening technique must be performed properly in order to obtain correct results and should not be considered a substitute for consulting with a physician.

## Learn How to Check Your Pulse

### Step 1

Turn your left hand palm-side up, then place the first two fingers of your right hand along the outer edge of your left wrist just below where your wrist and thumb meet.

### Step 2

Slide your fingers toward the center of your wrist. You should feel the pulse between the wrist bone and the tendon.

### Step 3

Press down with our fingers until you feel your pulse. Do not press too hard, or you will not be able to feel the pulsation. Feel free to move your fingers until the pulse is easiest to feel.

**Table 41.1.** Heart Beat Characteristics

| Regular Pulse-Beat or Heart-Beat | Irregular Pulse-Beat or Heart-Beat |
|---|---|
| Steady and even | Unsteady and uneven |
| Beats in a constant fashion | Not constant |
| Like the steady ticking of a clock | Ticks erratically |
| Even pattern of beats | Uneven pattern of beats |
| Uniform thumping | Many missed or extra beats |
| Same strength to each beat | Some beats are stronger and some are weaker |

*Step 4*

Continue to feel your pulse for a full minute. Concentrate on whether the beats are evenly spaced, or whether they are erratic, with missed beats, extra beats, or beats that are too close together.

## What Should I Do if I Can't Find It?

Sometimes the pulse is difficult to locate. Here are some tips that might help:

- Try holding your arm pointing down toward the floor, if you have been holding it up toward your face.

- Try using your fingertips to feel the pulse instead of laying your fingers across your wrist. Put your fingertips in different places stopping for about five seconds in each position to try to feel the pulse before moving to another location. Lift, place, and feel; lift, place, and feel, until you find a spot where you can feel the pulsations well.

- Try varying the pressure of your fingertips on your wrist. You may need to lighten up or press a little harder to feel the pulse.

- Try these steps on the other wrist.

- If you still have difficulty, ask a friend to follow the steps and find your pulse.

## Is Your Pulse Normal?

Checking your pulse is easy and most people are able to do it once they learn the proper technique. You may already be an experienced pulse-taker; perhaps you have checked your pulse while exercising, to tell how fast your heart is beating. However, the Take Your Pulse for Life™ technique is different from the way you have evaluated your pulse in the past.

## It's How Steadily Your Heart Beats, Not How Fast

When you check your pulse for an irregular heartbeat that may indicate AF, you don't count the beats. Instead, you pay attention to whether the beats are evenly spaced and steady, not how rapidly your heart is beating. A normal heartbeat is so regular and constant that

411

you can predict when the next beat will occur. In AF, there are many missed, skipped, or extra beats. There are irregular intervals between the beats; you can't predict when the next beat will occur.

This is the pattern of a regular pulse with the beats represented by dashes. Notice that the beats are steady and uniform, with even spacing between them.

‐ ‐ ‐ ‐ ‐ ‐ ‐ ‐ ‐ ‐ ‐ ‐ ‐ ‐ ‐ ‐ ‐ ‐ ‐ ‐ ‐ ‐ ‐ ‐ ‐

This is the pattern of an irregular pulse. Notice that the beats are unsteady and uneven. You can see where there have been missed beats and extra beats, and that the interval between beats is irregular and unpredictable.

‐ ‐ ‐ ‐ — ‐ ‐‐‐‐ ‐ ‐ — ‐

If your pulse feels irregular, unsteady, and uneven, you might have Atrial Fibrillation (or AF) and could be at increased risk for a stroke.

### *How Is Take Your Pulse for Life™ Technique Different from Checking My Pulse to See How Fast It Is Beating?*

You may already know how to take your pulse. Perhaps you have checked it while exercising, to see how fast your heart is beating. You may already know that one of the easiest places to find your pulse is at your wrist. However, there is something very different about the Take Your Pulse for Life™ technique, compared to the way you have always listened to your pulse-beat.

When you are checking your pulse for an irregular heartbeat that may indicate AF, you are *not* counting the beats. You will be feeling your pulse to see if it is steady and constant; feeling the rhythm and the pattern of the beats. You won't need to count how many beats occur each minute. You will pay more attention to the uniformity and constancy of the thumping. A pulse that beats in a steady pattern is called a regular pulse. A pulse that beats erratically, with many extra or missed beats, is called an irregular pulse and might mean you have AF.

### *What Should I Do?*

Even if your pulse is very irregular, it does not necessarily mean you have AF. By doing a simple, painless electrocardiogram (ECG), your doctor can tell for sure. AF is not an emergency, but if you think you have an irregular pulse, consult a physician soon.

The only way to completely confirm AF is by using an ECG. During the ECG, electrodes that detect electrical impulses from the heart are placed on the chest. The impulses appear on a television screen or a strip of paper called an ECG strip. By evaluating the pattern of the electrical impulses on the screen or the ECG strip, a doctor can determine whether a patient has AF.

## Is It an Emergency?

An irregular pulse is *not* an emergency. However, if you think you have an irregular pulse, consult a physician soon. Your doctor can determine if you have AF.

Keep in mind that the warning signs and symptoms of a stroke or heart attack are an emergency. Make a copy of the stroke and heart attack symptoms. Keep it handy (perhaps taped on your refrigerator?). If you experience one or more of the symptoms, call 911—seek emergency treatment immediately.

**Table 41.2.** Identifying an emergency.

| | | |
|---|---|---|
| Irregular pulse | Not an emergency | Consult a physician soon |
| Stroke symptoms | **Emergency!** | Call 911, Seek immediate treatment |
| Heart attack symptoms | **Emergency!** | Call 911, Seek immediate treatment |

## What Can I Do if I Have AF?

AF can be treated, reducing your risk of stroke. Many people continue to live normal lives after being diagnosed and given proper treatment for AF.

Whenever possible, your doctor will try to bring your heartbeat back to a normal, regular beat. Frequently, this can be done with medications or the use of electrical stimulation.

When these efforts do not work, AF treatment concentrates on protecting you from stroke-causing clots. To reduce the risk of stroke, your doctor may then prescribe a clot prevention drug called warfarin

(Coumadin®) or, in some cases, aspirin. Medications can greatly reduce the risk of stroke, but need to be taken properly and monitored. Be sure you understand all the risks and responsibilities before you begin any treatment.

## Check Every Month

Get into the habit of checking your pulse every month. AF can come and go and frequently has no symptoms. As you get older, your risk of having AF increases. So, getting into the habit of checking your pulse now is a good idea. Even if your pulse is regular now, check it once a month—particularly if you are over 55. Talk to your doctor about any sense you might have that your pulse is irregular.

## Start with the Basics: What Is a Stroke

A stroke is sometimes referred to as a brain attack, because the process that causes it is similar to what happens in a heart attack. Strokes occur when the blood flow to a part of the brain is blocked. If the blockage is not relieved, brain cells will die. The body functions that depend upon that part of the brain will suddenly be lost. The size of the stroke and the area of the brain where it occurs determine what the symptoms will be. A small stroke may produce mild weakness in one arm or one leg, and you may recover completely, while a larger stroke may paralyze an entire side of the body or leave you unable to communicate.

A stroke is an emergency, just like a heart attack. However, unlike a heart attack, a stroke is usually not painful. That's why it's important to learn the warning signs and symptoms of a stroke so you can react quickly.

Anyone who experiences any of the warning signs of stroke should call 911 and get to a hospital immediately. Stroke requires urgent treatment in order to have the best outcome. Do not wait to see whether the symptoms will get better. The longer you delay getting to a hospital, the more likely it is that the damage to your brain will be severe or permanent.

Stroke is the third leading cause of death in the United States. Strokes kill twice as many American women as breast cancer. Each year, 750,000 Americans suffer a stroke (one person every 45 seconds) and 160,000 have a fatal outcome. Of those who survive, many suffer permanent disability—stroke is the leading cause of disability in adults.

414

Stroke risk increases with age. After age 55, your chance of having a stroke doubles every ten years. Two-thirds of all strokes occur in people older than 65.

Risk factors for stroke are generally the same as those for heart attack—high blood pressure, smoking, high cholesterol, diabetes, family history, etc. But there is another risk factor for stroke—an abnormal heart rhythm called atrial fibrillation.

## What Is Atrial Fibrillation and How Can It Lead to a Stroke?

Atrial Fibrillation (often called A-fib or AF) is a relatively common disorder that affects more than two million Americans. Most of them don't know they have it. The risk of stroke is five times higher in people who have AF.

The heart has four chambers. The upper chambers are the atria (left atrium, right atrium), where blood enters the heart. The lower chambers are the ventricles, which pump blood out of the heart to the body.

A normal heartbeat involves coordinated movement of all four chambers. It begins with the atria and proceeds to the ventricles. In AF, instead of this normal synchronized movement, there is a disorganized twitching of the atria, called fibrillation. When that happens, a clot may form inside the heart. A piece of the clot may then break off, be pumped out of the heart, and travel to the brain, causing a stroke.

AF causes about 15-20% of all strokes. The good news is that these strokes can be prevented. If everyone with AF received proper treatment, we could prevent about 80,000 strokes every year.

## Who Has AF?

AF can develop in anyone, but becomes much more common as we grow older. About 5% of people age 65 have AF, while about 10% of people over 75 are affected. It can occur in otherwise healthy people, but is more common in those who have high blood pressure, heart disease, or lung disease.

## What Are the Symptoms of AF?

There may be no symptoms at all, and you may be completely unaware that you have AF. Some people can sense that their heartbeat

415

isn't quite right, with frequent missed, skipped, or extra beats. This is sometimes described as a fluttering, pounding, or racing sensation in the chest. Others may experience occasional dizziness, faintness, or light-headedness.

Whether you have any of these symptoms or not, you may be able to discover whether you have AF simply by checking your pulse.

## How Does AF Affect my Pulse?

Your pulse is caused by the surge of blood flow in your arteries each time your heart beats. A normal heartbeat begins in the atria, followed immediately by the more powerful beat of the ventricles, which produces the pulse you feel. Normally, the beats follow each other at regular intervals—they are evenly spaced and steady. In AF, the coordination between the atria and ventricles is lost, and the pulse becomes uneven, unsteady, and irregular.

## How Can I Discover Whether I Have AF?

You can discover whether your heartbeat is irregular by learning to take your own pulse. Its simple, free, requires no equipment, and we've proven that it works! If you detect an irregular pulse, you can check with your doctor to see whether it is due to AF or to some other condition.

Chapter 42

# The DASH Diet Lowers Blood Pressure and Stroke Risk

## NHLBI Study Finds DASH Diet and Reduced Sodium Lowers Blood Pressure for All

The DASH (Dietary Approaches to Stop Hypertension) diet plus reduced dietary sodium lowers blood pressure for all persons, according to the first detailed subgroup analysis of the DASH study results. The Dietary Approaches to Stop Hypertension study was supported by the National Heart, Lung, and Blood Institute (NHLBI).

The detailed analysis, published in the December 18, 2001, issue of the *Annals of Internal Medicine*, showed the blood pressure lowering effects of the DASH diet and reduced dietary sodium in a wide variety of population subgroups: persons with and without hypertension or a family history of hypertension, older and younger adults, men and women, African-American and other races, obese and nonobese, as well as people with higher or lower physical activity levels, larger or smaller waist circumferences, and higher or lower annual family income or education.

While the combination of the DASH diet and reduced dietary sodium produced the biggest reductions, each intervention also lowered blood pressure for all groups when used alone.

"NHLBI Study Finds DASH Diet and Reduced Sodium Lowers Blood Pressure for All," NIH News Release 12/17/2001, National Heart, Lung, and Blood Institute (NHLBI); and excerpts from "Facts about the DASH Diet," National Heart, Lung, and Blood Institute (NHLBI), NIH Publication No. 01-4082, updated May 2001.

417

The DASH diet is rich in fruits, vegetables, and low fat dairy foods and reduced in total and saturated fat. It also is reduced in red meat, sweets, and sugar-containing drinks. It is rich in potassium, calcium, magnesium, fiber, and protein. Prior studies found that the DASH diet lowers blood pressure and also lowers blood LDL-cholesterol (the bad cholesterol) and the amino acid homocysteine, which appears to increase the risk of heart disease. Prior studies also showed reducing dietary sodium lowers blood pressure, both with and without the DASH diet.

"This new study underscores the blood pressure-lowering effects of a reduced intake of salt and other forms of dietary sodium," said NHLBI Director Dr. Claude Lenfant. "Earlier research on the link between sodium and blood pressure had given conflicting results in various population groups. Now, we can say that cutting back on dietary sodium will benefit Americans generally and not just those with high blood pressure."

"The study's participants have blood pressures in the same range as half of adult Americans, including about 80 percent of those age 50 and older," said Dr. Frank Sacks, Professor of Cardiovascular Disease Prevention, Harvard School of Public Health and chair of the DASH Steering Committee. "Adopting these measures could help millions of Americans avoid the rise in blood pressure that occurs with advancing age."

High blood pressure, also called hypertension, is a major risk for heart disease and the chief risk factor for stroke.

The new data come from the DASH-Sodium study, a multicenter, 14-week randomized feeding trial in which all food was provided to participants. It involved 412 participants, aged 22 and older, and with systolic blood pressures of 120-160 mm Hg and diastolic blood pressures of 80-95 mm Hg.

Fifty-two percent of the participants were women and 48 percent men; 54 percent were African-American, 42 percent white, and 10 percent other races. Forty-one percent had hypertension and 59 percent did not.

For 3 months, participants ate either the DASH diet or a typical American diet. Weight was kept stable. During the study period, each group followed three different intakes of dietary sodium for 1 month each in random order. The sodium levels were 3,300 milligrams a day (the average level consumed by Americans), 2,400 milligrams a day (the upper limit currently recommended by the National High Blood Pressure Education Program), and 1,500 milligrams a day.

The largest blood pressure differences occurred for those on the DASH diet with a daily sodium intake of 1,500-milligrams compared with those on the control diet with a sodium intake of 3,300 milligrams.

Detailed analysis showed that the DASH diet and reduced sodium intake reduced blood pressure for all the population subgroups studied. The following list shows the average blood pressure reduction for key subgroups:

- For those with hypertension: 12/6 mm Hg (systolic/diastolic); for those without hypertension, 7/4 mm Hg.

- For those over age 45, 12/6 mm Hg; for those 45 or younger, 6/3 mm Hg.

- For women, 11/5 mm Hg; for men, 7/4 mm Hg.

- For African-Americans, 10/5 mm Hg; for other races, 8/4 mm Hg.

Other results include:

- Compared with the typical American diet, the DASH diet alone (at the higher sodium level) reduced blood pressure by about 6/3 mm Hg for African-Americans, and 6/2 mm Hg for other races.

- For those with hypertension, reductions from the DASH diet alone were 7/3 mm Hg; and for those without hypertension, the reductions were 5/3 mm Hg.

- The effects of sodium reduction appeared in all subgroups and were greater for those who ate the typical American diet, compared with those on the DASH diet. The effects from sodium reduction were particularly great for those with hypertension, African-Americans, women, and those over age 45. Sodium reduction in those eating the control diet resulted in lower systolic and diastolic pressures by 8.3 mm Hg and 4.4 mm Hg, respectively, in hypertensives, and 5.4 and 2.8 mm Hg, respectively, in non-hypertensives.

"Following the DASH diet and reducing the intake of dietary sodium are two non-drug approaches that work to control blood pressure," said Dr. Denise Simons-Morton, Leader of the NHLBI Prevention Scientific Research Group and a DASH co-author. "The blood pressure reductions achieved from this combination came in only 4 weeks and persisted through the duration of the study. Ideally, Americans should use both the DASH diet and reduced sodium approaches but, even if they do only one, they'll still reap significant health benefits.

"If the U.S. food supply were lower in sodium," added Simons-Morton, "it would help lower levels of blood pressure in the general population."

## *Facts about the DASH Diet*

Research has found that diet affects the development of high blood pressure, or hypertension (the medical term). Recently, two studies showed that following a particular eating plan—called the DASH diet—and reducing the amount of sodium consumed lowers blood pressure.

While each step alone lowers blood pressure, the combination of the eating plan and a reduced sodium intake gives the biggest benefit and may help prevent the development of high blood pressure.

Those with high blood pressure may especially benefit from following the eating plan and reducing their sodium intake. But the combination is a heart-healthy recipe that all adults can follow.

**Table 42.1.** Blood Pressure Categories for Adults*

|  | Systolic** | Diastolic** |
|---|---|---|
| Optimal | <120 mm Hg and | <80 mm Hg |
| Normal | <130 mm Hg and | <85 mm Hg |
| High-Normal | 130-139 mm Hg or | 85-89 mm Hg |
| High |  |  |
| Stage 1 | 140-159 mm Hg or | 90-99 mm Hg |
| Stage 2 | 160-179 mm Hg or | 100-109 mm Hg |
| Stage 3 | ≥180 mm Hg or | ≥110 mm Hg |

*Categories are for those age 18 and older and come from the NHBPEP. The categories are for those not on a high blood pressure medication and who have no short-term serious illness.

**If your systolic and diastolic pressures fall into different categories, your overall status is the higher category.

< means less than; ≥ means greater than or equal to.

## What Is High Blood Pressure?

Blood pressure is the force of blood against artery walls. It is measured in millimeters of mercury (mm Hg) and recorded as two numbers—systolic pressure (as the heart beats) over diastolic pressure (as the heart relaxes between beats). Both numbers are important.

Blood pressure rises and falls during the day. But when it stays elevated over time, then it's called high blood pressure. High blood pressure is dangerous because it makes the heart work too hard, and the force of its blood flow can harm arteries. High blood pressure often has no warning signs or symptoms. Once it occurs, it usually lasts a lifetime. If uncontrolled, it can lead to heart and kidney disease, and stroke.

High blood pressure affects about 50 million—or 1 in 4—adult Americans. High blood pressure is especially common among African-Americans, who tend to develop it at an earlier age and more often than whites. It also is common among older Americans—about 60 percent of those age 60 and older have high blood pressure.

High blood pressure can be controlled if you take these steps:

• maintain a healthy weight;

• be physically active;

• follow a healthy eating plan, which includes foods lower in salt and sodium;

• if you drink alcoholic beverages, do so in moderation; and,

• if you have high blood pressure and are prescribed medication, take it as directed.

All steps but the last also help to prevent high blood pressure.

## What Is the DASH Diet?

Blood pressure can be unhealthy even if it stays only slightly above the optimal level of less than 120/80 mm Hg. The higher blood pressure rises above optimal, the greater the health risk.

In the past, researchers tried to find clues about what in the diet affects blood pressure by testing various single nutrients, such as calcium and magnesium. These studies were done mostly with dietary supplements and their findings were not conclusive.

Then, scientists supported by the National Heart, Lung, and Blood Institute (NHLBI) conducted two key studies. The first was called

**Table 42.2.** Following the DASH Diet

The DASH eating plan shown is based on 2,000 calories a day. The number of daily servings in a food group may vary from those listed depending on your caloric needs. Use this chart to help you plan your menus or take it with you when you go to the store.

| Food Group | Daily Servings (except as noted) | Serving Sizes | Examples and Notes | Significance of Each Food Group to the DASH Eating Plan |
|---|---|---|---|---|
| Grains and grain products | 7-8 | 1 slice bread, 1 oz dry cereal*, ½ cup cooked rice, pasta, or cereal | whole wheat bread, English muffin, pita bread, bagel, cereals, grits, oatmeal, crackers unsalted pretzels, and popcorn | major sources of energy and fiber |
| Vegetables | 4-5 | 1 cup raw leafy vegetable, ½ cup cooked vegetable, 6 oz vegetable juice | tomatoes, potatoes, carrots, green peas, squash, broccoli, turnip greens, collards, kale, spinach, artichokes, green beans, lima beans, sweet potatoes | rich sources of potassium, magnesium, and fiber |
| Fruits | 4-5 | 6 oz fruit juice, 1 medium fruit, ¼ cup dried fruit, ¼ cup fresh, frozen, or canned fruit | apricots, bananas, dates, grapes, oranges, orange juice, grapefruit, grapefruit juice, mangoes, melons, peaches, pineapples, prunes, raisins, strawberries, tangerines | important sources of potassium, magnesium, and fiber |
| Low fat or fat free dairy foods | 2-3 | 8 oz milk, 1 cup yogurt, 1½ oz cheese | fat free (skim) or low fat (1%) milk, fat free or low fat butter-milk, fat free or low fat regular | major sources of calcium and protein |

422

| | | | | |
|---|---|---|---|---|
| Meats, poultry, and fish | 2 or less | 3 oz cooked meats, poultry, or fish | or frozen yogurt, low fat and fat free cheese<br><br>select only lean; trim away visible fats, broil, roast, or boil, instead of frying; remove skin from poultry | rich sources of protein and magnesium |
| Nuts, seeds, and dry beans | 4-5 per week | 1/3 cup or 1½ oz nuts, 2 Tbsp or ½ oz seeds, ½ cup cooked dry beans | almonds, filberts, mixed nuts, peanuts, walnuts, sunflower seeds, kidney beans, lentils, peas | rich sources of energy, magnesium, potassium, protein, and fiber |
| Fats and oils** | 2-3 | 1 tsp soft margarine 1 Tbsp low fat mayonnaise, 2 Tbsp light salad dressing, 1 tsp vegetable oil | soft margarine, low fat mayonnaise, light salad dressing, vegetable oil (such as olive, corn, canola, or safflower) | DASH has 27 percent of calories as fat, including that in or added to foods |
| Sweets | 5 per week | 1 Tbsp sugar, 1 Tbsp jelly or jam, ½ oz jelly beans, 8 oz lemonade | maple syrup, sugar, jelly, jam, fruit-flavored gelatin, jelly beans, hard candy, fruit punch, sorbet, ices | sweets should be low in fat |

*Equals ½–1¼ cup, depending on cereal type. Check the product's nutrition label.

** Fat content changes serving counts for fats and oils: For example, 1 Tbsp of regular salad dressing equals 1 serving; 1 Tbsp of a low fat dressing equals ½ serving; 1 Tbsp of a fat free dressing equals 0 servings.

DASH, for Dietary Approaches to Stop Hypertension, and it tested nutrients as they occur together in food. Its findings showed that blood pressures were reduced with an eating plan that is low in saturated fat, cholesterol, and total fat, and that emphasizes fruits, vegetables, and low fat dairy foods. This eating plan—known as the DASH diet—also includes whole grain products, fish, poultry, and nuts. It is reduced in red meat, sweets, and sugar-containing beverages. It is rich in magnesium, potassium, and calcium, as well as protein and fiber.

The DASH study involved 459 adults with systolic blood pressures of less than 160 mm Hg and diastolic pressures of 80-95 mm Hg. About 27 percent of the participants had hypertension. About 50 percent were women and 60 percent were African-Americans.

DASH compared three eating plans: A plan similar in nutrients to what many Americans consume; a plan similar to what Americans consume but higher in fruits and vegetables; and the DASH diet. All three plans used about 3,000 milligrams of sodium daily. None of the plans were vegetarian or used specialty foods.

Results were dramatic: Both the fruits and vegetables plan and the DASH diet reduced blood pressure. But the DASH diet had the greatest effect, especially for those with high blood pressure. Further, the blood pressure reductions came fast—within 2 weeks of starting the plan.

The second study was called DASH-Sodium, and it looked at the effect on blood pressure of a reduced dietary sodium intake as participants followed either the DASH diet or an eating plan typical of what many Americans consume. DASH-Sodium involved 412 participants. Their systolic blood pressures were 120-159 mm Hg and their diastolic blood pressures were 80-95 mm Hg. About 41 percent of them had high blood pressure. About 57 percent were women and about 57 percent were African-Americans.

Participants were randomly assigned to one of the two eating plans and then followed for a month at each of three sodium levels. The three sodium levels were: a higher intake of about 3,300 milligrams per day (the level consumed by many Americans); an intermediate intake of about 2,400 milligrams per day; and a lower intake of about 1,500 milligrams per day. Results showed that reducing dietary sodium lowered blood pressure for both eating plans. At each sodium level, blood pressure was lower on the DASH diet than on the other eating plan. The biggest blood pressure reductions were for the DASH diet at the sodium intake of 1,500 milligrams per day. Those with hypertension saw the biggest reductions, but those without it also had large decreases.

Those on the 1,500-milligram sodium intake, as well as those on the DASH diet, had fewer headaches. Other than that and blood pressure levels, there were no significant effects caused by the two eating plans or different sodium levels. DASH-Sodium shows the importance of lowering sodium intake—whatever your eating plan. But for a true winning combination, follow the DASH diet and lower your intake of salt.

## How to Lower Calories on the DASH Eating Plan

The DASH eating plan was not designed to promote weight loss. But it is rich in lower-calorie foods, such as fruits and vegetables. You can make it lower in calories by replacing higher-calorie foods with more fruits and vegetables—and that also will make it easier for you to reach your DASH goals. Here are some examples:

*To increase fruits*

- Eat a medium apple instead of four shortbread cookies. You'll save 80 calories.

- Eat ¼ cup of dried apricots instead of a 2-ounce bag of pork rinds. You'll save 230 calories.

*To increase vegetables*

- Have a hamburger that's 3 ounces of meat instead of 6 ounces. Add ½ cup serving of carrots and ½ cup serving of spinach. You'll save more than 200 calories.

- Instead of 5 ounces of chicken, have a stir-fry with 2 ounces of chicken and 1½ cups of raw vegetables. Use a small amount of vegetable oil. You'll save 50 calories.

*To increase low fat or fat free dairy products*

- Have a ½ cup serving of low fat frozen yogurt instead of a 1½ ounce milk chocolate bar. You'll save about 110 calories.

*And don't forget these calorie-saving tips*

- Use low fat or fat free condiments.

- Use half as much vegetable oil, soft or liquid margarine, or salad dressing, or choose fat free versions.

- Eat smaller portions—cut back gradually.

- Choose low fat or fat free dairy products to reduce total fat intake.

- Check the food labels to compare fat content in packaged foods—items marked low fat or fat free are not always lower in calories than their regular versions.

- Limit foods with lots of added sugar, such as pies, flavored yogurts, candy bars, ice cream, sherbet, regular soft drinks, and fruit drinks.

- Eat fruits canned in their own juice.

- Add fruit to plain yogurt.

- Snack on fruit, vegetable sticks, unbuttered and unsalted popcorn, or bread sticks.

- Drink water or club soda.

**Table 42.3.** Dash Eating Plan Number of Servings for Other Calorie Levels

| Food Group | Servings/Day | |
|---|---|---|
| | 1,600 calories/day | 3,100 calories/day |
| Grains and grain products | 6 | 12-13 |
| Vegetables | 3-4 | 6 |
| Fruits | 4 | 6 |
| Low fat or fat free dairy foods | 2-3 | 3-4 |
| Meats, poultry, and fish | 1-2 | 2-3 |
| Nuts, seeds, and dry beans | 3/week | 1 |
| Fat and oils | 2 | 4 |
| Sweets | 0 | 2 |

## Where's the Sodium?

Only a small amount of sodium occurs naturally in foods. Most sodium is added during processing. The Table 42.4 gives examples of varying amounts of sodium that occur in foods before and after processing.

**Table 42.4.** Amounts of Sodium That Occur in Foods before and after Processing

| Food Groups | Sodium (mg) |
|---|---|
| *Grains and grain products* | |
| Cooked cereal, rice, pasta, unsalted, ½ cup | 0-5 |
| Ready-to-eat-cereal, 1 cup | 100-360 |
| Bread, 1 slice | 110-175 |
| | |
| *Vegetables* | |
| Fresh or frozen, cooked without salt, ½ cup | 1-70 |
| Canned or frozen with sauce, ½ cup | 140-460 |
| Tomato juice, canned ¾ cup | 820 |
| | |
| *Fruit* | |
| Fresh, frozen, canned, ½ cup | 0-5 |
| | |
| *Low fat or fat free dairy foods* | |
| Milk, 1 cup | 120 |
| Yogurt, 8 oz | 160 |
| Natural cheeses, 1½ oz | 110-450 |
| Processed cheeses, 1½ oz | 600 |
| | |
| *Nuts, seeds, and dry beans* | |
| Peanuts, salted, 1/3 cup | 120 |
| Peanuts, unsalted, 1/3 cup | 0-5 |
| Beans, cooked from dried or frozen, without salt, ½ cup | 0-5 |
| Beans, canned, ½ cup | 400 |
| | |
| *Meats, fish, and poultry* | |
| Fresh meat, fish, poultry, 3 oz | 30-90 |
| Tuna canned, water pack, no salt added, 3 oz | 35-45 |
| Tuna canned, water pack, 3 oz | 250-350 |
| Ham, lean, roasted, 3 oz | 1,020 |

## Tips to Reduce Salt and Sodium

- Use reduced sodium or no-salt-added products. For example, choose low- or reduced-sodium, or no-salt-added versions of foods and condiments when available.

- Buy fresh, plain frozen, or canned with no-salt-added vegetables.

- Use fresh poultry, fish, and lean meat, rather than canned, smoked, or processed types.

- Choose ready-to-eat breakfast cereals that are lower in sodium.

- Limit cured foods (such as bacon and ham), foods packed in brine (such as pickles, pickled vegetables, olives, and sauerkraut), and condiments (such as MSG, mustard, horseradish, catsup, and barbecue sauce). Limit even lower sodium versions of soy sauce and teriyaki sauce-treat these condiments as you do table salt.

- Be spicy instead of salty. In cooking and at the table, flavor foods with herbs, spices, lemon, lime, vinegar, or salt-free seasoning blends. Start by cutting salt in half.

- Cook rice, pasta, and hot cereals without salt. Cut back on instant or flavored rice, pasta, and cereal mixes, which usually have added salt.

- Choose convenience foods that are lower in sodium. Cut back on frozen dinners, mixed dishes such as pizza, packaged mixes, canned soups or broths, and salad dressings—these often have a lot of sodium.

- Rinse canned foods, such as tuna, to remove some sodium.

## How Do I Make the DASH?

The DASH diet used in the studies calls for a certain number of servings daily from various food groups. The number of servings you require may vary, depending on your caloric need.

You should be aware that the DASH diet has more daily servings of fruits, vegetables, and whole grain foods than you may be used to eating. This makes it high in fiber, which can cause bloating and diarrhea in some persons. To avoid these problems, gradually increase your intake of fruit, vegetables, and whole grain foods.

Twenty-four hundred milligrams of sodium equals about 6 grams, or 1 teaspoon, of table salt (sodium chloride); 1,500 milligrams of sodium equals about 4 grams, or 2/3 teaspoon, of table salt. These amounts include all salt consumed—that in food products, used in cooking, and added at the table. Only small amounts of sodium occur naturally in food. Processed foods account for most of the salt and sodium Americans consume. So, be sure to read food labels to choose products lower in sodium.

You may be surprised at many of the foods that have sodium. They include soy sauce, seasoned salts, monosodium glutamate (MSG), baking soda, and some antacids—the range is wide.

Since it is rich in fruits and vegetables, which are naturally lower in sodium than many other foods, the DASH diet makes it easier to consume less salt and sodium. Still, you may want to begin by adopting the DASH diet at the level of 2,400 milligrams of sodium per day and then further lower your sodium intake to 1,500 milligrams per day.

Remember that some days the foods you eat may add up to more than the recommended servings from one food group and less from another. Similarly, you may have too much sodium on a particular day. But don't worry. Just be sure that the average of several days or a week comes close to what's recommended for the food groups and for your chosen daily sodium level.

One note: If you take medication to control high blood pressure, you should not stop using it. Follow the DASH diet and talk with your doctor about your drug treatment.

## Reducing Sodium when Eating Out

- Ask how foods are prepared. Ask that they be prepared without added salt, MSG, or salt-containing ingredients. Most restaurants are willing to accommodate requests.

- Know the terms that indicate high sodium content: pickled, cured, soy sauce, broth.

- Move the salt shaker away.

- Limit condiments, such as mustard, catsup, pickles, and sauces with salt-containing ingredients.

- Choose fruit or vegetables, instead of salty snack foods.

## Compare Food Labels

Read the Nutrition Facts on food labels to compare the amount of sodium in products. Look for the sodium content in milligrams and the % Daily Value. Aim for foods that are less than 5 percent of the Daily Value of sodium.

**Table 42.5.** Label Language

Food labels can help you choose items lower in sodium and saturated and total fat. Look for the following labels on cans, boxes, bottles, bags, and other packaging:

| Phrase | What it means |
| --- | --- |
| *Sodium* | |
| Sodium free or salt free | Less than 5 mg per serving |
| Very low sodium | 35 mg or less of sodium per serving |
| Low sodium | 140 mg or less of sodium per serving |
| Low sodium meal | 140 mg or less of sodium per 3½ oz (100 g) |
| Reduced or less sodium | At least 25 percent less sodium than the regular version |
| Light in sodium | 50 percent less sodium than the regular version |
| Unsalted or no salt added | No salt added to the product during processing |
| | |
| *Fat* | |
| Fat free | Less than 0.5 g per serving |
| Low-saturated fat | 1 g or less per serving |
| Low fat | 3 g or less per serving |
| Reduced fat | At least 25 percent less fat than the regular version |
| Light in fat | Half the fat than the regular version |

## Getting Started

It's easy to adopt the DASH eating plan. Here are some ways to get started:

**Change gradually.**

• If you now eat one or two vegetables a day, add a serving at lunch and another at dinner.

• If you don't eat fruit now or have only juice at breakfast, add a serving to your meals or have it as a snack.

• Gradually increase your use of fat free and low fat dairy products to three servings a day. For example, drink milk with lunch or dinner, instead of soda, sugar-sweetened tea, or alcohol. Choose low fat (1 percent) or fat free (skim) dairy products to reduce your intake of saturated fat, total fat, cholesterol, and calories.

• Read food labels on margarines and salad dressings to choose those lowest in unsaturated fat. Some margarines are now trans-fat free.

**Treat meat as one part of the whole meal, instead of the focus.**

• Limit meat to 6 ounces a day (2 servings)—all that's needed. Three to four ounces is about the size of a deck of cards.

• If you now eat large portions of meat, cut them back gradually—by a half or a third at each meal.

• Include two or more vegetarian-style (meatless) meals each week.

• Increase servings of vegetables, rice, pasta, and dry beans in meals. Try casseroles and pasta, and stir-fry dishes, which have less meat and more vegetables, grains, and dry beans.

**Use fruits or other foods low in saturated fat, cholesterol, and calories as desserts and snacks.**

• Fruits and other low fat foods offer great taste and variety. Use fruits canned in their own juice. Fresh fruits require little or no preparation. Dried fruits are a good choice to carry with you or to have ready in the car.

- Try these snacks ideas: unsalted pretzels or nuts mixed with raisins; graham crackers; low fat and fat free yogurt and frozen yogurt; popcorn with no salt or butter added; and raw vegetables.

Try these other tips.

- Choose whole grain foods to get added nutrients, such as minerals and fiber. For example, choose whole wheat bread or whole grain cereals.

- If you have trouble digesting dairy products, try taking lactase enzyme pills or drops (available at drugstores and groceries) with the dairy foods. Or, buy lactose-free milk or milk with lactase enzyme added to it.

- Use fresh, frozen, or no-salt-added canned vegetables.

Chapter 43

# Aspirin and Warfarin for Stroke Prevention

## Study Shows That Aspirin and Warfarin Are Equally Effective for Stroke Prevention

A study appearing in the November 15, 2001, issue of *The New England Journal of Medicine** shows that aspirin works as well as warfarin in helping to prevent recurrent strokes in most patients. The Warfarin versus Aspirin Recurrent Stroke Study (WARSS) was a 7-year double-blind, randomized clinical trial involving 2,206 patients at 48 participating centers—the largest trial to date comparing aspirin to warfarin for recurrent stroke prevention. The study was sponsored by the National Institute of Neurological Disorders and Stroke (NINDS).

"Treatment is far superior to no treatment and treatment with either aspirin or warfarin is safe under carefully monitored conditions," says J. P. Mohr, MD, director of the Stroke Unit at New York's Columbia University and lead investigator of the trial.

Both drugs slow clotting of the blood, and blood clots are involved in the final stages of the most common type of stroke due to blockage

---

This chapter includes "Study Shows That Aspirin and Warfarin Are Equally Effective for Stroke Prevention," Research Notebook, January-February 2002 *FDA Consumer*, U.S. Food and Drug Administration; "What Are Anticoagulants and Antiplatelet Agents?" reprinted with permission from the American Heart Association World Wide Web Site, www.americanheart.org. © 2002, Copyright American Heart Association; and "Two-Thirds of Elderly Stroke Survivors in Nursing Homes Are Not Receiving Medication to Prevent Further Strokes," *Research*, September 2001, Agency for Healthcare Research Quality (AHRQ).

of the vessels that supply oxygen-rich blood to the brain. Aspirin affects the blood platelets, while warfarin inhibits circulating clotting proteins in the blood. Aspirin has been used for over 100 years, but its beneficial effects to prevent stroke and heart attack only started to be recognized in the 1970s. Whether warfarin was superior to aspirin for stroke prevention was unclear prior to WARSS. Numerous previous studies have proven that use of aspirin reduces recurrent stroke by about 25 percent. Part of the controversy about aspirin versus warfarin for stroke prevention has been the thinking among clinicians that warfarin may be a better blood thinner than aspirin to prevent almost all forms of stroke, but that it has greater side effects, increased risk of hemorrhage, and higher costs due to the need for blood tests to monitor the treatment effect for patients.

An earlier NINDS trial, Stroke Prevention in Atrial Fibrillation Study (SPAF), cleared up some of the confusion by showing a distinct benefit of warfarin over aspirin in preventing recurrent stroke in patients whose stroke was related to atrial fibrillation (AF)—strokes caused by clots coming from the heart. About 15 percent of stroke patients have this heart rhythm abnormality, a condition in which the two upper chambers of the heart (the atria) do not have a rhythmic, forceful beat, and the pulse is irregular. Although the superior efficacy of warfarin versus aspirin in preventing recurrent stroke in patients with atrial fibrillation was confirmed in SPAF, greater insight was needed to determine optimal therapy in preventing recurrent stroke in the larger number of patients without clots in the heart, which was the purpose of the WARSS study.

"We had evidence that patients with AF should be taking warfarin, but we didn't know which medicine to recommend to stroke patients without AF," said John R. Marler, MD, Associate Director for Clinical Trials for the NINDS. "This scientifically sound definitive clinical trial provides important information in the fight against stroke. It supports the widespread use of aspirin and other antiplatelet drugs, but it demonstrates an equally efficacious alternative, appropriate for selected patients," he added.

To make the aspirin and warfarin arms of the study as unbiased as possible, the investigators matched both groups of patients for primary stroke severity, age, gender, education, and race/ethnicity. The two groups were also matched for stroke risk factors, including hypertension, diabetes, cardiac disease, smoking, alcohol consumption, and physical activity. The investigators used an aspirin dose of 325 mg/day and a warfarin dose specifically tailored to each individual patient, and a double-blind plan in which neither the treating doctor nor the patient knew which treatment was being received.

The study included patients who had strokes due to small vessel lacunar infarcts, the predominant type of stroke in people with diabetes; strokes due to large artery atherosclerosis (build-up of cholesterol plaques); and cryptogenic stroke of undetermined cause. The study excluded patients with atrial fibrillation, those with a blood clot in the heart, and those eligible for carotid endarterectomy surgery. For these patients, appropriate treatment guidelines already exist from earlier NINDS-sponsored clinical trials. For safety, patients with a history of severe bleeding from any cause and patients whose strokes were related to surgical procedures were not included in the trial.

Several subsets of patients seemed to show slight benefits from one of the two therapies, but neither of the treatments showed a difference greater than would be expected from chance alone. The lacunar infarct and small vessel disease subgroup seemed to fare better with aspirin, as did, to a lesser extent, the large artery disease subgroup. The cryptogenic subgroup appeared to fare better with warfarin, but investigators believe some of these patients have a tendency to form blood clots in the heart. Four parallel studies for WARSS are looking for groups of patients who might gain more benefit from warfarin or aspirin. Additional analysis of the WARSS data may point to differences in the ability of aspirin and warfarin to prevent stroke for some patients. Overall, there was no evidence of significant differences between the two drugs.

Stroke is the third leading cause of death in the United States and the leading cause of serious, long-term disability. Approximately 600,000 new strokes are reported in the United States annually and about 160,000 Americans die each year from stroke.

Bristol-Myers Squibb Company provided an unrestricted educational grant for this study.

* Mohr, J.P.; Thompson, J.L.P.; Lazar, R.M.; Levin, B.; Sacco, R.L.; Furie, K.L.; Kistler. J.P.; Albers, G.W.; Pettigrew, L.C.; Adams, H.P., Jr.; Jackson, C.M.; Pullicino, P.; and the WARSS Study Group. *The New England Journal of Medicine*, November 15, 2001, Vol. 345, pp. 1444-1445.

## What Are Anticoagulants and Antiplatelet Agents?

Both anticoagulants (an-ty-ko-AG-u-lants) and antiplatelet (an-ty-PLAYT-lit) agents are medicines that reduce blood clotting in an artery, a vein, or the heart. Such clots can block the blood flow to your heart and cause a heart attack. Clots also can break loose from the inner wall of the artery or heart and become stuck in smaller vessels, which also reduces vital blood flow.

## What Should I Know about Anticoagulants?

Anticoagulants (sometimes called blood thinners) are drugs that cause your blood to take longer to clot. They can keep harmful clots from forming in your heart, veins, or arteries. Clots like this can block the blood flow and cause a heart attack or stroke.

- Common names are warfarin, coumadin, and heparin.

- You must take anticoagulants just the way your doctor tells you.

- You will need blood tests regularly so your doctor can tell how they're working.

- You must tell other doctors and dentists that you're taking anticoagulants.

- Never take aspirin with anticoagulants unless your doctor tells you to.

- You must ask your doctor before taking anything else—such as vitamins, cold medicine, sleeping pills, or antibiotics.

- Tell your family how you take them and carry your emergency medical ID card with you.

## Could Anticoagulants Cause Problems?

If you do as your doctor tells you, there probably won't be problems. But you must tell your doctor right away if:

- Your urine turns pink or red.

- Your stools turn red, dark brown, or black.

- You bleed more than normal when you have your period.

- Your gums bleed.

- You have a very bad headache or stomach pain that doesn't go away.

- You get sick or feel weak, faint, or dizzy.

- You think you're pregnant.

- You often find bruises or blood blisters.

- You have an accident of any kind.

436

## What Are Antiplatelet Agents?

These drugs, such as aspirin, keep blood clots from forming. Many doctors now prescribe aspirin to heart patients for this reason.

## How Does Aspirin Help?

Aspirin is a medicine that can save your life if you have heart problems. You don't need a prescription to get it, but it's just as important as any other medicine your doctor tells you to take. You must use it just as you're told, and not in your own way. You should know that aspirin:

• Helps keep blood from clotting.

• Has been shown to reduce the risk of a second heart attack, stroke, or TIA.

• Should not be taken with anticoagulants unless your doctor tells you to.

• Must be used as your doctor orders—most often in small doses every day or every other day.

• Might not be taken while you're having surgery.

## How Can I Learn More?

Talk to your doctor, nurse, or healthcare professional. Or call your local American Heart Association at 1-800-242-8721. If you have heart disease, members of your family also may be at higher risk. It's very important for them to make changes now to lower their risk.

## Two-Thirds of Elderly Stroke Survivors in Nursing Homes Are Not Receiving Medication to Prevent Further Strokes

Stroke remains the third leading cause of death among Americans and the leading cause of nursing home placement. Unfortunately, two-thirds (67 percent) of stroke survivors in nursing homes do not receive anticoagulant or antiplatelet drug therapy to prevent further strokes, according to the findings of a study that was supported in part by the Agency for Healthcare Research and Quality (HS11256).

Those over 85 years of age were 14 percent less likely to be treated than those 65 to 74 years of age (odds ratio, OR 0.86). Black residents were 20 percent less likely to be treated than whites (OR 0.80), even though blacks have a greater risk of stroke. Residents with severe cognitive or physical impairment were about one-third less likely (OR 0.63 and 0.69, respectively) to receive treatment than those without impairments.

Patient contraindications to blood-thinning drugs, such as gastrointestinal bleeding and peptic ulcer disease, contributed to physicians' decisions not to treat them. However, they did not fully account for the large gap between recommended and observed levels of treatment, note Brown University researchers, Brian J. Quilliam, Ph.D., and Kate L. Lapane, Ph.D. Using the SAGE (Systematic Assessment of Geriatric drug use via Epidemiology) database, they obtained information on all residents diagnosed with stroke from 1992 to 1995 at Medicare/Medicaid-certified nursing homes in five States. They used logistic regression modeling to identify independent predictors of stroke prevention drug treatment, including aspirin, dipyridamole, ticlopidine, and warfarin alone or in combination with another drug.

Among those treated, most received aspirin alone (16 percent) or warfarin alone (10 percent). The prevalence of atrial fibrillation, which markedly elevates stroke risk, increased with age in these patients, but the use of warfarin decreased with advancing age. Perhaps doctors fear the increased risk of bleeding from warfarin among the elderly or feel they cannot adequately monitor high-risk patients, note the researchers. They suggest that pharmacist-run anticoagulant clinics might alleviate some of these concerns.

In conclusion, Drs. Quilliam and Lapane draw attention to their findings which indicate differential treatment along racial/ethnic lines. Because they did not have any information on educational level, income, or occupation, it was not possible for them to evaluate the effect of race/ethnicity within the context of socioeconomic position. They note that they are unaware of any physiological reasons justifying such differential treatment and voice concern about the underlying reasons for the disparities. The researchers call for further research to explore the effect of race/ethnicity within a social context on the decision to treat or not treat elderly stroke survivors.

## Additional Reading

"Clinical correlates and drug treatment of residents with stroke in long-term care," by Drs. Quilliam and Lapane, in the June 2001 *Stroke* 32, pp. 1385-1393.

Chapter 44

# Estrogen Doesn't Prevent Second Strokes

## Protective Effects of Hormone Replacement Therapy Challenged

Estrogen hormone replacement therapy does not reduce the risk of stroke or death in postmenopausal women who have already had a stroke or a transient ischemic attack (TIA), according to a report from the first randomized, controlled clinical trial of estrogen therapy for secondary prevention of cerebrovascular disease.

Previous observational studies have suggested that estrogen replacement therapy may reduce the risk of stroke and death in postmenopausal women. However, it was not clear whether the apparent benefits of estrogen among women in those studies were due to the hormone therapy or other factors. The new randomized, double-blind, placebo-controlled study, called the Women's Estrogen for Stroke Trial (WEST), was designed to resolve this question. The study, led by Ralph I. Horwitz, MD, of the Yale University School of Medicine, was funded by the National Institute of Neurological Disorders and Stroke (NINDS) and was published in the October 25, 2001, issue of *The New England Journal of Medicine.**

"Estrogen Doesn't Prevent Second Strokes: Protective Effects of Hormone Replacement Therapy Challenged," NIH News Release: Thursday, October 25, 2001, National Institute of Neurological Diseases and Stroke (NINDS); and excerpts from "Postmenopausal Hormone Therapy: WHI HRT Update: 2002," National Heart, Lung, and Blood Institute (NHLBI).

"The good news is that we have taken a lot of guesswork out of treating women with strokes. The benefits from estrogen that we hoped for are not there to balance the risks," says John R. Marler, MD, NINDS Associate Director for Clinical Trials.

Based on this finding, the investigators say, estrogen therapy should not be prescribed for the purpose of preventing a second stroke or death in postmenopausal women. Postmenopausal women who are already taking estrogen or who wish to take it for other reasons should seek the advice of their personal physicians to decide whether to continue or start therapy. Estrogen has rarely been prescribed specifically for stroke prevention, says Lawrence M. Brass, MD, of the Yale University School of Medicine, principal neurologist on the study. However, it has been widely prescribed for prevention of osteoporosis (thinning of the bones) and relief of menopausal symptoms such as hot flashes.

The researchers enrolled 664 postmenopausal women with an average age of 71 years who had experienced an ischemic stroke or a TIA within the previous 90 days. Ischemic strokes and TIAs result from blockages in the vessels that supply blood to the brain. Participants were given a number of initial assessments, including the NIH Stroke Scale (NIHSS) of neurological impairment and the Barthel index of functional ability in activities of daily living. In addition to the usual best care for patients who have had a stroke, women in the trial received either oral estrogen (estradiol 17-beta at the standard replacement dose of 1 mg daily) or a matching placebo. Patients were studied for an average of 2.8 years. They stopped receiving the estrogen or placebo if they had a stroke. The researchers found that there was no significant difference in the incidence of stroke or death in the women who were randomly assigned to receive estrogen instead of placebo. However, they found that the incidence of death due to stroke was higher in the estrogen group and that the non-fatal strokes in that group were associated with slightly worse neurological and functional impairments at 1 month after stroke. The risk of stroke within the first 6 months after enrollment in the study was also higher among women in the estrogen group. There were no significant differences between treatment groups in the number of TIAs or non-fatal heart attacks. However, participants receiving estrogen were more likely to experience gynecologic complications, particularly vaginal bleeding.

While this is the first controlled clinical trial to evaluate estrogen for stroke prevention, the results are similar to findings from the Heart and Estrogen/Progestin Replacement Study (HERS), the first placebo-controlled randomized clinical trial of hormone replacement therapy for prevention of heart disease in postmenopausal women who had pre-existing heart disease. The HERS results, published in 1998, showed that treating these women with a combination of estrogen and progestin did not reduce heart attacks or death from heart disease. That study also found no reduction in strokes among women who received the study drug.

While the WEST study provides important information about the use of estrogen in women with existing cerebrovascular disease, many questions remain to be answered, according to the investigators. They are planning additional analyses of their data to look at the effects of estrogen on cognition and physical function. The study results also may change researchers' understanding of how estrogen affects blood vessels and lead to new research in that area, says Dr. Horwitz.

## Women's Health Initiative (WHI) Hormone Replacement Therapy Update: 2002

The WHI Hormone Program is studying two types of hormone pills. One is estrogen plus progestin in women who had not had a hysterectomy before joining the WHI. The other is estrogen alone in women who already had a hysterectomy before joining.

The WHI Data and Safety Monitoring Board (DSMB) reviewed the health status of women in the Women's Health Initiative in 2002. Based on this review, the DSMB recommended that:

• Women in the study of estrogen plus progestin stop their study pills, because the risks now exceed the benefits.

• Women in the study of estrogen alone continue taking their study pills as before, because it remains uncertain whether the benefits outweigh the risks.

### How Many Women Were Affected?

Only 2.5% of women in the estrogen plus progestin study had these health events. These results tell us that during one year, for every 10,000 women taking estrogen plus progestin, we would expect:

• 7 more women with heart attacks. In other words, 37 women taking estrogen plus progestin would have heart attacks compared to 30 women taking placebo.

• 8 more women with strokes.

- 8 more women with breast cancer.

- 18 more women with blood clots.


These results also suggest that for every 10,000 women taking estrogen plus progestin we would expect:

- 6 fewer colorectal cancers.

- 5 fewer hip fractures.

- Fewer fractures in other bones.


In summary, more women taking estrogen plus progestin had a serious health event than did women taking placebo. We conclude that estrogen plus progestin does not prevent heart disease and is not beneficial overall.

*Viscoli, C. M.; Brass, L.M.; Kernan, W.N.; Sarrel, P.M.; Suissa, S.; Horwitz, R.I. "Estrogen Replacement after Ischemic Stroke: Report of the Women's Estrogen for Stroke Trial (WEST)." *The New England Journal of Medicine*, October 25, 2001, Vol. 345, No. 17, pp. 1243-1249.

Chapter 45

# Community-Based Interventions: Looking at the Stroke Belt Initiative

People choose behaviors that affect their health because of a number of factors, including social, financial, environmental, and cultural issues. Overcoming cultural barriers and other elements to change behavior in a specific population is an ongoing challenge for health care professionals. Another is intervening to persuade someone to change behavior when the payoff lies in the distant future and the current behavior has immediate rewards.

Over the past 20 years, the NHLBI has supported multidisciplinary studies to examine what impact interventions have on the social and environmental factors that have a positive influence on health behaviors or policies. On September 25-26, 1996, more than 100 scientists representing various disciplines gathered on the NIH campus to participate in an NHLBI-sponsored conference, "Community Trials for Cardiopulmonary Health: Directions for Public Health Practice, Policy, and Research." The conference focused on what has been learned from two decades of intervention research involving intact groups, as are found in schools, work sites, medical practices, religious organizations, and entire communities.

An understanding of the target population is essential to the effectiveness of an intervention program. This includes knowledge of how the population has been informed or misinformed about a particular

"Taking It to the Streets: Community-Based Interventions," *Heart Memo*, Summer 1997, National Heart, Lung, and Blood Institute (NHLBI), reviewed in November 2002 by David A. Cooke, MD, Diplomate, American Board of Internal Medicine.

disease. It also includes knowing whether people are aware of the risks and how they can minimize or increase their risk by lifestyle choices.

## The Tie That Binds the South

Getting recognition can be a tricky business. Take what happened in the southeastern United States. That part of the country is recognized for having high humidity, great college basketball, and uncommon hospitality. All acceptable characteristics. But almost two decades ago, the NHLBI recognized 11 States in the Southeast for having the highest death rates from stroke in the country—10 percent higher than average. Forget the humidity. Forget the basketball. Forget the hospitality. These States—Alabama, Arkansas, Georgia, Indiana, Kentucky, Louisiana, Mississippi, North Carolina, South Carolina, Tennessee, and Virginia—became known as the Stroke Belt.

The NHLBI responded to the recognition by creating a special initiative to lower the risk of stroke in these States through community-based education and prevention programs. "The initiative was unique in many ways," according to Mr. Glen Bennett, NHLBI project officer for the Stroke Belt Initiative.

Notably, the NHLBI's first step was to convene representatives from each State to hear their assessments of the problem and the need. "We realized that local health departments know their populations better than anyone else, and so we wanted to help them put their ideas to work," explained Bennett.

The NHLBI funding allowed States to implement activities in four categories: (1) problem assessment, (2) evaluation and data analysis, (3) educational interventions, and (4) community organization techniques. Most States selected one category, but some responded to multiple categories. Pilot projects for many States paralleled what they had described during the initial meeting.

The NHLBI provided phase I funding for 1-year pilot projects that demonstrated the States' capacity to design and implement projects aimed at reducing risk factors for stroke in their communities. The funding was directed to State health departments because they are ultimately responsible for addressing health concerns within the States. Phase II funding allowed States to deliver effective health education interventions, using the methods and materials from the pilot projects.

The projects, which lasted 2 to 3 years, were in one of four general education/intervention categories: (1) interventions in health department clinics and outreach services, (2) church-based risk factor intervention programs, (3) community education and intervention programs, or (4) public education campaigns using the mass media.

In spite of these and other best efforts, stroke or cerebrovascular disease remains the third leading cause of death in the United States. More than half a million Americans have a stroke each year—150,000 die as a result. High blood pressure is an established risk factor for stroke, and recently cigarette smoking and obesity have been identified as significant risk factors.

Principal investigators and key staff members for Stroke Belt Initiative projects convened May 9 and 10, 1996, at Morgan State University in Baltimore to review their accomplishments and reflect on lessons learned.

## Highlights of State Projects

**Alabama** used Stroke Belt Initiative funding to improve and expand existing detection, treatment, and follow-up interventions in health department clinics. The State was able to improve the quality of care and increase the number of people receiving care by using quality assurance (QA) audits and a patient recruitment program for county health department clinics with low patient loads. The State established clinical standards as well as administrative/environmental standards. QA teams visited clinics to review patient charts for compliance. A paid patient recruiter worked with clinics to increase clinic usage. Health departments offered blood pressure monitoring, free or low-cost medication, and patient counseling for Alabama's medically indigent population.

**Arkansas** formed planning groups or coalitions in the State's 10 counties with the highest stroke mortality. The coalitions were organized and convened by a project coordinator who was hired by the health department and who planned and implemented activities. Health fairs were the predominant sponsored activity, supplemented by church- or school-based programs such as nutrition workshops or hypertension screenings.

**Georgia** conducted a mass media campaign to encourage people with hypertension to remain on treatment. The centerpiece of the campaign, Strike Out Stroke (SOS), spotlighted activities during selected Atlanta Braves games. SOS also broadcast public service announcements and received live media coverage, including features on African-American gospel and talk radio programs. The print component

445

targeted small, local newspapers by issuing feature articles, health reports, human interest stories, and letters to the editor. Georgia installed automated equipment in State office buildings to measure blood pressure, pulse rate, and weight. Partnered with the Georgia Stroke Belt Consortium, the project developed easy-to-read materials; conducted screenings at churches, community centers, and State office buildings; and sponsored SOS contests in churches.

**Indiana** expanded its focus after the pilot to include smoking cessation in addition to hypertension control. The project targeted low-income populations at two health centers in Indianapolis and their adjacent housing projects. The smoking cessation component included community awareness and education. Smoking cessation participants also received nicotine replacement patches and behavior modification counseling. A health educator offered individual counseling and conducted onsite presentations and risk factor screenings. Health educators helped patients with high blood pressure set goals or lifestyle changes. The project also developed an electronic database for patient tracking and evaluation.

**Kentucky** developed a program for public health nurses in their function as educators and role models, as well as obesity, smoking cessation, and hypertension. The project also conducted smoking cessation classes to reduce the number of nursing staff members who smoke. Nurses were taught to give effective advice to patients on smoking cessation. They also led smoking cessation classes and support groups at health departments. Low-income smokers who attended support groups received free nicotine patches and follow-up counseling.

**Louisiana** focused on establishing hypertension prevention and control programs in African-American churches. Some churches also conducted weight loss and smoking cessation sessions. The project established programs in 26 churches in the New Orleans area during phase I. Phase II was a 2-year effort to involve churches in other areas of the State. Consultants were hired from the targeted communities to recruit churches and help them organize and establish the programs. The project provided a 4-hour training workshop for the health care ministry teams established in each participating church to plan and conduct the activities and a blood pressure measurement course for students. Several churches identified their best cooks, and a project nutritionist worked with them to make their favorite recipes heart healthy. The dishes were tested at church-sponsored food events and then published in a cookbook, *Soul Food Cooking the Heart Healthy Way*.

**Mississippi** conducted a stroke education and intervention program targeted for high-risk populations in medically underserved counties with an extremely high—41 percent—rate of poverty among African-Americans. The project installed automated equipment in the courthouse and public health clinic of each participating county to give free blood pressure readings. The machines displayed a message instructing persons with elevated results to see a doctor and displayed a toll-free telephone number for those without access to care. A project nurse answered the calls and helped patients find care, medication, nutrition counseling, and social services as needed. To augment the automated screenings, trained teams offered hypertension screenings at churches, community centers, civic organizations, health fairs, schools, banks and other businesses, and other community gatherings. The project staff wrote *The Angry Heart*, a one-act play for elementary school children that promoted healthy lifestyles.

**North Carolina** combined a mass media campaign with community outreach and professional education to address high blood pressure in African-Americans. Media representatives and local community leaders developed culturally appropriate educational messages. Staff members, health care professionals, and other volunteers were trained to give interviews on hypertension to local television and radio programs and newspapers. Community outreach activities included the dissemination of easy-to-read educational materials, poster and letter writing contests in churches, hypertension screenings at fast food restaurants and convenience stores, and risk factor reduction classes in community centers. The project also compiled the educational materials developed by the project into a resource guide to distribute to health agencies across the State.

**South Carolina** focused on African-Americans because they have more than twice the stroke mortality rates of whites—65.4 percent versus 31.8 percent per 100,000 population. The goal of the project was to improve hypertension awareness, treatment, and control while increasing the number of community-based programs. The project used three channels in the community: churches, the media, and beauty shops and barbershops. This capacity-building project developed training manuals to help health professionals and volunteers develop stroke prevention initiatives within each of these channels.

447

**Tennessee** targeted African-Americans in three metropolitan counties where nearly 70 percent of all African-Americans in the State reside. The project's goal was to enable each county to organize and develop stroke education and prevention activities. One of the three counties formed a coalition that provided leadership and community involvement to the project. The coalition also formed a Youth Mentor Program to carry out smoking education, prevention, and cessation activities for adults and youths. The State focused primarily on recruiting African-American churches to develop and carry out programs for their congregations on smoking cessation, nutrition education, and weight management. Many church teams used creative ways to communicate health messages to their congregations, such as children's letter writing campaigns, food tasting events, plays, and a youth mentor program.

**Virginia** formed a unique collaboration between the Virginia Department of Health (VDH) and the Baptist General Convention of Virginia (BGC), an association of more than 1,000 independent African-American churches in the State whose members total more than 200,000. The VDH and the BGC focused on three risk factors—high blood pressure, smoking, and obesity. The director of the BGC health care ministry worked with volunteer coordinators to recruit churches, train volunteers, and support church activities. The project developed training manuals for the hypertension component, including one for training trainers, and an educational piece for the congregation, *Stroke Busters*. The smoking cessation and obesity components used existing materials, cleverly redesigned around appropriate themes, such as "Thank God I'm Free (TGIF)" and "Taking Responsibility in Meal Management (TRIMM)."

## Lessons Learned

### Working with Churches

- Patience and time are required to organize and implement health programs in churches.

- No best way exists to recruit churches and sustain their participation.

- Support from the clergy is essential.

- The creativity of church teams to reach their congregations should be encouraged.

- The coordinator of a church health care ministry or team is critical to the motivation of the team members.

## *Working in the Community*

- Quality control audits can improve the level of care for patients with hypertension in health department clinics.

- Patient recruitment and outreach can increase the use of local clinics.

- Development of coalitions takes time.

- Programs that can be integrated into the health center's basic services and that gain the support of administrators and clinicians are likely to be sustained.

- Automated equipment can contribute to hypertension detection and control efforts.

## Additional Information

### *NHLBI Information Center*
P.O. Box 30105
Bethesda, MD 20824-0105
Toll-Free: 800-575-WELL (9355)
Tel: 301-592-8573
Fax: 301-592-8563
Website: www.nhlbi.nih.gov
E-mail: NHLBIinfo@rover.nhlbi.nih.gov

Chapter 46

# Stroke Treatment and Ongoing Prevention Act

February 6, 2002 the United States Senate passed the Stroke Treatment and Ongoing Prevention Act, S1274, the first comprehensive federal legislation to address stroke and the toll it takes on millions of Americans. The legislation, spearheaded by the National Stroke Association, will improve stroke care by providing resources for stroke education, research, and patient care programs across the country.

Specifically, the bill authorizes $40 million for a national education campaign to promote stroke prevention and increase the number of stroke patients who seek immediate treatment. Additionally, it establishes a grant program for states to develop statewide stroke care systems, providing $425 million in funding over the next five years.

Stroke is the third leading cause of death and the number one cause of adult disability in the United States. Each year stroke affects more than 750,000 Americans, kills 160,000 individuals, and costs the nation more than $45 billion in direct and indirect costs.

The legislation also authorizes funding for stroke research, professional development grants for stroke care, and maintenance of the Paul Coverdell National Acute Stroke Registry. The registry, named in honor of Sen. Coverdell who died from a stroke, is a clearinghouse of data and analysis of acute stroke patients, and will serve as a tool for health officials to track and improve the delivery of stroke care.

"Senate Passes Landmark Legislation to Improve Stroke Care Nationwide," News Release: Thursday, February 7, 2002, © National Stroke Association, reprinted with permission.

"The National Stroke Association believes that the STOP Stroke Act is historic, groundbreaking legislation," said Patti Shwayder, executive director/CEO. "We are pleased that the U.S. Senate recognizes that stroke is a preventable and treatable medical condition. I want to thank Sens. Kennedy and Frist for their leadership in raising this issue higher on the public health agenda, and we urge the House of Representatives to take swift action on this critical legislation," said Shwayder. A companion bill, H.R. 3431 sponsored by Representatives Capps and Pickering, has been introduced in the House with more than 90 co-sponsors.

Research shows that public awareness of the warning signs of stroke is alarmingly poor. In fact, nearly 40 percent of adults do not know that stroke occurs in the brain and more than 20 percent do not know how to prevent a stroke.

Based in Englewood, Colo., National Stroke Association is a leading independent national non-profit organization devoting 100 percent of its efforts and resources to stroke—including prevention, treatment, rehabilitation, and support for stroke survivors and their families.

## Additional Information

### National Stroke Association
9707 East Easter Lane
Englewood, CO 80112-3747
Toll-Free: 800-STROKES (800-787-6537)
Tel: 303-649-9299
Fax: 303-649-1328
Website: www.stroke.org

Chapter 47

# Stroke Initiatives and Current Research

## 2002 Stroke Testimony by Audrey S. Penn, MD

Mr. Chairman and Members of the Committee, I am Dr. Audrey Penn, Acting Director of the National Institute of Neurological Disorders and Stroke (NINDS). I am pleased to be here before you today to discuss our efforts in addressing stroke—the third leading cause of death in the United States after heart disease and cancer, and a leading cause of long-term disability. The National Institute of Neurological Disorders and Stroke at the National Institutes of Health (NIH) is the leading federal organization committed to research on improving stroke prevention, treatment, and recovery, through increased understanding of how to protect and restore the brain. Historically, NINDS has committed more funding to stroke research than to any other single disease or disorder within our mission. In Fiscal Year (FY) 2001, NINDS funding for stroke research was more than $117 million, and the NIH total was nearly $239 million. More importantly, our stroke programs impact all areas of scientific opportunity and public health priority—from stroke awareness to rehabilitation—and are advancing the state of cutting-edge knowledge about the ways to prevent, diagnose, treat, and educate the public and health professionals about stroke.

"2002 Stroke Testimony Statement of Audrey S. Penn, MD Acting Director National Institute of Neurological Disorders and Stroke before the House Committee on Energy and Commerce Subcommittee on Health," June 6, 2002, National Institute of Neurological Disorders and Stroke (NINDS).

## Background

As many of you know, a stroke is a brain attack caused by an interruption of blood flow to the brain. There are two different types of stroke—ischemic and hemorrhagic. Ischemic strokes occur when blood flowing to a region of the brain is reduced or blocked, either by a blood clot or by the narrowing of a vessel supplying blood to the brain. Approximately 80 percent of all strokes are ischemic. The remaining 20 percent of strokes are caused by the rupture of a blood vessel, and leakage of blood into the brain tissue. These hemorrhagic strokes can occur from the rupture of an aneurysm, which is a blood-filled sac ballooning from a vessel wall, or leakage from a vessel wall itself weakened by an underlying condition like high blood pressure.

At every conceivable level, stroke is a tremendous public health burden to our country. More than 600,000 people experience a stroke each year. Of the more than 4 million stroke survivors alive today, many experience permanent impairments of their ability to move, think, understand and use language, or speak—losses that compromise their independence and quality of life. Furthermore, stroke risk increases with age, and as the American population is growing older, the number of persons at risk for experiencing a stroke is increasing. Over the past several decades, NINDS has supported some of the most significant achievements in stroke research, which have contributed to reductions in the death rate from stroke. We continue to be committed to reducing this burden.

## Historical Progress in Stroke Prevention and Treatment

NINDS has a long and distinguished history of supporting productive clinical studies in the field of stroke prevention and acute treatment. Indeed, successes in prevention date back more than twenty years, and there has been remarkable progress in stroke prevention—which reflects sustained efforts of private organizations, NIH, and other government agencies. Stroke prevention is also highly cost-effective because it averts the direct costs of hospitalization and rehabilitation. As NINDS celebrated its 50th anniversary, the U.S. Centers for Disease Control and Prevention estimated that the age-standardized stroke death rate declined by 70 percent for the U.S. population from 1950 to 1996 [*MMWR Weekly* 48:649-56 1999], and the American Heart Association tallied a 15 percent decline just from 1988 to 1998. I would like to briefly summarize a few of the major NINDS-supported efforts, which have included dozens of clinical trials, which have contributed significantly to our knowledge of stroke.

Several early studies investigated medical management approaches to the prevention of recurrent strokes in people with atrial fibrillation (AF). This irregular heart rate and rhythm is a common disorder in older Americans, and a significant stroke risk factor. It has been estimated that two million Americans, primarily over the age of 60, have AF and are six times more likely to have a stroke as a result. The drugs aspirin and warfarin had been used to prevent recurrent stroke in these individuals, however their use was based on little hard scientific evidence. To address this issue, NINDS supported a series of three trials in Stroke Prevention in Atrial Fibrillation— referred to as the SPAF trials. The SPAF I, II, and III trials evaluated the use of aspirin and warfarin for stroke prevention in more than 3,800 human subjects. The SPAF I study reported in 1990 that both aspirin and warfarin were so beneficial in preventing stroke in patients with atrial fibrillation that the risk of stroke was cut by 50 to 80 percent. The results suggested that 20,000 to 30,000 strokes could be prevented each year with proper treatment. The SPAF II study results in 1994 identified the 60 percent of people with atrial fibrillation for whom a daily adult aspirin provides adequate protection against stroke with minimal complications. This group consists of those younger than 75 and those older than 75 with no additional stroke risk factors such as high blood pressure or heart disease. SPAF III, which included 1,044 patients at 20 medical centers in the U.S. and Canada, studied the remaining 40 percent of atrial fibrillation patients with additional risk factors for stroke and for whom warfarin had been shown to be effective. The study was stopped ahead of schedule in 1996 because early results clearly demonstrated the benefit of standard warfarin therapy over the combination therapy of aspirin and fixed-dose warfarin, in these high-risk patients. Other reports have estimated that the use of warfarin to prevent strokes in persons with AF costs as much as $1,000 annually, but a year of post-stroke treatment can cost $25,000. Based on these estimates, optimal use of standard warfarin therapy in the appropriate patients could prevent as many as 40,000 strokes a year in the U.S., and save nearly $600 million a year in health care costs.

Other studies supported by the Institute, such as the Warfarin Antiplatelet Recurrent Stroke Study, the Vitamin Intervention for Stroke Prevention Study, the African-American Antiplatelet Stroke Prevention Study, and the Women's Estrogen for Stroke Trial, build on these earlier findings, and continue to add to our knowledge about medical interventions that can affect the incidence of stroke in different at-risk groups.

The NINDS has also supported several major studies of surgical approaches to the secondary prevention of stroke. This work has particular significance for people with carotid artery stenosis, a narrowing of the major blood vessels that supply the brain. One definitive study in the late 1970s examined a procedure called extracranial/intracranial (EC/IC) bypass. EC/IC bypass had been used for several years as a means to restore blood flow to the brain. The NINDS-funded study of the procedure's effectiveness found that the data did not support its continued use in medical practice to prevent stroke. These findings were of significant benefit to patients, who could avoid the risks and costs of this surgery, and to researchers, who used this information to redirect their attention to other promising approaches. As a result, investigators explored an alternative surgical strategy, called carotid endarterectomy, which involves the removal of fatty deposits, or plaque, in the carotid arteries. In two NINDS-funded trials—the North American Symptomatic Carotid Endarterectomy Trial (NASCET), and the Asymptomatic Carotid Atherosclerosis Study (ACAS)—this approach was examined more extensively.

The results of the 12-year NASCET trial were reported in two stages. The investigators' early data led to a radical change in the recommended treatment for severe (70-99 percent) carotid stenosis, or blockage, when it was determined that, together with appropriate medical care, carotid endarterectomy for patients with severe blockage prevented more strokes than did medical treatment alone. NINDS responded to this finding by halting the part of the study involving patients with severe blockage, and issuing a nationwide alert to physicians asking them to consider the study results in making recommendations to their patients. The rest of the study focused on determining the efficacy of this surgery for symptomatic patients with moderate carotid stenosis (30-69 percent blockage). Those results showed that patients with the higher grades of moderate stenosis (50-69 percent) clearly benefit from surgery. There was no significant benefit for patients with less than 50 percent stenosis. As a result of the NASCET trial, patients with moderate stenosis are better able to decide whether to risk surgery in order to prevent possible future strokes.

In the ACAS trial, carotid endarterectomy was found highly beneficial for persons who are symptom-free, but have a carotid stenosis of 60 to 99 percent. In this group, the surgery reduces the estimated 5-year risk of stroke by more than one-half, from about 1 in 10 to less than 1 in 20.

To the long list of studies contributing to improvements in secondary stroke prevention, we can add a more recent NINDS-funded trial, which resulted in the first FDA-approved acute treatment for ischemic stroke, in 1996. This therapy—tissue plasminogen activator or tPA—dissolves blood clots and restores blood flow, if given intravenously within the first three hours after an ischemic stroke. Patients must be screened carefully before receiving tPA, since it is not appropriate for use in treating hemorrhagic stroke, and should not be given beyond the three-hour window. However, in carefully selected patients, use of tPA can achieve a complete recovery. Unfortunately many, indeed most, stroke patients do not receive tPA because they do not arrive at the hospital in time to be evaluated and treated within the crucial three-hour window of effectiveness. Or, in many cases, hospitals are not prepared to rapidly identify and treat these patients. It is this dual challenge that NINDS is actively pursuing through the development of model systems and through education and outreach efforts that are discussed later in my testimony.

## Recent Advances

Within the framework of these historical successes, NINDS continues to build its basic science and clinical stroke programs, and to reap the rewards of past investments. A sampling of these recent advances includes:

### The Use of Medical Therapy to Prevent Recurrent Stroke in People without Cardiac Risk Factors

As described, past clinical studies provided important information about preventing recurrent stroke in people with cardiac arrhythmia. However, it has been difficult for physicians to choose between aspirin and warfarin for patients who do not present with cardiac risk factors. To help address these questions, another large clinical trial—the Warfarin versus Aspirin Recurrent Stroke Study (WARSS) was initiated with NINDS support. More than 2000 individuals with a history of stroke unrelated to cardiac problems participated in this study, with equal groups receiving aspirin and warfarin. After two years of treatment, there was no significant difference in the prevention of recurrent stroke or death, or in the rate of brain hemorrhage, in the aspirin and warfarin groups. This finding will likely have a major impact on the standard of care for this group of stroke survivors, since aspirin is considerably less expensive, safer, and easier to administer than warfarin.

### The Use of the Warning Signs of Stroke to Aid in Prevention

Recently, NINDS-funded researchers evaluated the risk of stroke after a transient ischemic attack (TIA), or mini-stroke. The symptoms of TIAs pass quickly, within a day or even hours, and are often ignored. After following 1700 people with a TIA, the study found that these episodes warn of a dramatically increased likelihood of experiencing a stroke within the subsequent 90-day period. Other risk factors, such as advanced age, other health conditions, and severity of the TIA, also helped to predict stroke risk, and may be useful in determining whether patients should be hospitalized immediately and/or receive preventive interventions following a TIA.

### The Development of Clinical Tools that Can Be Used to Predict Stroke Recovery

In order to offer clinicians the best possible methods for evaluating patients after a stroke, intramural investigators at NINDS have explored the types of clinical measurements and diagnostic tools that might be used to predict how well a person will recover from a stroke. They found that the combined use of a unique type of magnetic resonance imaging, the score on the NIH Stroke Scale—a diagnostic tool developed at NINDS for evaluating stroke patients, and the time from the onset of symptoms to the brain scan, can effectively predict the extent of stroke recovery. Future studies will focus on the potential of computerized tomography (CT) scanning to predict recovery as this is a technology more commonly available in most hospitals. We expect that all of these tools will help physicians manage patients more efficiently and reduce distress and anxiety among patients and their families.

### Brain Plasticity

Over the last several years research has revealed the remarkable extent of brain plasticity—that is, the capacity of the brain to change in response to experience or injury. Scientists are now using brain imaging techniques that reveal the activity of brain cells, as well as structure, to understand why some patients recover lost abilities following stroke and others do not. In other efforts, researchers are trying to apply what has been learned about brain plasticity to encourage stroke recovery through a method called constraint-induced therapy. This therapy involves constraining an unaffected extremity while actively exercising the affected one, thereby inducing use-dependent brain reorganization.

458

## The Use of Stem Cells to Treat Stroke in Animal Models

Stem cells are immature cells that can multiply and form more specialized cell types. Recent animal studies have provided evidence that transplanted stem cells can help restore brain function after stroke. Other animal research suggests that the adult brain may itself have a latent capacity to regenerate new cells following stroke, which might be encouraged in efforts to repair the brain. The continuing efforts to develop these approaches to restoration of function in survivors of stroke build on active NINDS support to understand the basic biology of animal embryonic stem cells and adult human stem cells. Within the President's policy guidelines, the Institute is encouraging research to evaluate the capabilities of human embryonic stem cells.

## Current Stroke Initiatives

The generous appropriations provided by Congress have made it possible for us to expand our programs in stroke, and we are grateful for the opportunity. Since the doubling of the NIH budget began in FY 1999, the Institute has initiated many new clinical and basic science projects. Currently, the Institute is supporting 14 Phase III clinical trials in stroke, eight of which have been initiated since the start of the doubling effort. Even more importantly, the doubling effort has enabled NINDS to fund 17 Phase I and II clinical trials in stroke. These numbers are impressive and indicate that many novel prevention strategies, therapeutic interventions, and rehabilitation techniques for stroke are closer to the clinic as a result of the significant investments in NIH over the past several years. Areas of clinical research that are under exploration include the use of hypothermia to improve outcome following aneurysm surgery, the use of magnesium to treat stroke, and improvements in stroke imaging techniques. Several studies, including research in the NINDS intramural program at the NIH Clinical Center, are examining various strategies for rehabilitation after stroke including the use of constraint therapy, exercise, anesthesia, and electrical stimulation to improve functional recovery.

NINDS also continues to be committed to exploring stroke at the basic science level, and has provided funding for many new projects since the doubling effort began. These include studies of procedures and drugs that may protect the brain against further injury, a possible vaccine for stroke, the role of inflammation, the expression of genes and proteins in response to stroke, and pre-clinical testing of

459

therapies—just to name a few. Cellular communications between blood vessels, neurons, and glia, and the role of the blood-brain barrier, are also subjects of intense interest. In addition to studies specifically targeted to stroke, NINDS also provides support for many areas of basic neuroscience research that have broad applicability to stroke and other brain injuries. These include mechanisms of cell survival and death, neural growth factors, stem cell therapy, neuronal plasticity, and glial cell biology.

In addition to the investigator-initiated projects that make up the core of our grant programs, NINDS is constantly looking for understudied areas in stroke research that the Institute could address through the use of targeted initiatives. Several years ago, NINDS identified a need for acute stroke centers, and in May 2001, we issued a grant solicitation for Specialized Programs of Translational Research in Acute Stroke (SPOTRIAS). The goal of the SPOTRIAS program is to reduce disability and mortality in stroke patients, by promoting rapid diagnosis and effective interventions. It will support a collaboration of clinical researchers from different specialties whose collective efforts will lead to new approaches to early diagnosis and treatment of acute stroke patients. In its report language for the Institute's FY2001 appropriation, the Senate also encouraged the creation of acute stroke research or treatment research centers to provide rapid, early, continuous 24-hour treatment to stroke victims, and noted that a dedicated area in a medical facility with resources, personnel, and equipment dedicated to treat stroke, would also provide an opportunity for early evaluation of stroke treatments. The SPOTRIAS program is responsive to the recommendation highlighted by the Senate. Institutions supported under this program must be able to deliver rapid treatment for acute stroke and to conduct the highest quality translational research on the diagnosis and treatment of acute ischemic and hemorrhagic stroke. They will also help to recruit and train the next generation of stroke researchers. The SPOTRIAS initiative will facilitate the translation of basic research findings into clinical research, and ultimately, the incorporation of clinical research findings into clinical practice. The first two centers have recently been approved for funding under this program, and as more centers are added, it is expected that they will form a national network that will lead to significant changes in the care of stroke patients.

On a more local level, NINDS is also developing the Acute Brain Attack Research Program in the Baltimore-Washington Area. This effort has already established a 24-hour stroke research program in diagnosis and treatment at Suburban Hospital in Bethesda, Maryland, and our plan is to replicate this program in other medical facilities in the Baltimore-Washington metropolitan area, next targeting those serving predominantly inner city minority populations.

## *Stroke Research Planning*

While a significant knowledge base about stroke has been amassed through research supported by the NINDS, continually emerging discoveries and new technologies create constantly increasing research needs and scientific opportunities. Coupled with the increases in the NINDS budget as a result of the recent NIH doubling effort, it is necessary to identify clear scientific priorities, so that the Institute can determine the best uses for its resources. Such priorities will also serve as benchmarks for the broader scientific community against which progress can be measured. NINDS convened a Stroke Progress Review Group (Stroke PRG) to identify priorities in stroke research. The Stroke PRG had its origins in Fiscal Year 2001 report language from the House and Senate Appropriations Committees to the NINDS urging us to develop a national research plan for stroke. Following on the success of the Brain Tumor Progress Review Group, a joint collaboration between NINDS and the National Cancer Institute to identify priorities for research on brain tumors, NINDS decided to use a Progress Review Group to develop a plan for stroke research. Members of the Stroke PRG include approximately 140 prominent scientists, clinicians, consumer advocates—including leaders from the American Stroke Association and the National Stroke Association, industry representatives, and participants from other NIH Institutes. Together, these individuals represent the full spectrum of expertise required to identify and prioritize scientific needs and opportunities that are critical to advancing the field of stroke research.

At the Stroke PRG Roundtable meeting in July 2001, and in many subsequent discussions, the Stroke PRG report was developed—a comprehensive document that identifies the national needs and opportunities in the field of stroke research. The final draft of this report was submitted for deliberation and acceptance by the National Advisory Neurological Disorders and Stroke Council in February, and the final report was published in April 2002. The PRG report will be widely disseminated to the stroke community, and is available online at www.ninds.nih.gov (Search: Stroke PRG).

Several areas of scientific need are identified in the Stroke PRG report, but five consensus priorities emerged from the PRG:

- Identification of the genes and proteins that contribute to stroke;

- An improved understanding of the relationship of blood, blood vessels, and brain tissue;

- A better appreciation of how blood flow is regulated and how it can be improved after stroke;

- The development of combination therapies based on molecular and cellular pathways of injury; and

- A better understanding of the neural mechanisms that regulate recovery after stroke.

Participants also identified a number of scientific resource needs including:

- Access to new technologies that allow for large numbers of genes or proteins to be analyzed simultaneously;

- Improved animal models of stroke that better simulate the human disease;

- Improved methods of imaging the brain;

- Improvements in clinical trial design and methods;

- Development of a network of stroke centers;

- A national database that would capture information on the burden of stroke; and

- Better education and training for clinicians in the care of stroke patients.

The full PRG report expands on all of these issues, and provides in-depth analysis of the status of 15 different fields of stroke research. As we move forward from the planning process into the implementation phase, the Stroke PRG members will work with NINDS staff to map the Institute's current stroke research efforts to the recommendations of the report. Using this approach, we will be able to identify existing research gaps and resource needs, and to incorporate these into a formal implementation plan.

## Health Disparities in Stroke

NINDS recognizes that stroke is one of several neurological disorders that has a disproportionate effect on minority and underserved

462

populations. For example, African-Americans are twice as likely to die of stroke or complications from stroke as people in any other racial or ethnic group in the country, and Hispanics have a stroke rate two times higher than that of Caucasians. For this reason, we have identified stroke as a critical health disparities issue in several Institute planning efforts: health disparities in stroke was considered as an over-arching issue by the Stroke PRG panel; stroke is one of the top research priorities in the NINDS Five-Year Strategic Plan on Minority Health Disparities; and the Institute is also in the process of establishing a planning panel that will specifically address health disparities in stroke.

The NINDS is also working to establish prevention/intervention research networks throughout the extramural community, particularly in regions of the Stroke Belt, an area in the Southeastern U.S. with stroke mortality rates approximately 25 percent above the rest of the nation. The goal is to foster stronger linkages between investigators at minority and majority institutions and community-based organizations in order to improve minority recruitment and retention in clinical studies as one way of addressing health disparities. As part of this program, NINDS, working with the National Heart, Lung, and Blood Institute (NHLBI) and the National Center for Research Resources, is developing the Stroke and Cardiovascular Prevention-Intervention Research Program. The pilot phase of this program is at the Morehouse School of Medicine in Atlanta, Georgia.

In addition to these programs, NINDS supports a number of ongoing clinical projects that specifically address stroke in minority populations, including a new study that will examine the phenomenon of the Stroke Belt. In this study, the role of geographic and racial differences as contributors to differential mortality rates will be examined and risk factors estimated. We are also engaged in targeting special public education efforts to minority populations.

## Stroke in Women

In addition, we recognize that stroke is a major health problem for women. To address this critical research area, NINDS is supporting studies that will help us to better understand gender differences in stroke. Specific projects include a clinical study to determine if hormone replacement therapy affects stroke severity, and a study examining blood flow in the brain and the role of female hormones in protecting brain tissue during ischemia. In all clinical trials, we ensure that appropriate numbers of women are enrolled, and many of these trials involve specific analyses to examine the effects of the intervention tested in the female participants. For example, we are currently supporting a clinical study that is comparing the efficacy of two procedures—carotid endarterectomy and carotid stenting—that unblock a clogged carotid artery in the neck, a significant risk factor for stroke. Previous research has shown that women may not benefit from carotid endarterectomy as much as men do, so one facet of the trial will examine gender differences in these procedures.

## Education and Outreach Programs

NINDS recognizes that supporting research into new prevention strategies and treatment options is only part of the battle in reducing the health burden of stroke. Helping people to recognize that they are having a stroke, so that they can seek help immediately, is a critical first step. To address this problem, the NINDS directs an extensive health promotion effort to raise awareness of the signs and symptoms of stroke, the need for urgent action if experiencing a stroke, and the possibility of a positive outcome with timely hospital treatment.

In May 2001, the NINDS launched the "Know Stroke. Know the Signs. Act in Time" campaign, a multi-faceted public education campaign to educate people about how to recognize stroke symptoms, and then to call 911 to get to a hospital quickly for treatment. The campaign's target audiences are those most at-risk for stroke—primarily people over the age of 50—and their family members, caregivers, and health care providers. Because stroke attacks the brain, a stroke patient often cannot act alone to call 911 and seek medical treatment, so bystanders are integral to acting quickly and getting stroke patients to the hospital. For this activity, the NINDS developed a wide variety of public education materials including airport dioramas jointly sponsored with the National Stroke Association, billboard displays, an award-winning eight minute film, consumer education brochures, exhibits, and new radio and television public service announcements (PSAs). All indications are that the "Know Stroke" campaign has been extremely well-received and effective. The television PSA garnered more than 87 million viewer impressions and hundreds of thousands of dollars worth of free broadcast time; the radio PSAs received more than 46,000 broadcasts on 272 stations; the airport dioramas received more than 800 million annual impressions; and thousands of nursing homes, hospitals, senior centers, and other organizations have received consumer education materials.

All of our public education strategies are designed to increase awareness of stroke. However, since the problem of stroke is even more acute in the African-American and Hispanic communities, some are targeted to specific at-risk minority communities. These campaigns started with outreach to the media in May 2002 for Stroke Awareness Month, and in the coming months and years will include public service advertising and grassroots community education components. NINDS also co-sponsored a "Stroke Sunday" program in October 2000, with the American Stroke Association and the Black Commissioned Officers' Advisory Group of the U.S. Public Health Service. This program was led by the former U.S. Surgeon General, Dr. David Satcher, and I participated on behalf of the NINDS. Held at a Rockville, Maryland church, the event was designed to bring attention to the major impact of stroke in the African-American community and to help inform participants about reducing their stroke risk.

NINDS also participates in "Operation Stroke," a coalition of health care professionals, allied health providers, civic leaders, and representatives of community organizations for stroke education. This effort is being coordinated by the American Stroke Association, and is aimed at the public as well as medical professionals. An intramural investigator at NINDS, who is a stroke clinician, is chairing this coalition in the greater DC and Maryland suburban areas.

Finally, NINDS has held several meetings and workshops to help educate health care professionals about advancements in stroke research, like tPA. For example, our Institute held a major national scientific meeting after the publication of the tPA study that involved more than 400 medical professionals. We plan to convene another conference later this year to revisit stroke treatment, and to explore how more people can be encouraged to recognize stroke as an emergency medical situation. The Institute hopes to use this symposium to educate healthcare professionals about the benefits of early treatment for all stroke patients. In addition, NINDS scientists speak at medical meetings all over the country in order to educate physicians about effective stroke care, and our grantees produce educational videos and offer continuing medical education courses on proper administration of tPA. To complement these efforts, NINDS also distributes free copies of the NIH Stroke Scale.

## Partnerships

As part of our ongoing prevention efforts, we have formed collaborative relationships with other NIH Institutes and federal agencies, and numerous voluntary organizations. NINDS coordinates the Brain Attack Coalition—a group of professional, voluntary, and government groups dedicated to reducing the occurrence, disabilities, and death associated with stroke—to increase awareness of stroke symptoms. To encourage improvements in stroke care, the Brain Attack Coalition published an article in June 2000 designed to help physicians and hospitals set up stroke centers.

In February 2001, the NINDS signed a memorandum of understanding (MOU) with NHLBI, the Centers for Disease Control and Prevention (CDC), the HHS Office of Disease Prevention and Health Promotion, and the American Heart Association to foster cooperation in reaching the heart disease and stroke goals for the nation articulated in the Healthy People 2010 initiative. These goals include: the prevention of risk factors for cardiovascular disease (CVD) and stroke; the detection and treatment of risk factors; the early identification and treatment of CVD and stroke, especially in their acute phases; and the prevention of recurrent CVD and stroke, and their complications.

In order to achieve these goals, we will work with the participating partners on focused initiatives such as population- and community-based public education and health promotion programs; activities to bring about improvements in the nation's cardiovascular health care delivery systems; media-based public awareness campaigns about the warning signs and symptoms of heart attack and stroke; promoting professional education and training, and other activities. CDC has already used our public education materials in cooperation with their networks, and we are enthusiastic about this partnership, and anticipate that it will continue for the next several years.

NINDS is also participating in the development of a comprehensive National Action Plan for Cardiovascular Health—A Comprehensive Public Health Strategy to Combat Heart Disease and Stroke. This planning process was initiated last year by the CDC. It will chart a course for the CDC with the states, territories, and other partners—including public health agencies, health care providers, and the public—for achieving national goals for heart disease and stroke prevention over the next two decades. The pillars of this public health strategy incorporate the three core functions of public health: assessment, policy development, and assurance.

## Conclusion

NINDS has made, and continues to make, significant contributions to the achievements in stroke prevention, treatment, and rehabilitation, and we are extremely proud of our accomplishments. However, the incremental nature of progress in stroke prevention has confirmed that there is no easy route to success. There are still difficult challenges to be addressed, and we have invested more than a year in gathering recommendations from the best clinicians and researchers in the field, as well as our committed partners in the advocacy community, in order to help us make the best use of our resources.

Our planning efforts tell us we must continue to pursue, in parallel, several areas of basic, translational, and clinical research that may have an impact on stroke. We must find better ways to prevent strokes before they occur. We must improve upon and encourage acceptance of pioneering diagnostic tools and acute treatments for when stroke happens. We must capitalize on the prospect, for the first time, of actually repairing the brain damaged by stroke and recovering function. The broad portfolio of NINDS research on stroke offers a glimpse of what the future might bring—the possibility of vaccines, genetic tests to tailor preventive measures for each individual, studies that may link infections or inflammation within blood vessels to stroke, biological markers that could aid in the identification of stroke risk, and new information about how chronic stress and hormones may affect susceptibility to stroke damage. Encouraged by the recent progress in neuroscience, guided by extensive and inclusive planning, and enabled by the support from Congress, I assure you that NINDS is committed to pursuing all of these opportunities to alleviate the devastating effects of stroke on our society.

467

# Part Six

# Legal and Financial Information for Stroke Survivors

Chapter 48

# A Guide for Stroke Survivors with Disabilities Seeking Employment

There are more opportunities now than ever before for people who are receiving SSDI and SSI benefits to learn job skills and find permanent employment.

If you are seeking a job or are new to the workforce, you should become familiar with the *Americans with Disabilities Act* of 1990 (ADA), a federal civil rights law designed to prevent discrimination and enable individuals with disabilities to participate fully in all aspects of society. One fundamental principle of the ADA is that individuals with disabilities who want to work and are qualified to work must have an equal opportunity to work. This chapter answers questions you may have about your employment rights under the ADA.

## How Do I Know If I Am Protected by the ADA?

To be protected, you must be a qualified individual with a disability. This means that you must have a disability as defined by the ADA. Under the ADA, you have a disability if you have a physical or mental impairment that substantially limits a major life activity such as hearing, seeing, speaking, thinking, walking, breathing, or performing manual tasks. You also must be able to do the job you want or were hired to do, with or without reasonable accommodation.

"A Guide for People with Disabilities Seeking Employment," *Americans with Disabilities Act*, U.S. Department of Justice, October 2000; Publication Number ADA-0001, ICN 951750, updated March 2, 2001.

471

## What Are My Rights under the ADA?

The ADA protects you from discrimination in all employment practices, including: job application procedures, hiring, firing, training, pay, promotion, benefits, and leave. You also have a right to be free from harassment because of your disability, and an employer may not fire or discipline you for asserting your rights under the ADA. Most importantly, you have a right to request a reasonable accommodation for the hiring process and on the job.

## What Is a Reasonable Accommodation?

A reasonable accommodation is any change or adjustment to a job, the work environment, or the way things usually are done that would allow you to apply for a job, perform job functions, or enjoy equal access to benefits available to other individuals in the workplace. There are many types of things that may help people with disabilities work successfully. Some of the most common types of accommodations include:

- physical changes, such as installing a ramp or modifying a workspace or restroom;

- sign language interpreters for people who are deaf or readers for people who are blind;

- providing a quieter workspace or making other changes to reduce noisy distractions for someone with a mental disability;

- training and other written materials in an accessible format, such as in Braille, on audio tape, or on computer disk;

- TTYs for use with telephones by people who are deaf, and hardware and software that make computers accessible to people with vision impairments or who have difficulty using their hands; and

- time off for someone who needs treatment for a disability.

## What Should I Do If I Think I Might Need a Reasonable Accommodation?

If you think you might need an accommodation for the application process or on the job, you have to request one. You may request a reasonable accommodation at any time during the application process or any time before or after you start working.

## How Do I Request a Reasonable Accommodation?

You simply must let your employer know that you need an adjustment or change because of your disability. You do not need to complete any special forms or use technical language to do this. For example, if you use a wheelchair and it does not fit under your desk at work, you should tell your supervisor. This is a request for a reasonable accommodation. A doctor's note requesting time off due to a disability or stating that you can work with certain restrictions is also a request for a reasonable accommodation.

## What Happens after I Make a Request for a Reasonable Accommodation?

Once you have made a request for a reasonable accommodation, the employer should discuss available options with you. If you have a disability that is not obvious, the employer may request documentation from you demonstrating that you have a disability and explaining why you need a reasonable accommodation. You and the employer should work together to determine an appropriate accommodation.

## What Should I Do If I Think My ADA Rights Have Been Violated?

You should contact the nearest office of the Equal Employment Opportunity Commission (EEOC). Someone will help you determine whether you should file a charge of discrimination. Charges may be filed with the EEOC in person, by mail, or by telephone.

There are strict time frames for filing charges of employment discrimination. In most states, you have 300 days from the time the alleged discrimination occurred to file a charge, but in some states you may have only 180 days. The EEOC field office nearest you can tell you which time period applies to you. However, you should file a charge as soon as possible after you believe the discrimination occurred.

## Is There Any Cost to File a Charge?

No. There is no cost to file a charge.

473

## Do I Need a Lawyer to File a Charge?

No. You may file a charge on your own without a lawyer, though some people do choose to retain one. Your local bar association may be able to help you locate a lawyer, and many communities have organizations that can provide free legal services or legal services at a reduced rate to people who qualify for them.

## What Happens after I File a Charge with the EEOC?

- First, the EEOC notifies your employer that a charge has been filed.

- In some instances, the EEOC will suggest mediation as a way of resolving the charge. Mediation is a process by which an impartial party tries to help people resolve a dispute. Mediation is voluntary, free, and completely confidential.

- If a charge is not referred to mediation or if mediation is unsuccessful, and the EEOC determines that a violation has not occurred, your charge will be dismissed and you will be sent a letter telling you that you may file your own lawsuit.

- If the EEOC concludes that you were discriminated against, it will attempt to settle the claim informally. If this is unsuccessful, the EEOC will decide whether to bring a lawsuit or issue you a letter giving you the right to file a lawsuit on your own.

### Additional Information

*Social Security Administration*
Office of Public Inquiries
Windsor Park Building
6401 Security Blvd.
Baltimore, MD 21235
Toll-Free: 800-772-1213
Toll-Free TTY: 800-325-0778
Website: www.ssa.gov/work

If you have a problem, you should first contact your local SSA office or call the toll-free number. Please include your Social Security number and claim number anytime you write to SSA.

474

*Equal Employment Opportunity Commission (EEOC)*
1801 L Street N.W.
Washington, DC
Toll-Free: 800-669-4000
Toll-Free TTY: 800-669-6820
Tel: 202-663-4900
Website: www.eeoc.gov

*Department of Justice (DOJ)*
950 Pennsylvania Ave. N.W.
Washington, DC 20530
Toll-Free: 800-514-0301
Toll-Free TTY: 800-514-0383
Fax: 202-307-1198
Website: www.usdoj.gov/crt/ada
E-mail: askdoj@usdoj.gov

*Job Accommodation Network*
918 Chestnut Ridge Rd., Suite 1
West Virginia University
P.O. Box 6080
Morgantown, WV 26506-6080
Toll-Free: 800-526-7234 (voice/TTY)
Fax: 304-293-5407
Website: http://janweb.icdi.wvu.edu
E-mail: jan@jan.icdi.wvu.edu

Chapter 49

# Social Security Disability Benefits for Stroke Survivors

## Contents

# Section 49.1

# *Introduction to Disability and Social Security*

"Social Security Disability Benefits," Social Security Association (SSA), Publication No. 05-10029, ICN 456000, February 2002.

## *Who Should Read This?*

You should, if you want to know more about the various kinds of disability benefits available from Social Security. This chapter will tell you who may get benefits, how to apply, and what you need to know once benefits start.

Social Security Disability pays disability benefits under two programs: the Social Security disability insurance program and the Supplemental Security Income (SSI) program. For most people, the medical requirements for disability payments are the same under both programs and a person's disability is determined by the same process. While eligibility for Social Security disability is based on prior work under Social Security, SSI disability payments are made on the basis of financial need. And there are other differences in the eligibility rules for the two programs. This section deals primarily with the Social Security disability insurance program. For information on SSI disability payments, see Section 49.2.

Please note: This chapter provides a general overview of the Social Security disability insurance program. The information it contains is not intended to cover all provisions of the law. For specific information about your case, contact Social Security.

### *Social Security Administration*
Office of Public Inquires
Windsor Park Building
6401 Security Blvd.
Baltimore, MD 21235
Toll-Free: 800-772-1213
TTY: 800-325-0778
Website: www.ssa.gov

# Introduction to Disability and Social Security

Disability is something most people don't like to think about. But the chances of your becoming disabled are probably greater than you realize. Studies show that a 20-year-old worker has a 3-in-10 chance of becoming disabled before reaching retirement age.

It's a fact that, while most people spend time working to succeed in their jobs and careers, few think about ensuring that they have a safety net to fall back on should the unthinkable happen. This is where Social Security (SS) comes in. In general, SS pays cash benefits to people who are unable to work for a year or more because of a disability. Benefits continue until a person is able to work again on a regular basis, and a number of work incentives are available to ease the transition back to work.

# What Does Social Security Mean by Disability?

It's important that you understand how Social Security defines disability. That's because other programs have different definitions for disability. Some programs pay for partial disability or for short-term disability. Social Security does not.

Disability under Social Security is based on your inability to work. You will be considered disabled if you cannot do work you did before and we decide that you cannot adjust to other work because of your medical condition(s). Your disability also must last or be expected to last for at least a year or to result in death.

This is a strict definition of disability. The program assumes that working families have access to other resources to provide support during periods of short-term disabilities, including workers' compensation, insurance, savings, and investments.

# Who Can Get Disability Benefits?

You can receive Social Security disability benefits until age 65. When you reach age 65, your disability benefits automatically convert to retirement benefits, but the amount remains the same. Certain members of your family may qualify for benefits on your record. They include:

- Your spouse who is age 62 or older, or any age if he or she is caring for a child of yours who is under age 16 or disabled and also receiving checks.

- Your disabled widow or widower age 50 or older. The disability must have started before your death or within seven years after your death. (If your widow or widower caring for your children receives Social Security checks, she or he is eligible if she or he becomes disabled before those payments end or within seven years after they end.)

- Your unmarried son or daughter, including an adopted child, or, in some cases, a stepchild or grandchild. The child must be under age 18 or under age 19 if in high school full time.

- Your unmarried son or daughter, age 18 or older, if he or she has a disability that started before age 22. These children are considered disabled if they meet the adult definition of disability. (If a disabled child under age 18 is receiving benefits as the dependent of a retired, deceased, or disabled worker, someone should contact Social Security to have his or her checks continued at age 18 on the basis of disability.)

If you become the parent of a child (including an adopted child) after you begin receiving Social Security benefits, be sure to notify us so that we can determine if the child qualifies for benefits. For more information about disability benefits for children, ask Social Security for the booklet, *Benefits for Children with Disabilities* (Publication No. 05-10026).

Note: The Supplemental Security Income (SSI) program also pays benefits to needy disabled children under age 18.

## How Much Work Do I Need?

To qualify for Social Security disability benefits, you must have worked long enough and recently enough under Social Security. You can earn up to a maximum of four work credits per year. The amount of earnings required for a credit increases each year as general wage levels rise. Family members who qualify for benefits on your work record do not need work credits.

The number of work credits you need for disability benefits depends on your age when you became disabled. Generally you need 20 credits earned in the last 10 years ending with the year you became disabled. However, younger workers may qualify with fewer credits. The rules are as follows:

- Before age 24—You may qualify if you have six credits earned in the three-year period ending when your disability starts.

• Age 24 to 31—You may qualify if you have credit for having worked half the time between 21 and the time you become disabled. For example, if you become disabled at age 27, you would need credit for three years of work (12 credits) out of the past six years (between age 21 and age 27).

• Age 31 or older—In general, you will need to have the number of work credits shown in the chart shown below. Unless you are blind, at least 20 of the credits must have been earned in the 10 years immediately before you became disabled.

**Table 49.1.** Social Security Credits by Age

| Born After 1929, Become Disabled At Age | Credits You Need |
|---|---|
| 31 through 42 | 20 |
| 44 | 22 |
| 46 | 24 |
| 48 | 26 |
| 50 | 28 |
| 52 | 30 |
| 54 | 32 |
| 56 | 34 |
| 58 | 36 |
| 60 | 38 |
| 62 or older | 40 |

## Signing Up for Disability

### How Do I Apply?

You should apply at any Social Security office as soon as you become disabled. You may file by phone, mail, or by visiting the nearest office. Note that, while you may receive back benefits from the date you became disabled, they are limited to one year before the date you filed for benefits.

### How Can I Speed Up My Claim?

It generally takes longer to process claims for disability benefits than other types of Social Security claims—from 60 to 90 days. You can help shorten the process by bringing certain documents with you when you apply and helping us to get any other medical evidence you need to show you are disabled. These include:

- the Social Security number and proof of age for each person applying for payments including your spouse and children, if they are applying for benefits;

- names, addresses, and phone numbers of doctors, hospitals, clinics, and institutions that treated you and dates of treatment;

- names of all medications you are taking;

- medical records from your doctors, therapists, hospitals, clinics, and caseworkers;

- laboratory and test results;

- a summary of where you worked and the kind of work you did;

- a copy of your W-2 Form (Wage and Tax Statement), or, if you are self-employed, your federal tax return for the past year; and

- dates of prior marriages if your spouse is applying.

Do not delay filing for benefits just because you do not have all of the information you need. The Social Security office will be glad to help you.

## Who Decides If I Am Disabled?

After helping you complete your application, the Social Security office will review it to see if you meet the basic requirements for disability benefits. They will look at whether you have worked long enough and recently enough, your age, and if you are applying for benefits as a family member, your relationship to the worker. The office then will send your application to the Disability Determination Services (DDS) office in your state. The DDS will decide whether you are disabled under the Social Security law.

The DDS will consider all the facts in your case. They will use the medical evidence from your doctors and from hospitals, clinics, or institutions where you have been treated and all the other information they have. On the medical report forms, your doctors or other sources are asked for a medical history of your condition:

- what is wrong with you;

- when it began;

- how it limits your activities;
- what the medical tests have shown; and
- what treatment you have received.

They also are asked for information about your ability to do work-related activities, such as walking, sitting, lifting and carrying, and remembering instructions. They are not asked to decide if you are disabled.

The DDS may need more medical information before they can decide your case. If it is not available from your current medical sources, they may ask you to go to a special examination called a consultative examination. Your doctor or the medical facility where you have been treated is the preferred source to do this examination but it may be done by someone else. Social Security will pay for the examination and for certain travel expenses related to it.

SS rules for determining disability are different from the disability rules in other government and private programs. However, a decision made by another agency and the medical reports it obtains may be considered in determining whether you are disabled under Social Security rules.

Once a decision is reached on your claim, a letter will be sent to you. If your claim is approved, the letter will show the amount of your benefit and when payments start. If it is not approved, the letter will explain why and tell you how to appeal if you don't agree.

## How Does SSA Determine Disability?

You should be familiar with the process SS uses to determine if you are disabled. It's a step-by-step process involving five questions. They are:

### 1. Are you working?

If you are and your earnings average more than $780 a month, you generally cannot be considered disabled. If you are not working, they go to the next step.

### 2. Is your condition severe?

Your condition must interfere with basic work-related activities for your claim to be considered. If it does not, SS will find that you are not disabled. If it does, SS will go to the next step.

### 3. Is your condition found in the list of disabling impairments?

SS maintains a list of impairments for each of the major body systems that are so severe they automatically mean you are disabled. If your condition is not on the list, SS will have to decide if it is of equal severity to an impairment on the list. If it is, SS will find that you are disabled. If it is not, they go to the next step.

### 4. Can you do the work you did previously?

If your condition is severe, but not at the same or equal severity as an impairment on the list, then SS must determine if it interferes with your ability to do the work you did previously. If it does not, your claim will be denied. If it does, SS will go to the next step.

### 5. Can you do any other type of work?

If you cannot do the work you did in the past, SS will see if you are able to adjust to other work. They consider your medical conditions and your age, education, past work experience, and any transferable skills you may have. If you cannot adjust to other work, your claim will be approved. If you can, your claim will be denied.

## Rules for Blind Persons

You are considered blind under Social Security rules if your vision cannot be corrected to better than 20/200 in your better eye or if your visual field is 20 degrees or less, even with a corrective lens.

There are a number of special rules for persons who are blind. The rules recognize the severe impact of blindness on a person's ability to work. For example, the monthly earnings limit for people who are blind is generally higher than the $780 limit that applies to non-blind disabled workers. This amount changes each year. For current amounts and other information on special rules for persons who are blind, ask SS for the booklet, *If You Are Blind Or Have Low Vision: How We Can Help* (Publication No. 05-10052).

## If Your Claim Is Denied

If your claim is denied or you disagree with any part of the decision, you may appeal the decision. The Social Security office will help you complete the paperwork.

You have 60 days from the time you receive our letter to file an appeal. SS assumes that you received the letter with their decision five days after the date on it, unless you can show them that you received it later. For more information about appeals, ask for the fact sheet, *The Appeals Process* (Publication No. 05-10041).

## When a Claim Is Approved

### When Do Benefits Start?

If your application is approved, your first Social Security benefits will be paid for the sixth full month after the date your disability began. For example, if we find that your disability began on January 15, your first disability benefit will be paid for the month of July. Because Social Security benefits are paid in the month following the month for which they're due, you would receive your July benefit in August.

You also will receive a booklet, *What You Need to Know When You Get Disability Benefits* (Publication No. 05-10153), in case you have questions.

### How Much Will I Get from Social Security?

The amount of your monthly disability benefit is based on your lifetime average earnings covered by Social Security. If you would like an estimate of your disability benefit, you can request a Social Security Statement that displays your earnings record and provides an estimate of your disability benefit. It will also include estimates of retirement and survivors benefits which you and your family may be eligible to receive now and in the future. The request form is available by calling or visiting Social Security. You can also type www.ssa.gov to get the form from our Internet website.

## How Do Other Payments Affect Your Benefits?

Eligibility for other government benefits can affect the amount of your Social Security benefits. The following publications provide more information and are available from Social Security.

- *How Workers' Compensation and Other Disability Payments May Affect Your Benefits* (Publication No. 05-10018).
- *The Windfall Elimination Provision* (Publication No. 05-10045.)

- *Government Pension Offset* (Publication No. 05-10007), a law that affects spouse's or widow(er)'s benefits.

If you have additional questions, contact your local Social Security office, or call toll-free at 800-772-1213.

### Are Benefits Taxed?

Some people have to pay federal income taxes on their Social Security benefits. This usually happens only if your total income is high. At the end of the year, you will receive a Social Security Benefit Statement (Form SSA-1099) showing the amount of benefits you received. Use the statement to complete your federal income tax return if any of your benefits are subject to tax. For more information about this tax, ask the Internal Revenue Service for a copy of Publication 915. Also, you may choose to have federal taxes withheld from your benefits.

## Can I Get Medicare If I'm Disabled?

SSA will automatically enroll you in Medicare after you get disability benefits for two years.

Medicare has two parts—hospital insurance and medical insurance. Hospital insurance helps pay hospital bills and some follow-up care. The taxes you paid while you were working financed this coverage, so it's free. The other part of Medicare, medical insurance, helps pay doctors' bills and other services. You will pay a monthly premium for this coverage if you want it. Most people have both parts of Medicare.

### Help for Low-Income Medicare Beneficiaries

If you get Medicare and have low income and few resources, your state may pay your Medicare premiums, and in some cases, other out-of-pocket Medicare expenses such as deductibles and coinsurance. Only your state can decide if you qualify. To find out if you do, contact your state or local welfare office or Medicaid agency. For more general information about the program, contact Social Security and ask for the leaflet, *Medicare Savings Programs* (HCFA Publication No. 10126).

## Is My Case Reviewed?

In general, your benefits will continue as long as you are disabled. However, SS will review your case periodically to see if you are still disabled. The frequency of the reviews depends on the expectation of recovery.

- If medical improvement is expected, your case normally will be reviewed within six to 18 months.

- If medical improvement is possible, your case normally will be reviewed no sooner than three years.

- If medical improvement is not expected, your case normally will be reviewed no sooner than seven years.

## What Can Cause Benefits to Stop?

There are two things that can cause SS to decide that you are no longer disabled and to stop your benefits.

Your benefits will stop if you work at a level we consider substantial. Usually, average earnings of $780 or more a month are considered substantial.

Your disability benefits also will stop if we decide that your medical condition has improved to the point that you are no longer disabled.

You must promptly report any improvement in your condition, your return to work, and certain other events as long as you are receiving benefits. These responsibilities are explained in the booklet you will receive when benefits start.

## Going Back to Work

### Can I Receive Benefits While I Work?

If you're like most people, you would rather work than try to live on disability benefits. There are a number of special rules that provide cash benefits and Medicare while you attempt to work. We call these rules work incentives, or employment support programs. You should be familiar with these special rules so you can use them to your advantage.

For more information about Social Security work incentives, ask for a copy of the booklet, *Working While Disabled: How We Can Help* (Publication No. 05-10095).

*The Ticket to Work and Work Incentives Improvement Act of 1999* substantially expands opportunities for people with disabilities who want to work. For information on this law, call 1-800-772-1213 and ask for the fact sheet, *Ticket to Work and Work Incentives Improvement Act of 1999* (Publication No. 05-10060). The fact sheet also is available on the SSA website at www.ssa.gov/work.

# Section 49.2

# *You May Be Able to Get SSI*

"You May Be Able to Get SSI," Social Security Administration, Publication Number 05-11069, ICN 480390, February 2002.

## What Is SSI?

SSI stands for Supplemental Security Income. It's a program run by Social Security. It pays monthly checks to the elderly, the blind, and people with disabilities who don't own many things or have much income.

If you get SSI, you usually get food stamps and Medicaid, too. Medicaid helps pay doctor and hospital bills.

To get SSI, you must be *elderly* or *blind* or have a *disability*.

- Elderly means you are 65 or older.

- Blind means you are either totally blind or have very poor eyesight. Children, as well as adults, can get benefits because of blindness.

- A disability means you have a physical or mental problem that is expected to last at least a year or result in death. Children, as well as adults, can get benefits because of disability.

## How Much Can You Get from SSI?

The basic monthly SSI check is the same in all states. It is:

- $545 for one person; or
- $817 for a couple.

Not everyone gets this exact amount. You may get more if you live in a state that adds to the SSI check. Or you may get less if you or your family have other money coming in each month. Your living arrangements also make a difference in eligibility and the amount you can get.

## Things You Own and Your Income

To get SSI, the things you own and your income must be below certain amounts.

### Things You Own

SSA doesn't count everything you own when deciding if you can get SSI. For example, they don't count your home. Usually, they don't count your car. They do count cash, bank accounts, stocks, and bonds.

You may be able to get SSI if the things they count are no more than:

- $2,000 for one person; or
- $3,000 for a couple.

### Your Income

Your income includes earnings, Social Security payments, pensions, and non-cash items you receive, such as food or shelter.

The amount of income you can have each month and still get SSI depends on where you live. In some states you can have more income than in others.

**If you don't work**, you may be able to get SSI if your monthly income is less than:

- $565 for one person; or
- $837 for a couple.

**If you work**, you can have more income each month. If all of your income is from working, you may be able to get SSI if you make less than:

- $1,175 a month for one person; or
- $1,719 a month for a couple.

489

However, if you're applying for SSI disability benefits and are earning $780 or more a month, you probably won't be eligible for benefits. Remember: they don't count all of your income, so you may be able to get SSI even if you have more income, especially if you live in a state that adds money to the SSI checks.

## Where You Live

To get SSI checks, you must live in the U.S. or Northern Mariana Islands and be a U.S. citizen or national. (Certain non-citizens also may be eligible for SSI. A Social Security representative can tell you if you qualify.)

## How to Sign Up for SSI

Call to set up an appointment with a Social Security representative.

### Social Security Administration
Toll-Free: 800-772-1213 (7 a.m.-7 p.m. on business days)
TTY: 800-325-0778 (7 a.m.-7 p.m. on business days)
Website: www.ssa.gov

At the SS website you can get answers to many questions and for special services. You can download forms and publications, get replacement Social Security and Medicare cards, subscribe to eNews, their free electronic newsletter, and apply for retirement benefits online.

The Social Security Administration treats all calls confidentially— whether they're made to the toll-free numbers or to one of the local offices. SS also wants to ensure that you receive accurate and courteous service. That is why they have a second Social Security representative monitor some incoming and outgoing telephone calls.

Section 49.3

# How to Apply for Social Security Disability Benefits

"Applying for Disability Benefits," Social Security Administration, found at www.ssa.gov/disability.html.

## When to Apply for Social Security Disability Benefits

You should apply as soon as you become disabled. If you apply for

- Social Security, disability benefits will not begin until the sixth full month of disability. The Social Security disability waiting period begins with the first full month after the date they decide your disability began.

- Supplemental Security Income (SSI), SS pays SSI disability benefits for the first full month after the date you filed your claim, or, if later, the date you become eligible for SSI.

## How to Apply

You can apply for Disability benefits online, or if your prefer, you can apply by calling the toll-free number, 800-772-1213. SS representatives there can make an appointment for your application to be taken over the telephone or at any convenient Social Security office. People who are deaf or hard of hearing may call the toll-free TTY number, 800-325-0778, between 7 a.m. and 7 p.m. on Monday through Friday.

## What You Need

The claims process for disability benefits is generally longer than for other types of Social Security benefits, from 60 to 90 days. It takes longer to obtain medical information and to assess the nature of the disability in terms of your ability to work. However, you can help shorten the process by bringing certain documents with you when you

491

apply and helping us to get any other medical evidence you need to show you are disabled. These include:

1. your Social Security number;

2. your birth certificate or other evidence of your date of birth;

3. your military discharge papers, if you were in the military service;

4. your spouse's birth certificate and Social Security number if he or she is applying for benefits;

5. your children's birth certificates and Social Security numbers if they are applying for benefits; and

6. your checking or savings account information, so your benefits can be directly deposited;

7. names, addresses, and phone numbers of doctors, hospitals, clinics, and institutions that treated you and dates of treatment;

8. names of all medications you are taking;

9. medical records from your doctors, therapists, hospitals, clinics, and caseworkers;

10. laboratory and test results;

11. a summary of where you worked in the past 15 years and the kind of work you did;

12. a copy of your W-2 Form (Wage and Tax Statement), or if you are self-employed, your federal tax return for the past year;

13. dates of prior marriages if your spouse is applying

The documents presented as evidence must be either originals or copies certified by the issuing agency. SS cannot accept uncertified or notarized photocopies as evidence since they cannot verify their authenticity. Do not delay filing for benefits just because you do not have all of the information you need. The Social Security office will be glad to help you.

If you do not have a birth certificate, you may request one from the State where you were born.

If you are applying for Supplemental Security Income benefits you also need the following:

- information about the home where you live, such as your mortgage or your lease and landlord's name;

- payroll slips, bank books, insurance policies, car registration, burial fund records, and other information about your income and the things you own.

## How SSA Determines Disability

You should be familiar with the process they use to determine if you are disabled. It's a step-by-step process involving five questions. They are:

1. Are you working? If you are and your earnings average more than $700 a month, you generally cannot be considered disabled.

2. Is your condition severe? Your impairments must interfere with basic work-related activities for your claim to be considered.

3. Is your condition found in the list of disabling impairments? SS maintains a list of impairments for each of the major body systems that are so severe they automatically mean you are disabled. If your condition is not on the list, they have to decide if it is of equal severity to an impairment on the list. If it is, your claim is approved. If it is not, they go to the next step.

4. Can you do the work you did previously? If your condition is severe, but not at the same or equal severity as an impairment on the list, then SS must determine if it interferes with your ability to do the work you did in the last 15 years. If it does not, your claim will be denied. If it does, your claim will be considered further.

5. Can you do any other type of work? If you cannot do the work you did in the last 15 years, they then look to see if you can do any other type of work. SS considers your age, education, past work experience, and transferable skills, and they review the job demands of occupations as determined by the Department of Labor. If you cannot do any other kind of work, your claim will be approved. If you can, your claim will be denied.

# Section 49.4.

# *Working While Disabled*

"Working While Disabled—How We Can Help,"
Social Security Administration, Publication Number 05-10095,
ICN 468625, March 2002.

## *Why SSA Wants to Help You Return to Work*

If you are receiving Social Security disability insurance benefits or Supplemental Security Income (SSI) disability benefits, but still want to work, this section provides information to help you treat your disability as a bridge, not the end of the road. The decision to work and earn as much as you can is yours, of course. However, many people see their work as more than just extra cash. They cite the satisfaction they get from overcoming a disability through their abilities, making new friends and getting back in the mainstream. Most find that their earnings gradually increase to the point where they are better off working than not working.

### *A National Policy*

Helping people with disabilities to lead independent and fuller lives is a national policy affecting both the government and the private sector. Most of the rules discussed in this section are the result of laws passed in 1980 and 1987. In addition, Congress passed the Americans with Disabilities Act in July 1990, which prohibits discrimination against people with disabilities who wish to work. Most recently, Congress passed the Ticket to Work and Work Incentives Improvement Act of 1999, which substantially expands opportunities for people with disabilities.

The new law establishes the Ticket to Work and Self-Sufficiency Program, which is being phased in nationally over a three-year period. It provides beneficiaries with disabilities a ticket they can take to an employment network for rehabilitation and employment services. The ticket program will start in 13 states and more states will be added as we gain experience in administering the program. The

494

first 13 states to get the ticket program are: Arizona, Colorado, Delaware, Florida, Illinois, Iowa, Massachusetts, New York, Oklahoma, Oregon, South Carolina, Vermont, and Wisconsin.

If you live in one of these states, you may receive a ticket with an instruction booklet explaining how to use the ticket from the ticket program manager, MAXIMUS, Inc. The number is 866-968-7842 (TTY 866-833-2967). If you do not live in a ticket state but would like more information about the law, you may call the toll-free number, 800-772-1213, and ask for the fact sheet, The Ticket to Work and Work Incentives Improvement Act of 1999.

## How SSA Can Help You Work

Social Security disability insurance benefits are paid to people with disabilities or to individuals who are blind and who have worked under Social Security and to their dependents. SSI disability benefits are paid to people with disabilities or to individuals who are blind who have little income and few resources. Social Security beneficiaries with low income and few resources also may qualify for SSI. Although there are differences between Social Security and SSI, the work incentives under both programs are designed to accomplish the same objective: to provide support and assistance while you attempt to return to work or as you enter the workforce for the first time.

If you're like most people, you would rather work than stay home. But working is a big step for a person with a disability, and you probably have many fears and questions about what could happen to your monthly benefits. "How will my benefits be affected?" "Will I lose my Medicare or Medicaid?" "What about the extra cost of working because of my disability?" Social Security and SSI have special rules called "work incentives" to help you overcome some of these fears and problems. These work incentives include:

- cash benefits while you work;

- Medicare and/or Medicaid while you work;

- help with any extra work expenses you may have as a result of your disability; and

- help with education, training, and rehabilitation to start a new line of work.

495

# What You Should Know about Social Security Work Incentives

## Work Incentive Rules at a Glance

Following is a brief description of the rules that will help you work while you get Social Security disability benefits.

**Trial Work Period**—If you return to work for nine months (not necessarily consecutive), your earnings will not affect your Social Security benefit. If the nine months of trial work do not fall within a 60-month period, you may have even longer to test your ability to work.

**Extended Period Of Eligibility**—For at least 36 months after a successful trial work period, if you continue to work while disabled, you may receive a benefit for any month your earnings fall below the substantial gainful activity level (in 2002, $780 a month for people with disabilities, $1,300 a month for people who are blind).

**Expedited Reinstatement of Benefits**—If you become unable to work again because of your medical condition within 60 months after your extended period of eligibility has ended, and your benefits were stopped because of your earnings, you may request reinstatement of benefits without filing a new disability application.

**Continuation of Medicare**—If you have premium-free Medicare hospital insurance and you start working, you may have at least 8½ years of extended coverage (including the nine-month trial work period). After that, you can buy Medicare coverage by paying a monthly premium.

**Impairment-Related Work Expenses**—Certain expenses for things you need because of your impairment in order to work may be deducted when counting earnings to determine if you are performing substantial work.

**Recovery during Vocational Rehabilitation**—If you medically recover while participating in a vocational rehabilitation program that is likely to lead to becoming self-supporting, benefits may continue until the program ends.

**Special Rules for Persons Who Are Blind**—If you are blind, several special rules will help you work.

**Help For Low-Income Medicare Beneficiaries**—If you get Medicare and have low income and few resources, your state may pay your Medicare premiums and, in some cases, other out-of-pocket Medicare expenses such as deductibles and coinsurance. Only your state can decide if you qualify. To find out if you do, contact your state or local welfare office or Medicaid agency. For more general information about the program, contact Social Security and ask for a copy of the leaflet, *Medicare Savings Programs* (HCFA Publication No. 10126).

## Answers to Most Commonly Asked Questions

### How Long Will Social Security Continue While I Work?

Generally, you'll receive your full monthly Social Security benefit for a year after you return to work. If you continue to work beyond that while still disabled, your eligibility for monthly cash benefits will continue for at least another 36 months. Here's how it works:

You usually can have a trial work period of nine months (not necessarily consecutive) during which your benefits will not be affected by your earnings regardless of how much you earn. A trial work month is any month in which your total earnings are more than $560 or, if you are self-employed, you earn more than $560 (after expenses) or spend more than 80 hours in your own business. When nine trial work months are successfully completed within 60 months, we review your work to see if your earnings are substantial. (Generally, more than $780 per month is considered substantial earnings.) If they are, your benefits would continue for a three-month grace period and then stop.

However, if you are still medically disabled and continue to work in spite of your disability, your benefits can be reinstated anytime during the next 36 months. During this time, you will receive your full Social Security benefit for any month your earnings fall below $780. Benefits would continue as long as you remain disabled and your earnings do not exceed $780 a month.

### How Much Can I Earn before I Start Losing Benefits?

Usually, earnings of more than $780 a month are considered substantial. If your earnings average less than $780 a month, your benefits generally would continue indefinitely.

If your earnings average more than $780 a month, this is considered an indication of your ability to work.

During the trial work period, there are no limits on your earnings. During the 36-month extended period of eligibility, the $780 level is the cutoff point. But, under another work incentive rule explained in the next answer, the work expenses you have as a result of your disability are deducted when SS counts your earnings to see if they affect your benefits. This means your earnings could be substantially higher than $780 before they affect your benefits.

### *What Kind of Help with My Work Expenses Can I Expect?*

SS deducts work expenses related to your disability from your earnings before they determine your continued eligibility for benefits. These expenses may include the cost of any item or service you need to work, even if the item or service also is useful to you in your daily living. Examples include a seeing-eye dog, prescription drugs, transportation to and from work (under certain conditions), a personal attendant or job coach, a wheelchair or any specialized work equipment.

If you also receive SSI payments, there is a special rule called a plan for achieving self-support (PASS) that permits you to set aside funds and resources for a specific work goal.

### *What Happens If I Lose My Job?*

If you lose your job during a trial work period, your benefits are not affected. If you lose your job during the 36-month extended period of eligibility, call SS and your benefits will be reinstated as long as you are still disabled. You do not have to reapply for benefits or undergo any waiting period as you did when you first applied for disability benefits.

If you become unable to work due to your disability within 60 months after you complete the extended period of eligibility, your benefits could be reinstated immediately without a new application or waiting period.

### *How Long Would Medicare Continue Once I Start Working?*

Your Medicare coverage will continue through the trial work period and may continue for at least 93 months after the trial work period if you are still disabled. During this period, your hospital insurance coverage is free. When your Medicare coverage runs out after this period and you are still disabled, you may purchase the same coverage for a monthly premium.

## What about Help with Rehabilitation, Training, or Education?

If you are likely to benefit from rehabilitation, you are referred to a state rehabilitation agency or private organization for rehabilitation services. Social Security pays for the services if you are successfully rehabilitated. If you recover from your disability while in an approved rehabilitation or training program that is likely to result in your becoming self-supporting, benefits will continue until the program is over.

For example, if you were in a nurse's aide training program and your condition improved so that you were no longer disabled, benefits ordinarily would stop. But if you have contacted Social Security and we are aware of your participation in the program and have approved it, then your benefits would continue until the program is over. For more information on Social Security and vocational rehabilitation, ask for the special leaflet, *How Social Security Can Help with Vocational Rehabilitation* (Publication No. 05-10050).

## How Do I Find Out If I Can Work Again?

Just notify any Social Security office that you want to start working on a trial basis. If a periodic review of your condition was scheduled, we will put it off until your trial work period is over.

## Are There Special Rules for Workers Who Are Blind?

If you are a blind person who works while receiving Social Security benefits, special rules apply to you.

* You can earn up to $1,300 a month in the year 2002 before your earnings affect your benefits.

* If your earnings are too high to receive disability benefits, you are still eligible for a disability freeze. This means that those years in which you had low or no earnings because of your disability will not be counted in figuring your future benefits, which are based on your average earnings over your worklife.

* If you are age 55 to 65, a more lenient rule is used to determine your inability to work. It says that you can receive disability benefits if you cannot do the same or similar work you did before you reached age 55 or became blind, whichever is later.

(The regular rule requires that a disabled person be unable to do any type of work in the general economy.) For more information on special rules for blind persons, ask Social Security for the booklet, *If You Are Blind Or Have Low Vision—How We Can Help* (Publication No. 05-10052).

## Example of What Happens when You Work under Social Security While Disabled

Pamela Watson, age 24, was receiving disability benefits of $557 a month based on a childhood condition that made it difficult for her to walk. She wanted to work but was afraid of losing her benefits and Medicare. When she discussed this with a Social Security representative, she was told about disability work incentives under which she could work and still get cash benefits and Medicare. She found out that for the first nine months of work, her benefits would not be affected no matter how much she earned. Pamela started working in a local laundry part time and earned $850 a month. Here's how her income changed:

| | |
|---|---|
| Gross earnings | $850 |
| Social Security check | + 557 |
| Total income | $1,407 |

At the end of the nine months of work, Social Security evaluated Pamela's work to see if it was substantial. Since she was earning more than $780, her work was considered substantial. Her benefits continued for three more months and then stopped. However, because she still was disabled, her benefits could be reinstated anytime during the next 36 months if her earnings dropped below $780. During the first year after her trial work period, her company relocated outside the city, where there were no bus lines. She hired a neighbor to drive her to work and paid a co-worker to take her home. Her transportation expenses totaled $120 a month.

In addition, she purchased a special motorized wheelchair so she could get around the new suburban plant. This cost $75 a month. Let's figure Pamela's countable earnings after deducting her impairment-related work expenses:

| | |
|---|---|
| Gross earnings | $850 |
| Subtract work expenses | −195 |
| Countable earnings | $655 |

Because her countable earnings are less than $780, Pam's Social Security checks were reinstated. Her total net income now is:

| | |
|---|---|
| Countable earnings | $655 |
| Social Security check | + 557 |
| Total income | $1,212 |

After a year, she paid off the motorized chair and she received a $340 raise. Her earnings increased to $990 a month. Her countable earnings now are:

| | |
|---|---|
| Gross earnings | $990 |
| Subtract work expenses | −120 |
| Countable earnings | $870 |

Because her countable earnings now exceed the substantial level ($780), her Social Security benefits will stop. As you can see, at each point in her working life, Pamela's income was greater than it would have been if she had not worked. In addition, her Medicare coverage continued for 93 months following the trial work period.

# What You Should Know about SSI Work Incentives

## Work Incentive Rules at a Glance

Following is a brief description of the rules that will help you work while you get SSI benefits. More detail is included in the pages that follow.

**Continuation of SSI**—If you work, you may continue to receive payments until the income SS counts exceeds the SSI limits.

**Expedited Reinstatement of Benefits**—If your SSI disability benefits have ended because of earnings from work and you again become unable to work because of your medical condition, you have 60 months during which you may request reinstatement of benefits without filing a new application.

**Continuation of Medicaid Eligibility**—Your Medicaid will usually continue even if you earn over the SSI limits if you cannot afford similar medical care and depend on Medicaid in order to work.

**Plans for Achieving Self-Support**—You may set aside income and resources toward an approved plan for achieving self-support (PASS).

501

**Work Expenses Related to Your Disability**—Certain work expenses you have because of your impairment may be subtracted from your earnings when SS determines your eligibility and payment amount. If you are blind, the work expenses need not be related to the impairment.

**Recovery during Vocational Rehabilitation**—If you recover while participating in a vocational rehabilitation program that is likely to lead to becoming self-supporting, benefits may continue until the program ends.

**Students with Disabilities**—Most scholarships or grants used to pay for tuition, books, and other expenses directly related to getting an education don't count as income if you go to school or are in a training program. You also may exclude up to $1,320 of earnings a month (up to a maximum of $5,340 a year).

**Help for Low-Income Medicare Beneficiaries**—If you get Medicare and have low income and few resources, your state may pay your Medicare premiums and, in some cases, other out-of-pocket Medicare expenses such as deductibles and coinsurance. Only your state can decide if you qualify. To find out if you do, contact your state or local welfare office or Medicaid agency. For more general information about the program, contact Social Security and ask for a copy of the leaflet, *Medicare Savings Programs* (HCFA Publication No. 10126).

## Answers to Most Commonly Asked Questions

### How Long Will My SSI Benefits Continue after I Go Back to Work?

It depends on how much you earn. The amount of your SSI check is based on how much other income you have. When your other income goes up, your SSI check usually goes down. So when your earnings push your income over the SSI limits, your checks will stop for those months. (We discuss these limits in the answers to the next two questions.) But, your checks will start up again without a new application for any month your income drops below the SSI limits. If you're off both SSI and Medicaid for 12 months or more, and your disability ended because of earnings from work, you have 60 months to request a reinstatement of benefits without a new application.

## How Do Earnings Reduce My Payments?

If your only income besides SSI is the money you make from your job, then we don't count the first $85 in earnings you get each month. One-half of what you earn over $85 is deducted from your SSI check.

If you have other income besides earnings (such as a Social Security check), then we don't count the first $65 in earnings you get each month. One-half of what you make over $65 is deducted from your SSI payments. But, $20 of your other income, such as your Social Security check, is not counted either.

## How Much Can I Earn before I Lose All My Benefits?

If you have no other income besides earnings, you may earn up to $1,174 a month in 2002 before losing your entire federal SSI payment. But if you live in a state that adds money to your federal SSI payment, you may earn more. If you have other income, such as Social Security benefits, the amount you can earn before losing any payment may be lower. However, when you apply for SSI disability payments, SS will consider earnings of $780 or more an indication that you are able to do substantial work and you would not qualify for SSI on the basis of disability.

## What Happens If I Lose or Quit My Job?

If you lose your job while you still are getting SSI, your payments will be increased because of your reduced income.

If you lose your job within 60 months after your payments stopped because your earnings were too high, and you are still disabled, your benefits will start again without an application.

## How Long Will Medicaid Continue While I'm Working?

In general, your Medicaid coverage will continue, even after your SSI payments stop, until your income reaches a certain level. That level varies with each state and reflects the cost of health care in your state. (Your Social Security office can tell you the Medicaid level for your state.) However, if your health care costs are higher than this level, you can have more income and keep your Medicaid.

Also, for Medicaid to continue, you must:

• need it in order to work;

• be unable to afford similar health insurance coverage without SSI;

- continue to have a disabling condition; and
- meet all nondisability requirements other than earnings.

If you qualify for Medicaid under these rules, SSA will review your case to see if you are still disabled or blind.

### How Can SSI Help Me with My Work Expenses?

The rules work the same as if you were receiving Social Security benefits. Work expenses that are related to your disability are deducted from your earnings when SS figures if they are high enough to affect your benefits. These expenses may include work equipment, such as a special typewriter or desk, or modifications to your car or home to help you get to and from work. This means you can earn well over the SSI income limits and still continue to get payments.

### What about Training and Rehabilitation Help?

Under SSI, there's a special rule called a plan for achieving self-support, or PASS. A PASS permits you to put aside money and assets toward a plan designed to help you support yourself. The money set aside won't reduce your SSI payment. The goal of your plan may be to start a business or get a job.

If you have too much income to get SSI, a PASS may help you qualify. You may set aside the necessary income and assets to accomplish a work goal, and these funds will not count when we decide if you are eligible for SSI or how much SSI you receive. In addition, as under Social Security, if you recover from your disability while you are in an approved vocational rehabilitation program, your SSI payments will continue until you have completed the program. For more information on vocational rehabilitation opportunities, ask for the special leaflet, *How Social Security Can Help With Vocational Rehabilitation* (Publication No. 05-10050).

### How Do I Get Started on a PASS?

Anyone can help you with a PASS, including your vocational rehabilitation worker, employer, or the Social Security office. In general, the following rules apply:

- the PASS must state a clear and realistic work goal;
- your goal must be a job or business that will produce sufficient income to reduce your dependency on SSI payments;

- the PASS must state the amount and sources of income or resources that will be set aside;

- the PASS must state how you will spend the money; you must be able to achieve the goal of the PASS within a specified period of time; and

- the PASS must be approved by Social Security.

For more information about setting up a PASS, ask for the leaflet, *Working While Disabled—A Guide to Plans for Achieving Self-Support* (Publication No. 05-11017).

### *Are There Special Rules for Persons Who Are Blind?*

If you are blind, most work expenses you have (not just those related to your disability) may be deducted from your income when SS decides if you are eligible for SSI. For example, special clothes needed on the job or special equipment needed to work can be deducted. For more information on special rules for blind persons, ask Social Security for the booklet, *If You Are Blind Or Have Low Vision—How We Can Help* (Publication No. 05-10052).

## What and How You Should Report to Social Security

Whether you're receiving Social Security or SSI disability payments, it's important that you stay in touch with Social Security while you're working. The people there will be able to help you plan your work effort and to show you how you can use other work incentives to achieve your work goals. You should immediately notify Social Security to report the following:

- improvement in your health;

- change in employment status;

- change of address;

- change in the number of people in your household;

- marriage or divorce;

- change in income;

- change in savings or investments, including selling your home, real estate, car, or personal property;

- change in work expenses;

- travel outside the United States;

- development or change in a PASS;

- or admission to or release from a hospital or other institution.

Also contact Social Security if you start receiving worker's compensation (including Black Lung) or a public disability benefit or if the amount of these benefits changes.

Chapter 50

# Advance Directives and Living Wills Assist Families of Stroke Victims

## Your Life, Your Choices

There's only one person who is truly qualified to tell health care providers how you feel about different kinds of health care issues—that's you. But, what if you get sick, or injured so severely that you can't communicate with your doctors or family members? Have you thought about what kinds of medical care you would want? Do your loved ones and health care providers know your wishes?

Many people assume that close family members automatically know what they want. But studies have shown that spouses guess wrong over half the time about what kinds of treatment their husbands or wives would want. You can help assure that your wishes will direct future health care decisions through the process of advance care planning.

### *What Should We Do for Dad?*

"We got the kind of call we'd feared. Dad had been in declining health for months. Then he fell asleep at the wheel and was in a bad car accident. Three weeks later he was still in a coma. A breathing machine pumped air into his lungs because he could not breathe on

---

Excerpted from "Your Life, Your Choices: Planning for Future Medical Decisions," by Robert Pearlman, MD MPH; Helen Starks, MPH; Kevin Cain, PhD; William Cole, PhD; David Rosengren, PhD; and Donald Patrick, PhD MSPH., U.S. Department of Veterans Affairs.

his own. The doctors thought his chances of coming out of the coma were slim. They talked with Mom and me about turning off the breathing machine and allowing Dad to die naturally.

I felt terrible. I didn't think Dad would want to be kept alive like this. But I knew Mom would feel guilty for the rest of her life if we told the doctors to 'pull the plug' while there was still even the slightest hope. We weren't sure what we should do because Dad never told us what he would have wanted. I really wish we'd talked about this before."

## What Do You Need to Do to Guide Your Future Health Care?

### 1. Figure Out What You Want

**Think.** You need to understand what kinds of situations you might face and the options for care.

### 2. Communicate This to Others

**Talk.** Tell your loved ones and health care providers about your strongly-held beliefs and what kinds of care you would want in different situations.

**Write.** Write down your wishes so your loved ones will have a record of what you told them. This also helps if no one is around who can speak for you.

## Why Do You Need to Think Now about Future Health Care Decisions?

Whether you are young or old, healthy or sick, there may come a time when an important decision needs to be made about your health care. And whether it's tomorrow or five years from now, there's no guarantee that you will be able to express your wishes for yourself at that time.

Consider the Larsen family: Chris Larsen never told his family what kind of medical measures he'd want if he became critically ill. He is in a nursing home after having suffered a severe stroke 9 months ago. He is paralyzed and unable to take care of himself or communicate in any way. Now he has pneumonia and will probably die unless he goes to the hospital to receive intravenous antibiotics. He also may need to be on a breathing machine for a week or so. The doctor says that his chances of returning to normal are remote, but that he has a fair chance of getting over the pneumonia. His family members disagree about what they should do. His son Bill says, "Dad was never a quitter. He'd want to fight to the very end, as long as there was the slightest hope." His daughter Trudy disagrees. "Sure, Dad wasn't a quitter, but he wanted to die naturally—he would be horrified to be kept alive this way."

In fact, Trudy's views were the closest to Mr. Larsen's true opinion. But the family never had a way to find this out. They treated his pneumonia and he lived another year in the nursing home without recovering his ability to communicate or care for himself.

This story shows why it is so important to discuss your wishes. Talking with your family and health care providers ahead of time can prevent confusion and help ease the burden on them.

## Do You Have Any Strongly Held Beliefs That Should Guide Your Care?

Think ahead. Imagine being in a critical condition—one in which you were unable to communicate your wishes. If medical decisions could mean the difference between life and death, what would you want your loved ones and health care providers to do?

Your strongly held beliefs can guide these choices because they help others understand what you value about life. But be sure to explain your beliefs because people often use the same words to mean very different things. Consider the cases of Mrs. Santini and Mrs. Johnson, both deeply religious women.

"I want to be kept alive as long as possible," Maria Santini has said on many occasions. "Life is sacred and has meaning, no matter what its quality."

"When my time comes, keep me comfortable." Irene Johnson also believes life is sacred. However, she has often said, "I've lived a long and full life. I don't want anything done just to keep me alive."

Because Mrs. Santini and Mrs. Johnson both believe that life is sacred, many people would assume that their views on being kept alive would been the same. But, as you've seen, it's not that simple.

Here's another example. Have you ever heard anyone say, "If I'm a vegetable, pull the plug"? What does this mean to you? What's a vegetable? What's a plug? Even people who live together can have very different ideas about what the same words mean without knowing it. The story of May and John Williams shows how important it is to be specific about what you mean.

509

When you say, "pull the plug" it could mean a variety of things:

- Stop the breathing machine
- Remove the feeding tube
- Don't give me antibiotics
- Stop everything

"I'd never want to live like a vegetable." Both May and John Williams have always shared this belief during their fifty years of marriage. But when they were talking about their advance care plans, they learned that they had very different views about what that meant. For May, it's when she can't take care of herself. John was surprised. For him, being a vegetable is much worse. "It's when my brain's not working but my body is being kept alive by machines."

People have very different notions of what it means to be a vegetable. Here are some more examples:

- "You sit in a chair and don't do anything all day."
- "You can't read anymore."
- "You're just a body with some life in it."

## *If You Couldn't Speak for Yourself, What Would You Want Done for You?*

Think about the following statements. Do you agree with any of them? Discussing your answers with others can help them understand what is important to you and where you stand with respect to health care decisions.

- My life should be prolonged as long as it can, no matter what its quality, and using any means possible.

- I believe there are some situations in which I would not want treatments to keep me alive.

- I'd want my religious advisors to be consulted about all medical decisions made on my behalf to make sure they are in keeping with my religious teachings.

- My personal wishes would not be as important as what my family thinks is best for me.

510

- I'd want to have my pain controlled, even if the medications make me sleepy or make it difficult to have conversations with my family.

## Who Will Speak for Me If I Can't Speak for Myself?

For people with close family members, choosing a spokesperson may seem simple. If you are married, your health care providers will ask your spouse to speak for you. If you are not married, other relatives usually are consulted. However, if these people disagree, it can be very difficult for health care providers to know whom to listen to.

Sometimes your closest next-of-kin is not the person you would like to speak for you. In that case, you can formally appoint the person of your choice to be your voice. You can give this person the legal authority to make health care decisions for you using a *durable power of attorney for health care*. The following story shows why this is so important.

Larry Roberts assumed his doctor would listen to his closest friend, Mrs. Alice Jergen, for advice about his wishes for medical treatment. She'd been visiting him daily since he entered the final stages of lung cancer and they talked about it often. Three days ago, he developed an infection and became delirious with a high fever. Before making a decision about whether to start him on antibiotics, Mr. Roberts' doctor felt it was appropriate to consult his next-of-kin. This turned out to be his brother Frank, who lives in another state. Frank and Mrs. Jergen disagreed about what medical treatment Mr. Roberts should have. Mr. Roberts never talked about this with his brother. But because Mrs. Jergen was not related to Mr. Roberts and had no legal authority, the doctor followed his brother's advice.

A durable power of attorney for health care ensures that the right person will speak for you when you can't speak for yourself.

## Common Questions about Choosing a Spokesperson.

If you are married, your spouse will be recognized as the person to make decisions on your behalf, unless you have a durable power of attorney for health care that appoints someone else.

### What Happens If I Don't Appoint a Spokesperson?

Health care providers will consult with someone close to you. They will usually contact your next-of-kin, starting with your spouse. If you are married and want your spouse to be your proxy, then doing nothing is probably okay. If you are separated from your spouse but not divorced, health care providers will still ask your spouse to make decisions for you.

### Can a Friend Be My Spokesperson?

Yes, but unless you appoint your friend as your spokesperson, using a durable power of attorney for health care, he or she may not be consulted or may be overruled by family members.

### What Happens If Some Family Members Don't Agree with My Spokesperson about What's Best for Me?

Health care providers usually will give treatment while they try to reach agreement about what to do. The best way to prevent disagreements is to communicate with everyone ahead of time to let them know who you've picked and what you want.

### Who Is the Best Person to Be My Spokesperson?

Think about the people in your life and ask yourself the following questions.

- Who knows me well?
- Who would do a good job representing me?
- Who is available to come to my side if needed?

### What If I Don't Know Anyone Who I Want to Be My Spokesperson?

Your best choice is to write down your wishes and give a copy to your health care provider. Fill out a legal form, such as a living will, with as much detail as possible. Include a personalized statement to provide a better understanding of your wishes.

### Do I Need to Talk to My Spokesperson Now?

Yes, because you need to make sure they are willing, and to tell them about your wishes so they'll know what to do for you.

## What Else Can I Do to Make My Wishes Known?

It is good idea to write down your wishes for future health care because it gives others the most complete picture of how you feel and what you would want. You can do this by signing an advance directive, which can be either a formal, legal document, or an informal statement of your wishes. There are two types of formal directives: proxy and instructional.

**A proxy directive** uses a legal document called a *durable power of attorney for health care* to appoint a spokesperson who can make health care decisions on your behalf. It goes into effect when health care decisions need to be made for you and you can't communicate or make health care decisions for yourself.

**Instructional directives**, such as a *living will* or *directive to physicians*, are written instructions to physicians in the event you cannot speak for yourself. They usually tell health care providers which treatments you would not want if you become terminally ill or end up in a permanent coma.

**A personalized statement** lets you express what is most important to you. In addition to talking with loved ones and health care providers, you can make this statement by writing a letter to your loved ones or making an audio or video tape.

## Which Directive Is Best?

It depends on your situation. You could complete either a proxy or instructional directive, both, or just a personal statement. Most health care providers like proxy directives best because it means they will have someone to talk with who knows you well. But not everyone has a proxy to represent them. In that case, an instructional directive will help your health care providers decide what's best for you. Either way, adding a personalized statement helps others feel more confident that they are doing what you would have wanted them to do.

There are 3 steps to advance care planning:

1.  Think through your preferences

2.  Talk about your wishes with others

3.  Document your wishes

Completing an advance directive or writing a personalized statement are ways to accomplish the third step.

## Common Questions about Advance Directives.

### Why Should I Complete an Advance Directive?

Advance directives are legal documents that help you keep control over future health care decisions. They can also relieve your loved ones of the burden of making life and death decisions on your behalf.

### When Do Advance Directives Go into Effect?

Only if you become unable to understand your medical treatment options or are unable to communicate your wishes for medical treatment.

### What's the Difference between a Living Will and a Regular Will?

A living will, like all advance directives, is restricted to decisions about your health care. It goes into effect while you are still alive but unable to communicate. A regular will pertains to your estate and property. It goes into effect after your death.

### What Should I Do with My Advance Directive after I've Signed It?

You should give a copy to each person whom you want to be informed of your wishes, including your health care providers. Keep a list of their names. Put the original in a place where others can easily find it. Do not put your only copy in a safe-deposit box because it may not be easy to get if someone needs it. You can also fill out a wallet card to let people know where they can find a copy.

### What If I Change My Mind about What I Want after I've Completed an Advance Directive?

You can always change your directive. Either write the changes on your existing directive (initial and date the changes), or destroy the old one and write a new one. Be sure to give revised copies to everyone who has a copy of your older version.

### I Have Homes in Two States. Is My Advance Directive Valid in Both Places?

States often have different laws and different forms. It may be best to complete separate forms for each state. Check with your health care providers in each place.

## What Situations and Decisions Do People Commonly Face?

There are many situations in which people are not able to talk or communicate their wishes because of illness or injury. The following stories describe the kinds of decisions family members, friends, and health care providers must make when people can't speak for themselves. As you read these stories, try to think about how you would value the quality of your life in each situation and whether you would make the same kinds of decisions for yourself.

* The percent of people with dementia increases with age. At age 65, it's about 5%, at age 75, it's 10-20%, and at age 85, it's about 35%.

* With Alzheimer's disease the mind fails before the body—many people are otherwise healthy.

* In the advanced stages of dementia, people typically do not know where they are or recognize family members. They frequently stop eating, even with help from others.

### *Dementia*

Lily Chen, an elderly widow, was diagnosed 4 years ago with Alzheimer's disease, a common form of dementia. Over time she has gradually been losing her ability to think clearly and make decisions. Now she doesn't remember where she is and she can no longer recognize her daughter who visits her every day. For the last 8 months, she has been completely dependent on nurse's aides to bathe and feed her. Recently, she stopped eating altogether. Her daughter has power of attorney for health care and has to decide whether to have a long-term feeding tube surgically placed into her mother's stomach. The surgery is quick and won't cause much pain, but the real issue is guessing how Mrs. Chen would value her current life. If they place the feeding tube, Mrs. Chen could live for many more years in the same or worse condition. If they don't, she will die in about 2 weeks or less, and probably won't feel hungry or thirsty.

### *Coma*

* People in a coma don't feel pain or any other sensations.

* Comas can be caused by injury, illness, drug overdoses, and heart stoppage. Predicting the outcome of coma depends on what caused it, how long the person has been in coma, and age.

- Doctors say that it can take 3-4 weeks to see whether a person will come out of coma or go into a related condition—persistent vegetative state or PVS.

Tom Rice was 29 years old when he was hit by a car as he was riding his bicycle. He was taken to the hospital where he went into a coma. He lay in bed with his eyes closed—it looked as if he were asleep, except that he didn't respond when people talked to him and he didn't wake up. He was put on a ventilator, or breathing machine, that pumped air into his lungs because he couldn't breathe on his own. He also had a feeding tube down his throat so liquid food and fluids could go straight into his stomach.

Tom was single so his parents were asked to decide whether to continue the treatments that were keeping him alive. His doctors thought Tom might come out of it but that it could take anywhere from one week up to a year. They said that the longer Tom remained in a coma, the less likely it was that he would ever wake up. They thought that if he did come out of the coma, he would probably have severe brain damage. He would need help taking care of himself and would not be able to live alone.

Tom had never said anything about what he would want if he were in an accident. His parents kept him hooked up for weeks and weeks to give him every chance. After 2 months, they decided it was hopeless since he hadn't changed in all that time. They stopped all treatment and Tom died that same day.

### Stroke

- Risk factors for stroke include being over age 55, high blood pressure, heart disease, diabetes, smoking, high cholesterol, and family history.

- Stroke is the #1 cause of adult disability. Impairments can be mild, moderate, or severe, depending on what part of the brain is affected.

- Most recovery of lost sensations or function occurs within the first 3-6 months after a stroke.

- People who've had a stroke have a 5-10% chance of having another one. The first few months after their first stroke is the time when they are at greatest risk.

Flora Park woke up one day and couldn't move her left arm. Her vision was blurred and she was having difficulty talking. Her husband called her doctor who told her to go to the hospital—he suspected a stroke. After a long day of tests, the doctors agreed it was a stroke. They started her on medication and rehabilitation therapy. After a few more days, her sight improved and she was talking clearly again. After two months, she could move her arm, but it was still a little clumsy and weak. Her therapist taught her ways to make the most of her weak arm. She was adjusting to her new situation, but she worried constantly about what would happen if she had a more serious stroke.

She talked about this with her husband and their children. She said, "This stroke has made me think long and hard about what's important to me. The doctor said that even with my medications, I could have another stroke and I might not be able to tell you what I want. So I'm telling you now. I love life and don't want to give up. That's why I'd be willing to go to the hospital and start rehab again to see whether I can get better. But if I get to a point where I'll never be able to feed myself or do anything on my own, then I don't want anything done to prolong my life. That means no CPR if my heart stops and no machines. My biggest fear is that I won't be able to talk with you or enjoy your company. I'd rather die quickly than suffer a long, slow decline."

## *Terminal Illness*

- With terminal illness, the underlying disease can no longer be cured. Most people with a terminal illness are expected to die within 6 months.

- Comfort care includes medications for pain and other symptoms, and keeping the person clean and dry. Sometimes treatments such as blood transfusions, antibiotics, or chemotherapy are used to provide comfort by relieving symptoms.

- People who are close to death often go in and out of awareness, being alert only part of the time.

Carlos Ruiz had severe heart disease for years. His doctor said, "Your heart is much worse and it will continue to get weaker. Now we need to make some decisions about your goals for care. One approach would be to concentrate on supporting your heart, lungs, and other vital organs to extend your life as long as possible. Another option would be to make relief of pain and discomfort our highest priority, even if it meant you might not live as long. Which of these approaches sounds right for you?"

517

Mr. Ruiz said, "I've lived with this bad heart for a long time. I'm tired of fighting, but I'm not quite ready to give up. I'd try simple treatments, especially if I can be at home with my family. I'd rather be comfortable than live a long time."

Mr. Ruiz' doctor gave him a referral to a hospice nurse who started visiting him at home. He got a few lung infections which made it hard to breathe. He cured them by taking antibiotic pills at home. Then he got another infection that didn't get better, despite taking antibiotic pills. He had a high fever and was so sick that his wife had to decide what to do. His doctor and hospice nurse said they could put him in the hospital to treat his infection which would relieve his symptoms and might prolong his life. Or he could stay at home with additional comfort measures until he died.

Mrs. Ruiz sent him to the hospital because she thought he might get better and could return home for a little while longer.

## Telling Others What You Want

Your loved ones and health care providers need to know how you feel if they are to carry out your wishes in the future.

Raising this topic is not always easy. If your family members and friends are uncomfortable talking or even thinking about these issues, consider these ideas to get a discussion started:

- Begin on a positive note by talking about how much you value them and their willingness to listen to you.

- Share one of these stories to show how planning in advance can ease the burden on family members.

- Remind them that accidents can happen to anyone at any time and that you just want to be prepared.

Including others in a discussion about what you want can also help clarify your wishes in your own mind. Consider the story of Mr. Nakamura.

Kenji Nakamura wanted to appoint his daughter Suzy to be his spokesperson. The first time he tried to talk to her about this she said, "Dad, you're going to live to be 100 years old! We don't need to talk about this now." The next time she came over he eased into the conversation by talking about the things he was thankful for, including his health. Then he asked her to look at the statement of his wishes that he'd been writing. Suzy was surprised to learn that her dad never wanted to be kept alive by machines. She said, "What if you only needed a breathing machine for a few days?" After talking about it they both had a clearer understanding of his wishes—he didn't want to be kept alive on a ventilator forever, but a short time would be OK.

## Writing It Down

Even if you've talked about your wishes, when the time comes, stress and strong emotions can cause your loved ones to forget what you told them or wonder if they are making the right decision. A written document can help keep things straight.

You may document your preferences formally using advance directives.

Some people are more comfortable documenting their wishes informally in a letter or an audio or video tape. It seems more personal. You can also personalize formal advance directives by attaching informal statements

Either way, writing it down means you've left a record of your wishes that everyone—family, friends, and health care providers—can use as a general guide or as explicit instructions. You won't have to worry that your wishes will be forgotten or misunderstood.

"What you say is in the air, what you write is always there."

Suzy was glad her dad had written his wishes down when Mr. Nakamura fell and broke his hip. While he was in the hospital, he got pneumonia and became confused. His doctors asked Suzy whether they should put him on a ventilator if he had trouble breathing. She shared his advance directive with the doctors and explained her father's fears of being kept alive forever by a machine. As a result, they decided to start antibiotic treatment, and if needed, they would put Mr. Nakamura on a breathing machine for only a short period of time. If he didn't seem to be improving, they would stop the breathing machine and focus their attention on keeping him comfortable. Suzy was thankful that her father had insisted on discussing his wishes. Including others in a discussion about what you want can also help clarify your wishes in your own mind.

## What's Next?

### Talk about It

Now that you've read through the basics of advance care planning, you may feel ready to talk about your wishes with your family and health care providers.

## Write about It

Sometimes it helps to have a few thoughts on paper. Don't worry about making them perfect—the important thing is to get started.

# More Information about Health Conditions and Treatments

## Coma

*What Is It?*

Coma is a state of unconsciousness that persists for some time. It may be caused by a head injury, a severe stroke, bleeding in the head, or a severe illness. A person who is unconscious shows little or no movement or response to stimulation. It usually looks as though they were asleep. A related and more serious condition is called persistent vegetative state (PVS). A person in PVS is unconscious but sometimes opens his or her eyes and may have unintentional movements such as yawning, and random movements of the head or limbs. PVS usually develops after about a month in a coma.

*What Is It Like?*

People who have been in a coma (and then come out of it) usually say they have no memory of any awareness at all during the coma. These people generally report no memory of pain or discomfort. Those few people who say they were aware of things going on around them or hearing what was being said near them were not in a true coma. Observation of coma patients typically shows no sign that the patient is in any pain or distress. People in coma do not get out of bed, or communicate in any way. They are usually cared for in a hospital or nursing home because they need to have all of their personal care done for them including being fed through a tube, having their body wastes cleaned up, and being turned every few hours to prevent bed sores.

*What's Likely to Happen?*

Just after a person goes into a coma, it is very hard to predict what will happen. If and when the person comes out of a coma depends on his or her age, what caused it, and his or her overall health. People have very little chance of ever coming out of coma that was caused by illness after about 3 months, or one that was caused by a head injury after about 12 months. There are stages of coma. A person in a lighter stage of coma has a better chance of coming out of it than someone in deeper stages.

### What Are the Key Things to Think About?

- Would you want to be kept alive after the point in time when your doctors think that you probably won't ever come out of the coma?

- Would you want to be kept alive if the doctors felt sure that if you were to come out of the coma, you would have permanent brain damage or other severe limitations?

## Dementia

### What Is It?

Dementia is a condition in which there is a loss of memory and other mental functions, serious enough to affect interacting with other people. The most common types of dementia are due to Alzheimer's disease, AIDS, and multiple strokes. Other types of dementia can occur as a result of head injury, heavy use of alcohol, or thyroid problems. With the most common forms of dementia, mental functions get worse over time. These include memory, thinking, talking, problem solving, and perception.

### What's It Like?

Some people in the early stage of Alzheimer's disease may be aware of their forgetfulness, but as the dementia progresses, they will become totally unaware of the forgetfulness and other mental deficits. They will lose the ability to concentrate. Later, there may be mood changes whereby they may lose interest in things around them, or become agitated or violent on occasion even with family members. In still later stages, they become less active, less talkative. In the latest stages, they may no longer recognize close family or friends, lose their sense of day and night, and wander around the house at odd hours.

### What's Likely to Happen?

Most types of dementia are irreversible and will get worse over time. Exceptions include dementia caused by thyroid problems, as well as memory problems due to depression which are treatable and may be reversible. The speed of deterioration is unpredictable, but severe dementia from Alzheimer's usually occurs within 5-10 years from the first signs of memory loss. In later stages, people with dementia become incontinent, losing control of their bowels and bladder. They often require nursing home care because they need daily help with feeding, dressing, and bathing and this is often more than most families can handle. As they lose interest in eating, complications of malnutrition such as infections and skin ulcers can lead to death.

*What Are the Key Things to Think About?*

• If you had severe dementia and then became ill with a reversible illness, such as pneumonia, would you want treatment even though the treatment would not help your memory problems? What if treatment included going to the hospital?

• If you were unable to eat enough and were severely demented would you want to receive your nutrition and fluids through a feeding tube placed directly into your stomach?

• Some people with dementia seem happy while others seem sad or upset. If you were severely demented, how much should other people pay attention to your mood when making decisions about what it best for you?

**Stroke**

*What Is It?*

Someone who has sustained an injury to a part of the brain, either because of a blockage in the blood vessels, or a burst blood vessel, is said to have had a stroke. Strokes rank third among all causes of death and are a major cause of long-term disability, but not all strokes cause disability. The kind of disability a person develops depends on what part of the brain is damaged and how severely. A stroke is also known as a cerebrovascular accident, or a CVA.

*What's It Like?*

The most common effects of a stroke are: (1) weakness or loss of movement and sensation in an arm, a leg, or both on one side of the body, (2) difficulty speaking, (3) partial loss of sight in one or both eyes,(4) trouble swallowing, and (5) problems understanding what other people are saying. Some people experience changes in their mood or personality. Depression is common among people who have had a stroke, often because of injury to the brain.

## *What's Likely to Happen?*

With the most minor of strokes, a person has a loss of feeling or ability to move a part of the body for less than a few days. With moderate strokes, a person may lose the ability to use one arm, need to walk with the assistance of a cane or walker, and have some slurring of speech. With serious strokes, a person might lose the use of one entire side of the body, need assistance to get out of bed and into a chair, or may not be able to speak or understand others at all. With the most severe strokes, a person often loses consciousness and falls into a coma. Most recovery from strokes happens within the first few days up to about 3 months, though modest improvements may continue up to 12 months. After that, whatever disability remains is likely to be permanent.

## *What Are the Key Things to Think About?*

Every stroke is different and so is a person's ability to adapt to losses in function and disability. Many people find that with time and help they can adjust to their new circumstances after a stroke. If you had a stroke, what level of disability do you think you would want to live with? Are there some situations that you would find unacceptable? If so, what are they?

## *Terminal Illness*

### *What Is It?*

Every illness that causes death has a terminal stage. That stage is defined as the point when treatments can no longer work to reverse the illness or keep the disease from getting worse. No matter what treatments are given, the person is going to die within a short time. It is very hard to predict exactly how much time a person has to live at this stage, but most doctors expect they will live about six months or less.

### *What's It Like?*

During a terminal illness people often lose strength and become confined to bed either in their own home, or if they need more help, in a hospital, nursing home, or hospice. Their bodies will begin to shut down. This may or may not be accompanied by pain. Some terminal illnesses, such as the later stages of cancer, can be painful, although medications can control the pain. Appetite usually diminishes. As people get closer to death they will almost certainly think and communicate less clearly.

### What's Likely to Happen?

Near death there are times when people are not able to express their wishes clearly. Some people experience short periods of mental confusion, for example, they drift in and out of awareness over the course of a day. Many people lapse into a coma just before they die. For example, they may become dehydrated or develop an infection that, if it is not treated, could cause death more quickly than their primary terminal illness. If the treatments for these conditions are successful, they would postpone the moment of death and might prolong any suffering or discomfort associated with the terminal illness.

### What Are the Key Things to Think About?

- If you had a terminal illness, what would be the most important thing for you: relieving suffering or prolonging life?

- What would be your goals for treatment of any other problems if you had a terminal illness? Treatment for secondary problems (such as an infection) would not cure the primary terminal illness (such as cancer or heart disease).

## Treatments

### CPR—Cardiopulmonary Resuscitation

#### What's the Problem?

During a life-threatening illness or a heart attack, your heart may suddenly stop beating and you may stop breathing. Or your heart may beat so irregularly that it no longer effectively pumps blood to your brain. These events mostly occur for people with heart disease, but can also occur without any known cause. Soon after blood stops moving to your brain you will lose consciousness and not be aware of anything going on around you.

*What's CPR?*

CPR involves vigorous pressing on your chest to keep blood circulating while electrical shock is applied to your chest to jump start your heart. Mouth-to-mouth breathing is used to restart your own breathing, or a breathing tube is placed into your windpipe and air is pumped into your lungs to help you breathe. You receive medications through a tube placed in one of your veins. Typically, all this goes on for about 15-30 minutes.

*What Happens If I Decide Not to Get CPR?*

With or without CPR, you will almost immediately lose consciousness. Without CPR, death will follow in about five to ten minutes.

*What Are the Good Points of Getting CPR?*

If you are in relatively good health when you need CPR, it can return you to roughly the same state you were in when your heart stopped. For people with some types of heart disease, CPR can restore an irregular heartbeat. Pain or discomfort is not an issue while you receive CPR because you are not conscious during the process.

*What Are the Bad Points of Getting CPR?*

After CPR, however, you could have a sore chest or broken ribs because of the electrical shocks and vigorous massage. In addition, the chest compressions could result in a collapsed lung, which would require additional treatment. Most people who need CPR need a mechanical ventilator to support their breathing afterwards.

The success rate for CPR depends on many things: your overall health when you need it, where you get it (in the community or in the hospital), your age, and how quickly it starts after your heart stops beating. If you are under age 65, the success rate ranges between 25-40%. If you are over age 65, this rate drops to between 1-4%. CPR is rarely successful if you already have a chronic illness that affects your vital organs, such as your heart, lungs, liver, or kidneys. Less than ten out of 100 hospitalized patients respond to CPR by returning to the state they were in before their heart stopped. Of those who survive, many continue to live, but in a weaker state or with significant brain damage because blood could not get to their brain in time. CPR could keep you from dying, but you might live in a coma or be unable to think clearly.

## Feeding Tubes—Artificial Delivery of Nutrition and Fluids

### What's the Problem?

You may find yourself unable to swallow food. This could happen after an accident that damages your throat. It could also happen if you are unconscious or have some kinds of brain damage. When this happens you will be unable to take in enough food and water by mouth to keep yourself alive.

### What's a Feeding Tube?

A feeding tube is used to carry liquid nutrition and fluids into your body. One kind of tube goes up your nose, down your throat, and into the stomach. This is called a nasogastric tube. It is about 1/8 of an inch in diameter. Another kind of tube is surgically placed into the wall of your stomach. The operation is quick and safe and you will feel little discomfort. Once the tube is in place it is painless.

### What Happens If I Decide Not to Get a Feeding Tube?

If you don't receive any nutrition or fluids you will fall into a state much like a deep sleep. This will take about one to three weeks, during which time, you will be kept comfortable. For example, ice chips on your lips will help keep them moist. Usually, after several days, you will no longer experience thirst or hunger. Also, you will not feel pain as easily as you do now. Within a day or two after you enter this deep sleep, your heart will fail, and death will follow within five to ten minutes.

### What Are the Good Points of Getting a Feeding Tube?

A feeding tube can provide your nutritional and fluid needs. With adequate nutrition, you will be less likely to get bedsores. A feeding tube is not painful, although the kind that goes down your nose (nasogastric tube) can be uncomfortable. The surgically placed stomach tube is easy to manage without help from others as long as you can take care of yourself. With this kind of tube, you can pour the liquid nutrition into the tube, move about, and bathe, all on your own. This tube is placed under your clothes, so other people would not know you have one.

### What Are the Bad Points of Getting a Feeding Tube?

Having a tube down your throat will feel somewhat uncomfortable and unpleasant, although not truly painful. You could aspirate liquid (get it into your lungs) which can cause pneumonia. With either tube, you will not be able to taste anything. Receiving fluids might make it harder for you to control urination if you are confined to a bed.

If you are already in the terminal stage of an illness, a feeding tube will likely postpone your death. Tube feeding also makes it possible (in some cases) to keep people alive who are in a coma, have severe strokes, or severe dementia for a long time, even if they might not have wanted it.

## *Mechanical Ventilators (Breathing Machines)*

### *What's the Problem?*

You may not be able to breathe on your own for a number of reasons. Perhaps you have been in an accident that has damaged your airways. You might have a serious lung disease, or maybe you have suffered brain damage. You need a machine to breathe for you, either for the short term (a few hours to a few days) or for the long term (the rest of your life). It may be impossible to tell how long you will need it.

### *What's a Mechanical Ventilator?*

Mechanical ventilators (also called breathing machines or respirators) completely take over the task of breathing. A tube is placed into your windpipe, either through your mouth or nose or through a small surgical incision at the base of your neck. The tube is about 3/4 of an inch in diameter, about as big as a dime. The tube will make it hard or impossible to talk. Most patients on a mechanical ventilator are in a hospital, usually in an intensive care unit. They are usually not able to get out of bed. In some situations, a portable ventilator allows a patient who is completely paralyzed to get around in a specially-equipped wheelchair.

### *What Happens If I Decide Not to Get a Mechanical Ventilator?*

Without some external breathing assistance, you will die quickly. If you stop breathing, you will die within five minutes. You could be given medications that will sedate you. These medications help you relax so you will not panic or feel like you are struggling for breath.

### *What Are the Good Points of Getting a Mechanical Ventilator?*

Mechanical ventilation is a painless, although often uncomfortable, way to continue your life. It is often needed for only a short time, for example, just long enough to let your body recover from a serious illness. In some cases, it can relieve the discomfort of feeling breathless. If you need a ventilator for a long time, it can sustain your life indefinitely when you might otherwise die.

*What Are the Bad Points of Getting a Mechanical Ventilator?*

Even if you are conscious, you will not be able to talk very well or at all. You will likely be confined to bed. You will also be dependent on others to bathe, feed, and dress you and to take care of your bowels and bladder. Nurses will also need to suction your lungs to keep them clear of mucous. It may be hard to tell how long you will need to be on a ventilator. If you have a terminal illness, a mechanical ventilator will only prolong dying.

## Talking about Your Wishes

Perhaps the single most important step in advance care planning is talking about your wishes with whomever might be called upon to speak for you. Whether or not you complete a formal advance directive, you still need to express your preferences clearly to your loved ones and health care providers.

Talking with your loved ones and health care providers can also help you think about what you want. Often they will ask you questions or tell you things that will make you think about your wishes in another way. The more thoroughly and clearly you communicate, the easier it will be for everyone to do the right thing.

### Starting the Discussion

There is no right way to start this conversation. Nor is there a right time. The best thing to do is make a time and get started. But what if loved ones resist? What if they make excuses like, "You've got a lot of life left in you—why do we have to talk about this now?" Here are some suggestions for getting started:

- **Relate a story from this chapter.** If there was a story from the first part of this chapter that got your attention, it may also get the attention of the person you want to talk to. Share this story with them to let them know what you are concerned about and why this is important to you.

- **Remind them of a situation someone else experienced.** Another way to introduce the topic is to think about stories of friends or relatives who experienced an illness and faced a difficult situation. You could start the conversation saying, "Do you remember what happened to so-and-so and what his family went through? I don't want you to have to go through that with me. That's why I want to talk about this now, while we can."

- **Be firm and straightforward.** If someone puts you off out of their own discomfort, you could say, "I know this makes you feel uncomfortable, but I need you to bear with me and hear what I have to say because it's very important to me."

- **Point out the possible consequences of not talking now.** Someone may be more willing to talk if you start by saying something like, "If we don't talk about this now, we could both end up in a situation that is even more uncomfortable. I'd really like to avoid that if I could."

- **Use a letter, tape, or video recording.** It may be easier for people to hear what you have to say initially if you aren't there. So you could ask them to read a personal letter, listen to a tape, or watch a video in which you express your feelings and preferences. Afterwards, they may be more ready to sit down and talk with you.

### Asking Someone to Be Your Spokesperson

When you ask someone to be your spokesperson, you are asking them to assume a big responsibility that you both want to be comfortable with. To ease into the conversation, you might ask questions like: "Would you be willing to represent my views about medical decisions if I can't speak for myself?" "Can you make decisions for me that are based on my values, preferences, and wishes—even if they're not like yours?"

You do not want this person to agree to be your spokesperson if they really have strong misgivings about it. So be sure to tell them that you will not be offended or hurt if they feel they cannot do this for you.

If the person agrees to be your spokesperson, you can reassure them that you are not expecting them to be superhuman or all-knowing. Give them explicit permission to make decisions for you, especially for those situations that you haven't discussed or couldn't predict.

### Who Else Should You Talk To?

Think about the people who play an important part in your life. Then try to imagine a time when you are either seriously ill or injured and unable to communicate. Who would you want to be around at such a time? These are the people you should make a point of sharing your feelings with now. They might include:

- Your spokesperson
- Family
- Health care providers
- Friends
- Other caregivers
- Clergy

You do not need to speak to everyone at the same time. However, it can be helpful to talk to your family as a group so that they all hear what you have to say in the same way.

### What If You Don't Have Close Family or Friends?

Your best option is to write down your wishes, either in an advance directive or personalized statement, or both. You could also make a tape or video recording of your wishes. Then be sure to share it with your health care providers.

## Nine Important Issues to Discuss

Talk about the following issues. Discussing them will help avoid confusion, conflict, and hurt feelings between loved ones and care providers.

### 1. Your Choice of a Spokesperson

Let your loved ones and care providers know who you have chosen to be your spokesperson—and why. This is especially important if your spokesperson is not a member of the family. You might say something like this: "I've asked so-and-so to be my spokesperson in case I need medical care but can't speak for myself. My choice is not a reflection of my relationship with you. But after careful thought, I feel that he/she is the right person to handle this responsibility for these reasons..."

### 2. Your Beliefs

Tell those close to you what it is that makes life worth living, as well as what would make it unbearable—and why. If you have fears about being a burden, explore these feelings with those who will care for you. Family members often view caring for loved ones as an honor—not a burden.

### 3. Health Conditions

Share how you feel about being kept alive in conditions that could leave you unable to speak for yourself.

### 4. Life-Sustaining Treatments

Share how you'd feel about different medical treatments, including hospice, and under what circumstances you would or would not want to receive them.

### 5. Your Vision of a Good Death

If you hope to die in a certain way—whether it's at home, in your sleep, with family by your side, or free of pain—tell people.

### 6. Organ Donation

If you'd like others to benefit from your healthy organs after your death, make sure you family understands this because they must give their permission.

### 7. Funeral Arrangements

Share your thoughts about what you want to be done with your remains. If you have ideas about what you would like for a memorial service or how you'd like an obituary to read, talk about that too.

### 8. Documentation of Your Wishes

If you've decided to complete an advance directive or write a personalized statement, tell people where they can find this information in the future.

### 9. Helping Others Use Your Personalized Directive

Instructional directives and personal statements can be understood either as specific instructions, or as general guidelines. You can help others interpret your written wishes by including something like this in your document:

531

- "I would like the statements in my personalized directive followed to the letter."

- "I would like the statements in my personalized directive to be used as a general guide."

- "I want those statements that I've marked with a star (*) followed to the letter because I feel very strongly about them. Use the rest of my statements as a general guide."

## Talking to Your Health Care Providers

Here are a few reasons why it is important to talk to your health care providers about advance care planning:

- They need to know that you've documented your wishes in an advance directive or personalized statement. Without this knowledge, your health care providers could make treatment decisions that may not agree with your wishes.

- You want to be sure that they will interpret your wishes or your advance directive in the way you intend. If they believe your words mean one thing, while your spokesperson or family members interpret it differently, you'll probably get treatment until they can resolve their differences.

- Your health care providers can answer questions you may have about different health conditions, treatments, and your prognosis.

### Make a Special Appointment

To make sure you've got their attention, make a special appointment with your health care provider to talk about this. Health care providers are people too—some are uncomfortable talking about end-of-life issues, or have other things on their mind. You don't want to be in a hurry when you have this conversation.

If your health care provider wants to just file your advance directive in your chart without discussing it, don't let that happen! Make sure they know why you feel the way you do. This will make it easier for them to understand and follow your wishes.

### What to Say

To help you organize your thoughts and cover all the important issues, bring a copy of your advance directive. Also, during this appointment, you may want to ask some or all of these questions:

- "Given my current health, am I at risk of facing a situation when I might not be able to communicate?"

- "Is there anything about my current health that would compromise the likelihood of success of different treatments?"

- "Can I count on you to respect my wishes and contact my spokesperson if I'm unable to speak for myself?"

- "What if you're not the health care provider who's there when I need care? How will the other health care providers know about my wishes?"

## Reviewing Your Wishes

With all the advances in medicine and health care, it's a good idea to review your wishes from time to time. Values and preferences for health care often change with age or when there are changes in your health condition. When and how often you review your wishes depends on your circumstances.

### Changes in Your Family Situation

If your spokesperson moves, you get a divorce, or a family member dies, you may need to rethink who will speak for you.

### When You Are Healthy

When you're healthy, a periodic review prepares you and your family for emergency situations, such as a car accident or a sudden illness. Here are some ideas about good times to schedule these reviews.

- Just before an annual check-up with your health care provider. You'll refresh your memory about what you said last year, and then be ready to talk about new questions or concerns at your appointment.

- Special anniversary dates. Some people pick dates such as a birthday or the first day of spring. By picking the same date every year, it gets on your to do list and becomes a part of your routine.

- Holidays or other family gatherings. Others like to do this during these times so they can take advantage of having everyone together in the same place. This makes it easier to share their views with everyone all at once.

## *When Your Health Changes*

Another important time to think about your wishes is if your health condition changes, especially if it takes a turn for the worse. Here are some things to think about in these circumstances.

- Adjusting to new limitations. People often think that if they had physical or mental limitations their life would be terrible. But some people adjust to limitations and disability and find that life still has a lot to offer them.

- Concerns about being a burden. It's normal for people with new limitations to feel like they are a burden because they need more help from others. But be sure to ask your family members what it means to them to be a burden before you spare them. You may be taking away their chance to return the gift of the love and care that you've given them.

## *When You Are Dying*

After people learn they are dying, they often rethink their priorities. Their attention often shifts to making the most of the time they have left. You need to focus on what's important at this time.

# Legal and Ethical Issues of Advance Care Planning

## *What Do I Need to Do to Make Sure My Advance Directive Is a Legal Document?*

Generally speaking, you need to sign your advance directive and have it witnessed.

## *Will My Advance Directive Be Legal in All 50 States?*

The laws vary from state to state, but most states will recognize the intent of an advance directive. If you have a home in more than one state, check with your health care provider or a lawyer in each state—one form might work for all places.

## *Do Health Care Providers Have to Follow My Advance Directive?*

Yes, but if they disagree with the preferences you indicate in your advance directive, they should refer your care to another provider. In a minority of cases, providers have overruled patient directives because they felt that the circumstances at the time did not match what was written.

### What If Family Members and/or Providers Disagree about How to Interpret My Directive?

Most health care facilities have an Ethics Committee who can help resolve disagreements between family members or family members and providers. Talking with your caregivers ahead of time can help avoid future conflicts.

### Is Withdrawing Treatment Considered Suicide?

Most people would say no. Withdrawing or stopping a treatment after it has been started, is one way that patients can exercise their right to refuse treatment especially if the treatment does not seem to be achieving the desired goal. However, some religions believe otherwise. You may want to check with your religious advisor to be sure.

### What Is the Difference between Withholding and Withdrawing Treatment?

From an ethical and legal standpoint, there is no difference between these two: both are ways to stop unwanted or ineffective treatments. However, not all religions agree with this view—again, you should check with your clergy. Also, some people feel it is harder to withdraw treatment once it is started than to withhold it. But having the option to withdraw treatments means that doctors can give treatments a try, then stop them if they aren't working.

### Can I Specify That I Want Assisted Suicide in My Directive?

No. Assisted suicide is currently illegal. However, even if it becomes legal, the person making the request would have to be competent and able to change their mind at the time of the suicide. Advance directives only go into effect when you are no longer competent to make decisions.

## Additional Resources

### Choice in Dying
1035 30th Street N.W.
Washington, DC 20007

## Choice in Dying, continued
Toll-Free: 800-989-9155
Tel: 202-338-9790
Website: www.unitedwaydenver.org
E-mail: cid@choices.org

## National Hospice and Palliative Care Organization
Department 929
Alexandria, VA 22334
Tel: 703-837-1500
Fax: 703-525-1233
Website: www.nhpco.org
E-mail: memberservice@nhpco.org

## National Funeral Directors Association
13625 Bishops Drive
Brookfield, WI 53005-6607
Toll-Free: 800-228-6332
Tel: 262-789-1880
Fax: 262-789-6977
Website: www.nfda.org
E-mail: nfda@nfda.org

## Neptune Society (cremation)
Corporate Headquarters
4312 Woodman Ave., 3rd Floor
Sherman Oaks, CA 91423
Toll-Free: 888-637-8863
Tel: 818-953-9995
Fax: 818-953-9844
Website: www.neptunesociety.com
E-mail: info@neptunesociety.com

# Part Seven

# Additional Help and Information

Chapter 51

# Glossary: Speaking the Language of Stroke

**Activities of daily living (ADL):** Basic daily living activities such as eating, grooming, toileting, and dressing.

**Ambulation:** The act of walking.

**Aneurysm:** A permanent abnormal balloon-like bulging of an artery's wall. The bursting of an aneurysm in a brain artery or blood vessel causes a hemorrhagic stroke.

**Anticoagulant agents:** Drugs used in stroke prevention therapy to prevent blood clots from forming or growing. Anticoagulants interfere with the production of certain blood components necessary for clot formation.

**Antihypertensive agents:** Drugs used in stroke prevention therapy to reduce high blood pressure. Various antihypertensives work in different ways some decrease the volume of plasma in the blood or slow the rate of blood flow through your body, while others relax the heart by affecting the passage of certain elements in the blood.

**Antiplatelet agents:** Drugs used in stroke prevention therapy to prevent blood clots from forming or growing. Antiplatelet agents attack the very beginning of the clot formation process by inhibiting an important enzyme necessary for platelet adhesion and activation.

---

"Speaking the Language of Stroke," © 2000 National Stroke Association (NSA), reprinted with permission.

539

**Aphasia:** A general term for communication problems, which may include the loss or reduction of the ability to speak, read, write, or understand, due to dysfunction of brain centers.

**Apoplexy:** Latin word for stroke, derived from the Greek word *plesso*. Apoplexy was defined as a stroke of God's hands.

**Apraxia:** A disorder of learned movement unexplained by deficits in strength, coordination, sensation, or comprehension.

**Arrhythmia:** An irregular or unpredictable heart beat.

**Atherosclerosis:** A hardening or build up of cholesterol plaque and other fatty deposits in the arteries.

**Aspiration:** The act of inhaling solid or liquid materials into the lungs.

**Ataxia:** A disorder in which muscles fail to move in a coordinated fashion.

**Atrial fibrillation (AF):** A heart disease in which the upper left chamber of the heart beats out of rhythm with the other three chambers. Atrial fibrillation increases a person's stroke risk by six times. AF is generally treatable with medication.

**Brain attack:** A term that more accurately describes the effect and action of stroke on the brain.

**Brain stem:** The stem-like part of the brain that connects the brain's right and left hemispheres with the spinal cord. Responsible for non-thinking activities such as breathing, blood pressure, and coordination of eye movements.

**Brain stem stroke:** A stroke that strikes the brain stem, which controls involuntary life-support functions such as breathing, blood pressure, and heart beat. Stroke in the brain stem can be particularly devastating.

**Bruit:** A distinctive rushing sound heard in the carotid arteries where plaque build up is present.

**Caregiver:** A person who provides direct support for a stroke survivor, usually in the home.

**Carotid artery:** The arteries on each side of the neck which carry blood from the heart to the brain. Each artery divides into internal and external carotid arteries. Each external carotid artery supplies blood to the neck and face. Each internal carotid artery supplies blood to the front part of the brain.

**Carotid endarterectomy:** The surgical removal of atherosclerotic plaque blocking or reducing blood flow in a carotid artery. It is performed when the artery is moderately to significantly diseased or blocked (more than 50 percent blockage).

**Carotid stenosis:** Narrowing of the carotid arteries caused by a buildup of plaque.

**Cerebellar stroke:** A stroke that strikes the cerebellum area of the brain, which controls balance and coordination.

**Cerebellum:** The second largest portion of the brain, responsible for coordinating voluntary muscle movements.

**Cerebral edema:** Swelling of the brain caused by an increase in intracellular water.

**Cerebrovascular accident:** A term traditionally used for stroke; also called CVA. The term is falling into disuse as we learn more about stroke's preventability and treatability. Stroke is no longer viewed as an accident.

**Cerebrovascular disease:** Known as CVD, cerebrovascular disease encompasses all abnormalities of the brain resulting from pathologies of its blood vessels. Stroke is the dominant, but not the only, form of CVD. Because of this dominance, the terms stroke and cerebrovascular disease are used interchangeably throughout literature. Examples of CVD outside of stroke include fibromuscular dysplasia, spontaneous dissecting carotid aneurysms, Moyamoya disease, and various inflammatory diseases of brain arteries.

**Compensation:** The ability of an individual with impairments from stroke to perform a task (or tasks) either using the impaired limb with an adapted (different) approach or using the unaffected limb to perform the task.

**Continence:** The ability to control bodily functions, especially urinary bladder and bowel functions.

541

**Contracture:** A condition of fixed, high resistance to passive stretching that results from fibrosis and shortening of tissues that support muscles or joints.

**CT or CAT scanner:** A specialized form of x-ray that allows physicians to see the internal structure of the brain in precise detail.

**Dysarthria:** A motor disorder that results in difficulty in motor speech mechanisms.

**Dysphagia:** Inability and/or difficulty in swallowing.

**Epidemiology:** The study of factors that influence the frequency and distribution of a disease in a population.

**Embolic stroke:** A stroke resulting from the blockage of an artery by a blood clot (or embolus).

**Emotional lability:** Instability or changeability of the emotions. In stroke survivors, emotional lability usually takes the form of inappropriate laughing or crying for no obvious reason.

**Forced use:** Use of an impaired limb encouraged by restraining the unaffected limb and hence, preventing it from taking over performance of required tasks.

**Functional limitation:** Reduced ability or lack of ability to perform an action or activity in the manner or within the range considered to be normal.

**Hemiplegia:** Paralysis of one side of the body.

**Hemorrhagic stroke:** A stroke caused by a ruptured blood vessel and characterized by a hemorrhage (bleeding) within or surrounding the brain.

**Hypertension:** Elevated blood pressure.

**Hypoxia:** Often mistaken for stroke, hypoxia refers to a lack of oxygen, in contrast to the lack of blood flow caused by stroke. Although the symptoms are similar to stroke, hypoxia is characterized by gait and speech disturbances, tremors, and weakness. The brain may suffer from hypoxia even if blood flow and blood pressure are normal. Causes include chronic pulmonary disease, pulmonary emboli, alveolar hypotension, anemia, and carbon monoxide poisoning.

**Incidence:** Describes the frequency with which new and recurrent cases of a specific disease occur during a certain period of time in a quantitatively undefined population (e.g., annual stroke incidence in the United States is 750,000).

**Incidence rate:** The number of new and recurrent cases of a disease that occur during a specified period of time per a defined number of individuals in a reference population (e.g., annual stroke incidence rate in African-Americans is 288 per 100,000).

**Incontinence:** Lack of control over excretory functions (urination, bowels).

**Infarct:** The immediate area of brain cell death caused by a stroke. When the brain cells in the infarct die, they release chemicals that set off a chain reaction that endangers brain cells in a larger surrounding area, known as the penumbra.

**Interdisciplinary treatment:** Treatment delivered to a patient by two or more medical or rehabilitative disciplines working collaboratively.

**Intracerebral hemorrhage:** A stroke caused by bleeding within the brain.

**Ischemia:** An interruption or blockage of blood flow to the brain.

**Left hemisphere:** The left half of the brain. Controls actions of the right side of the body, as well as analytic abilities, such as calculating, speaking, and writing.

**Mortality:** Describes the number of individuals who die from a specific disease during a certain period of time in a quantitatively undefined population (e.g., annual stroke mortality in the United States is 157,000).

**Mortality rate:** The number of persons dying from a specific disease within a specific population during a certain period of time (e.g., stroke mortality rate in the United States is 58.9 per 100,000).

**Motor control:** Ability to control movements of the body.

**Neglect:** A lack of awareness of actions or objects on the left or right side of the body, caused by damage to the other side of the brain. For example, a stroke survivor with left-side neglect may forget about food on the left side of the dinner plate.

**Neuroprotective agents:** Acute stroke interventional drugs which promise to protect brain cells, interrupting the process of secondary injury. Several neuroprotectives are in clinical trials. As of April, 1997, none is yet approved for acute stroke treatment. Most experimental neuroprotective drugs must be administered within a six-hour window of opportunity to limit damage following stroke symptoms.

**Penumbra:** An area of brain cells surrounding the initial site of brain damage from stroke. The brain cells in the penumbra are threatened by ischemic injury, but not irreversibly damaged.

**Platelets:** A component of blood that sticks together to form a plug, or clot, when certain substances beneath the blood vessel lining are exposed to circulating blood.

**Plesso:** Greek word meaning to be struck with violence or to be thunderstruck. The ancient Greeks used this word to describe the condition now known as a stroke.

**Prevalence:** The total number of individuals with a disease within a population group (e.g., stroke prevalence in the United States is 4 million).

**Randomized controlled trial:** A study in which subjects are assigned to the experimental or control (RCT) group by a random selection procedure before data collection begins.

**Right hemisphere:** The right half of the brain. Controls the actions of the left side of the body.

**Secondary injury:** Damage or death of brain cells in the larger area surrounding the infarct. Secondary injury is caused by a chain reaction of electrical and chemical events. Because this damage does not occur at the time of stroke, but in the hours following a stroke, it is critical to seek immediate medical treatment for stroke.

**Spasticity:** Abnormally increased tone in a muscle.

**Shock:** Colloquial term for stroke; used predominantly in the northeastern part of the country.

**Stenosis:** Reduction in the size of a vessel or other opening.

**Stroke:** The sudden interruption of blood flow to a part of the brain that kills brain cells within the area. As a result, body functions controlled by the affected area may be impaired or lost.

**Subarachnoid hemorrhage:** A stroke caused by bleeding under the thin, delicate membrane surrounding the brain.

**Thrombolytic agents:** Acute interventional drugs which work directly to break up or dissolve stroke-causing clots. Thrombolytics were first used successfully to treat heart attacks. Many other thrombolytic drugs are in clinical trials. TPA (tissue plasminogen activator) is the only FDA-approved acute stroke treatment.

**Thromboembolism:** An embolus that originates in and breaks away from a clot on one vessel to become lodged in another vessel.

**Thrombosis:** The clotting of blood within a vessel.

**Thrombotic stroke:** A stroke resulting from the blockage of a blood vessel by accumulated deposits, with blockage made complete when a clot develops or lodges on top of the deposits, preventing the free flow of blood.

**Transient ischemic attack:** Called TIAs, transient ischemic attacks are temporary interruptions of the blood supply to an area of the brain, typically caused by carotid stenosis. During a TIA, a person experiences a sudden onset of stroke symptoms. By definition, a TIA can last up to 24 hours, but most last only a few minutes and cause no permanent damage or disability. Sometimes called mini-strokes, TIAs must be taken seriously because they are usually a precursor to full strokes.

**Unilateral neglect:** A disturbance of a person's awareness of space on the side of the body opposite a stroke-causing lesion; often referred to as hemi-inattention.

**Vertebrobasilar arteries:** The two arteries in the back of the neck which supply blood to the brain stem and cerebellum.

Chapter 52

# Directory of Stroke Resources

## Government Agencies and Organizations

### Administration on Aging
1 Massachusetts Ave., NW
Washington, DC 20001
Toll-Free: 800-677-1116
Tel: 202-619-0724
Website: www.aoa.gov
E-mail: aoainfo@aoa.gov

### Brain Resources and Information Network (BRAIN)
P.O. Box 5801
Bethesda, MD 20824
Toll-Free: 800-352-9424
Tel: 301-496-5751
Fax: 301-402-2186
Website: http://ninds.nih.gov

### Eldercare Locator
National Association of Area
Agencies on Aging
927 15th St. N.W., 6th Floor
Washington, DC 20005
Toll-Free: 800-677-1116
Website: www.eldercare.gov
E-mail:
eldercare_locator@aoa.gov

### Equal Employment Opportunity Commission (EEOC)
1801 L Street N.W.
Washington, DC
Toll-Free: 800-669-4000
Toll-Free TTY: 800-669-6820
Tel: 202-663-4900
Website: www.ecoc.gov

This chapter includes resource listings compiled from sources deemed reliable and "Associations and Agencies," © NAA, reprinted with permission of the National Aphasia Association. Contact information was verified and updated in November 2002.

547

*National Heart, Lung, and Blood Institute Information Center*

Building 31, Room 5A52
31 Center Drive, MSC 2486
Bethesda, MD 20892
Tel: 301-592-8573
Fax: 301-592-8563
TTY: 240-629-3255
Website: www.nhlbi.nih.gov
E-mail:
NHLBIinfo@rover.nhlbi.nih.gov

*National High Blood Pressure Education Program*

NHLBI Information Center
P.O. Box 30105
Bethesda, MD 20824-0105
Tel: 301-592-8573
Fax: 301-592-8563
Website: www.nhlbi.nih.gov/
about/nhbpep

*Social Security Administration*

Office of Public Inquires
Windsor Park Building
6401 Security Blvd.
Baltimore, MD 21235
Toll-Free: 800-772-1213
Toll-Free TTY: 800-325-0778
Website: www.ssa.gov/work

## Private and Non-Profit Organizations

*American Heart Association/American Stroke Association*

7272 Greenville Avenue
Dallas, TX 75231-4596
Toll-Free: AHS: 800-242-8721
Toll-Free: ASA: 888-478-7653
Website:
www.americanheart.org

*Brain Aneurysm Foundation, Inc.*

12 Clarendon Street
Boston, MA 02116
Tel: 617-723-3870
Fax: 617-723-8672
Website: http://bafound.org
E-mail:
information@bafound.org

*National Rehabilitation Information Center*

4200 Forbes Blvd., Suite 202
Lanham, MD 20706
Toll-Free: 800-346-2742
Tel: 301-459-5900
Website: www.naric.com
E-mail:
naricinfo@heitechservices.com

*National Stroke Association*

9707 East Easter Lane
Englewood, CO 80112-3747
Toll-Free: 800-STROKES (787-6537)
Tel: 303-649-9299
Fax: 303-649-1328
Website: www.stroke.org

**Stroke Clubs International**
805 12th Street
Galveston, TX 77550
Tel: 409-762-1022
E-mail: strokeclub@aol.com

**Children's Hemiplegia and Stroke Association. (CHASA)**
Suite 305, PMB 149
4101 West Green Oaks Blvd.
Arlington, TX 76016
Tel: 817-492-4325
Website: www.hemikids.org
E-mail: support@chasa.org

## National Aphasia Association Listing of Associations and Agencies

***American Academy of Neurology***
1080 Montreal Ave.
St. Paul, MN 55116
Toll-Free: 800-879-1960
Tel: 651-695-1940
Fax: 651-695-2791
Website: www.aan.com
E-mail: memberservices@aan.com

Search for licensed neurologists in your community.

***American Academy of Physical Medicine and Rehabilitation***
Suite 2500
One IBM Plaza
Chicago, IL 60611-3604
Tel: 312-464-9700
Fax: 312-464-0227
Website: www.aapmr.org
E-mail: info@aapmr.org

Professional organization of physicians who are specialists in rehabilitation medicine (physiatrists).

## American Congress of Rehabilitation Medicine

Suite B-205
6801 Lake Plaza Drive
Indianapolis, IN 46220
Tel: 317-915-2250
Fax: 317-915-2245
Website: www.acrm.org
E-mail: acrm@acrm.org

Professional organization representing diverse professional disciplines interested in rehabilitation.

## American Heart Association—National Headquarters

7272 Greenville Avenue
Dallas, TX 75231
Toll-Free: 800-242-8721
Tel: 214-373-6300
Website:
www.americanheart.org

The AHA offers several free and low-cost publications of interest to persons with aphasia and their families, including the Stroke Connection and Stroke of Luck newsletters. They will also refer callers to local stroke support groups, and match them with pen pals with similar situations.

## American Occupational Therapy Association

4720 Montgomery Lane
P.O. Box 31220
Bethesda, MD 20814-3425
Tel: 301-652-2682
TDD: 800-377-8555
Fax: 301-652-7711
Website: www.aota.org

## American Physical Therapy Association

1111 N. Fairfax St.
Alexandria, VA 22314-1488
Toll-Free: 800-999-2782
Tel: 703-684-2782
Fax: 703-684-7343
Website: www.apta.org

Callers will be referred to their state chapter of the APTA for information about local therapists.

## American Psychological Association (Office of Public Information)

750 First Street, N.E.
Washington, DC 20002-4242
Toll-Free: 800-374-3120
Tel: 202-336-5500
Fax: 202-336-5549
Website: www.apa.org
E-mail: journals@apa.org

Callers will be referred to their state associations for local psychologists.

**American Speech-Language-Hearing Association (ASHA)**
10801 Rockville Pike
Rockville, MD 20852
Toll-Free: 800-638-8255
Tel: 301-897-5700
Website: www.asha.org.
E-mail: actioncenter@asha.org

ASHA will refer callers to Speech-Language Pathologists who specialize in aphasia (ask for adult neurogenic disorders), and other specialties. ASHA also sends free and low cost literature on a number of topics such as how to make a decision about which augmentative communication device is best for you, the *Americans with Disabilities Act*, and other topics.

**American Stroke Association**
7272 Greenville Ave.
Dallas, TX 75231
Tel: 888-478-7653
Fax: 214-706-5231.
Website:
www.strokeassociation.org

The American Stroke Association, a division of American Heart Association, is a non-profit organization dedicated to decreasing the impact of stroke through specifically targeted programs, products and services for healthcare professionals, consumers and stroke survivors focusing on stroke awareness, stroke prevention,

stroke treatment, and stroke rehabilitation.

**Association for Driver Rehabilitation Specialists (ADED)**
711 S. Vienna Street
Ruston, LA 71271
Toll-Free: 800-290-2344
Tel: 318-257-5055
Fax: 318-255-4175
Website: www.driver-ed.org
E-mail: webmaster@driver-ed.org

Will assist individuals in finding programs in their area. Can serve as a resource for equipment and where to get it.

**Brain Injury Association**
105 N. Alfred St.
Alexandria, VA 22314
Toll-Free Family Helpline: 800-444-6443
Tel: 703-236-6000
Fax: 703-236-6001
Website: www.biausa.org
E-mail:
familyhelpline@biausa.org

BIA also publishes a magazine and other literature for survivors of traumatic brain injuries and their families. Call for information about local chapters and support groups. The toll-free family helpline is answered by highly trained information and resource managers who answer all inquiries and send out packets of general information and direct callers to state and local resources.

## CARF... The Rehabilitation Accreditation Commission (CARF)

4891 East Grant Rd.
Tucson, AZ 85712
Tel: 520-325-1044
Fax: 520-318-1129
Website: www.carf.org
E-mail: info@carf.org

Send a self-addressed, stamped envelope along with your request for a listing of accredited rehabilitation facilities in a specific location. CARF does not accept requests for information by phone.

## Friend's Health Connection

P.O. Box 114
New Brunswick, NJ 08903
Toll-Free: 800-483-7436
Tel: 732-418-1811
Fax: 732-249-9897
Website: www.48friend.org
E-mail:
info@friendshealthconnection.org

Connects people who are currently experiencing or who have overcome the same disease, illness, handicap, or injury in order to communicate for mutual support.

## HEAD Injury Hotline

Brain Injury Resource Center
212 Pioneer Bldg.
Seattle, WA 98104-2221
Tel: 206-621-8558
Website: www.headinjury.com
E-mail: brain@headinjury.com

Provides hard to find information about head injury.

## HEATH Resource Center

National Clearinghouse on Post-Secondary Education for Individuals with Disabilities
American Council on Education
2020 K Street, N.W., Suite 220
Washington, DC 20037
Toll-Free: 800-544-3284
Tel: 202-973-0904 (Voice/TTY)
Fax: 202-973-0908
Website: www.heath-resource-center.org
E-mail:
askheath@heath.gwu.edu

Serves as an information exchange about educational support services, policies, procedures, adaptations and opportunities on American campuses, vocational-tech schools, adult education programs, independent living centers, transition, and other training entities after high school.

## Job Accommodation Network (JAN)

918 Chestnut Ridge Rd., Suite 1
West Virginia University
P.O. Box 6080
Morgantown, WV 26506-6080
Toll-Free: 800-526-7234 (Voice/TTY)
Tel: 304-293-7186
Fax: 304-293-5407
Website: http://janweb.icdi.wvu.edu
E-mail: jan@jan.icdi.wvu.edu

JAN provides information about job accommodation and the employability of people with functional limitations.

*Joint Commission on Accreditation of Healthcare Organizations (JCAHO)*
One Renaissance Blvd.
Oakbrook Terrace, IL 60181
Tel: 630-792-5000
Fax: 630-792-5005
Website: www.jcaho.org
E-mail: customerservice@jacho.org

JCAHO accredits hospitals, homecare facilities, ambulatory care facilities, long-term care facilities, laboratories, and networks (HMO's, affiliated clinics, etc.). They will provide verification that a specific facility is accredited, and they will also (for about $30.00) provide a summary of their on-site performance reports for specific organizations. Lists of all the accredited facilities within an area are expensive.

*Lending Library, Recordings for the Blind and Dyslexic*
20 Roszel Rd.
Princeton, NJ 08540
Toll-Free: 800-221-4792 or 866-RFBD-585
Tel: 609-452-0606
Website: http://rfbd.org
E-mail: custserv@rfbd.org

Approximately 83,000 books on audiotapes for people who have reading-related disabilities, including aphasia. Registration is $75.00 for first year and $25.00 in subsequent years.

*National Aphasia Association*
29 John St., Suite 1103
New York, NY 10038
Toll-Free: 800-922-4622
Fax: 212-267-2812
Website: www.aphasia.org
E-mail: naa@aphasia.org

*National Association of Social Workers*
Suite 700
750 First St., N.E.
Washington, DC 20002
Toll-Free: 800-638-8799
Tel: 202-336-8387
Website: www.naswdc.org
E-mail: membership@naswdc.org

Social workers seek to enhance or improve the psychosocial functioning of people through direct services or assistance in obtaining services such as housing, transportation, meals, healthcare, and caregivers support.

*National Brain Tumor Foundation*
Suite 700
414 13th St.
Oakland, CA 94612-2603
Toll-Free: 800-934-2873
Tel: 510-839-9777
Fax: 510-839-9779
Website: www.braintumor.org
E-mail: nbtf@braintumor.org

The NBTF provides educational information, support systems, and research concerning brain tumors.

## National Center for Learning Disabilities

381 Park Ave., South; Suite 1401
New York, NY 10016
Toll-Free: 888-575-7373
Tel: 212-545-7510
Fax: 212-545-9665
Website: www.ncld.org

NCLD's mission is to promote public awareness and understanding of children and adults with learning disabilities.

## National Easter Seal Society

230 West Monroe, Suite 1800
Chicago, IL 60606
Toll-Free: 800-221-6827
Tel: 312-726-6200
TTY: 312-726-4258
Fax: 312-726-1494
Website: www.easter-seals.org

Services differ a great deal, depending on the community served. Some affiliates are adult rehabilitation centers and have groups that offer support and information for people with aphasia and their families.

## National Family Caregivers Association

10400 Connecticut Ave., Suite 500
Kensington, MD 20895-3944
Toll-Free: 800-896-3650
Tel: 301-942-6450
Fax: 301-942-2302
Website: www.nfcacares.org
E-mail: info@nfcacares.org

## National Health Information Center

P.O. Box 1133
Washington, DC 20013-1133
Toll-Free: 800-336-4797
Tel: 301-565-4167
Fax: 301-984-4256
Website: www.health.gov/nhic
E-mail: info@nhic.org

## National Information Center for Children and Youth with Disabilities (NICHCY)

P.O. Box 1492
Washington, DC 20013
Toll-Free: 800-695-0285
Fax: 202-884-8441
Website: www.nichcy.org
E-mail: nichcy@aed.org

Focuses on children and youth (birth to age 22) by providing information on disabilities and disability-related issues. Can provide state resource sheet.

## National Institute on Deafness and Other Communication Disorders Clearinghouse (NIDCD)

1 Communication Avenue
Bethesda, MD 20892-3456
Toll-Free: 800-241-1044
TTY: 800-241-1055
Website: www.nidcd.nih.gov
E-mail: nidcdinfo@nidcd.nih.gov

NIDCD is a branch of the National Institutes of Health and will send low-cost and free materials about aphasia. They will also conduct literature searches on research about aphasia and related disorders.

### National Stroke Association (NSA)
9707 E. Easter Lane
Englewood, CO 80112-3747
Toll-Free: 800-787-6537
Tel: 303-649-9299
Fax: 303-649-1328
Website: www.stroke.org

The NSA offers several free and low-cost publications of interest to persons with aphasia and their families. They will also refer callers to local stroke survivor support groups.

### Parent Advocacy Coalition for Educational Rights (PACER)
8161 Normandale Blvd.
Minneapolis, MN 55437
Toll-Free: 800-537-2237
Tel: 952-838-9000
TTY: 952-838-0190
Fax: 952-838-1090
Website: www.pacer.org.
E-mail: pacer@pacer.org

PACER's mission is to improve and expand opportunities that enhance the quality of life for children and young adults with all disabilities.

### Office of Disability Employment Policy (ODEP)
U.S. Department of Labor
200 Constitution Avenue, N.W.
Washington, DC 20210
Toll-Free: 866-4-USA-DOL
Tel: 202-376-6200
TTY: 202-376-6205
Website: www.dol.gov/odep

The Presidents' Committee is an independent federal agency whose mission is to facilitate the communication, coordination, and promotion of public and private efforts to empower Americans with disabilities through employment.

### Rosalynn Carter Institute for Human Development,
Georgia Southwestern St. Univ.
800 Wheatley St.
Americus, GA 31709
Tel: 229-928-1234
Fax: 229-931-2663
Website: http://rci.gsw.edu
E-mail: rci@rci.gsw.edu

Advocates public awareness and policy changes which enhance the lives of caregivers.

### The Well Spouse Foundation
63 West Main Street, Suite H
Freehold, NJ 07728
Toll-Free: 800-838-0879
Tel: 732-577-8899
Fax: 732-577-8644
Website: www.wellspouse.org
E-mail: info@wellspouse.org

## The Well Spouse Foundation, continued

Support for spouses or partners of those who are chronically ill or disabled.

## Stroke Research Centers

To find better ways to prevent, diagnose, and treat stroke, the NINDS research program supports a broad spectrum of studies by investigators at leading biomedical research institutions across the country. Key components of this program are Stroke Research Centers. Information on research activities at these centers, possible clinical trials, and patient eligibility may be obtained from the principal investigators at these centers.

**Department of Neurosciences**
School of Medicine
University of California, San Diego
9500 Gilman Drive
La Jolla, CA 92093-0624
Tel: 858-534-3377
Fax: 858-534-8242
Website: http://medicine.ucsd/edu/neurosci
E-mail: neurograd@ucsd.edu

**Department of Medicine**
School of Medicine
University of California, Los Angeles
Los Angeles, CA 90024-1682
Toll-Free: 800-UCLA-MD1
Website: www.mednet.ucla.edu

**Department of Neurology**
School of Medicine
University of Southern California
1510 San Pablo Street
Suite 268
Los Angeles, CA 90033
Tel: 213-342-5710
Website: www.usc.edu/health/uscp/dept/neurology.htm

**Department of Neurology**
Veterans Affairs Medical Center
Mail Code V127
4150 Clement Street
San Francisco, CA 94121
Tel: 415-750-2011
Website: www.sf.med.va.gov

## Department of Neurosurgery

Stanford University School of Medicine
Boswell Building, A301
300 Pasteur Drive
Stanford, CA 94305-2015
Tel: 650-723-7093
Fax: 650-725-0390
Website: www.Stanford.edu/edpt/neurosurgery
E-mail: ims@medcenter.stanford.edu

## Department of Neurology

University of Miami School of Medicine
1150 N.W. 14th St., Suite 700
Miami, FL 33136
Tel: 305-243-7400
Website: www.Miami.edu

## University of Iowa College of Medicine

200 CMAB
Iowa City, IA 52242
Tel: 319-335-6707
Website: www.medicine.uiowa.edu

## Department of Anesthesiology

The Johns Hopkins University
720 Rutland Avenue
Baltimore, MD 21205
Tel: 410-955-8157
Website: www.hopkinsmedicine.org/anesthesiology

## Epidemiology and Preventive Medicine

University of Maryland Medical Center
Suite 109 Howard Hall
660 W. Redwood Street
Baltimore, MD 21201
Tel: 410-706-4576
Fax: 410-706-4581
Website: http://medschool.umaryland.edu/epidemiology

## Department of Anatomy and Neurology

Boston University School of Medicine
L-1004
715 Albany Street
Boston, MA 02118
Tel: 617-638-4200
Fax: 617-638-4216
Website: www.bumc.bu.edu

## Departments of Neurology and Neurosurgery

Massachusetts General Hospital
55 Fruit Street
Boston, MA 02114
Tel: 617-726-6000
Website: http://massgeneral.org

## Department of Neurology

Henry Ford Health Science Center
2799 West Grand Blvd.
Detroit, MI 48202
Tel: 313-876-2644
Fax: 313-916-5117
Website: www.henryfordhealth.org

*Department of Health*
*Sciences Research*
Mayo Clinic and Foundation
200 First Street, S.W.
Rochester, MN 55901
Tel: 507-284-1101
Website: www.mayo.edu/
research

*Washington University*
*School of Medicine*
660 South Euclid Avenue
St. Louis, MO 63110
Tel: 314-362-5000
Website: http://
medicine.uwstl.edu

*Department of Neurology*
Washington University School of
Medicine
660 South Euclid Avenue
Box 8111
St. Louis, MO 63110
Tel: 314-362-7177
Fax: 314-362-2826
Website: http://
medicine.uwstl.edu

*Department of Neurology*
Wake Forest University Baptist
Medical Center
Medical Center Boulevard
Winston-Salem, NC 27157-1078
Tel: 336-716-2338
Fax: 336-716-5477
Website: www.wfubmc.edu/
neurology

*Department of Neurology*
Hospital of the University of
Pennsylvania
Johnson Pavilion (G1)
Room 429
36th and Hamilton Walk
Philadelphia, PA 19104
Tel: 215-662-4000
Website: www.uphs.upenn.edu/
neuro
E-mail:
neuro@mail.med.upenn.edu

*Department of Neurology*
University of Pittsburgh School
of Medicine
446 Crawford Hall
Pittsburgh, PA 15260
Tel: 412-624-5043
Website: www.www.pitt.edu/
~neurosci

*Division of Hematology/*
*Oncology*
University of Texas Health
Science Center
6431 Fannin Street
Houston, TX 77030
Tel: 713-792-5450
Website: www.uthouston.edu
E-mail: info@uthouston.edu

# Index

# Index

Page numbers followed by 'n' indicate a footnote. Page numbers in *italics* indicate a table or illustration.

## A

AAPM&R *see* American Academy of Physical Medicine and Rehabilitation
Academy of Neurologic Communicative Disorders and Sciences, contact information 323
Ackerman, Sandra J. 93n
Activase thrombolytic agent 221
activities of daily living (ADL)
    defined 539
    dementia 181
    stroke recovery 266–67, 325–41, 358
A.D.A.M., Inc., publications
    atherosclerosis 101n
    hemorrhagic stroke 35n
    stroke risk tests 191n
    stroke secondary to carotid dissection 48n
    transient ischemic attack 40n
Adaptability, contact information 338
ADEAR *see* Alzheimer's Disease Education and Referral Center

ADED *see* Association for Driver Rehabilitation Specialists
ADL *see* activities of daily living
Administration on Aging, contact information 271, 314, 547
"Adult Aphasia: Recent Research" (NIDCD) 315n
advance directives 513–14
    *see also* living wills
aerobic capacity, described 300
AF *see* atrial fibrillation
After Therapy Catalog, contact information 338
age factor
    cholesterol levels 405–7
    heart attack 175–76
    hypertension 149
    stroke secondary to carotid dissection 48
    stroke statistics *10, 14,* 27
Agency for Healthcare Research and Quality (AHRQ)
    contact information 288n
    publications
        anticoagulants 433n
        discharge planning 265n, 355n
        gender factor, stroke risk 101n
        recurrent strokes 187n
        transient ischemic attack 40n

561

Aggrenox 44
agitated saline, described 208
AHA Stroke Connection, contact information 271, 314
AHRQ *see* Agency for Healthcare Research and Quality
Alabama
  community-based initiatives 445
  stroke belt 28
  stroke statistics *16*
Alaska, stroke statistics *16*
alcohol use
  anticoagulants 354
  balance 294
  hypertension 152
  stroke prevention 386
Alexandrov, Andrei 225–26
Alteplase 221
Alzheimer's Association, contact information 183
Alzheimer's disease 177, 180, 183
Alzheimer's Disease Education and Referral Center (ADEAR), contact information 183
ambulation, defined 539
American Academy of Neurology, contact information 549
American Academy of Physical Medicine and Rehabilitation (AAPM&R)
  contact information 264, 305, 549
  publications
    family, stroke recovery 261n
    stroke rehabilitation 291n
American Congress of Rehabilitation Medicine, contact information 550
American Diabetes Association, contact information 145
American Dietetic Association, contact information 272
American Heart Association
  contact information 287, 548, 550
  publications
    anticoagulants 433n
    caregivers 369n
    childhood stroke 53n
    dementia 177n
    hypertension 147n
    stroke diagnosis 201n
    stroke risk tests 191n

American Heart Association, continued
  publications, continued
    surgical stroke treatment 253n
    transient ischemic attack 40n
    women, strokes 171n
American Occupational Therapy Association
  contact information 314, 550
  occupational therapists publication 307n
American Parkinson Disease Association, stroke recovery publications 325n
American Physical Therapy Association (APTA)
  contact information 305, 550
  stroke recovery publication 291n
American Psychological Association, contact information 550
American Self-Help Clearinghouse, contact information 272
American Speech-Language-Hearing Association (ASHA), contact information 288, 323, 551
American Stroke Association
  contact information 184, 287, 390, 548, 551
  described 45
Americans with Disabilities Act (1990) 471–75, 494
analgesics, stroke treatment 38
Anchor Audio, Inc., contact information 341
anemia, stroke prevention 387
aneurysm, defined 539
angina, described 397
angiography *see* digital subtraction angiography; magnetic resonance angiography (MRA)
animal tests, stroke research 459
ankle-foot orthosis, described 346
anomic aphasia, described 317
"Another Reason to Avoid a Sugar High: Study Links High Blood Sugar to Mortality after Stroke" (Zeigler) 129n
anoxia, described 33
antianxiety medications, stroke treatment 38

atrial fibrillation (AF), continued
research 455
stroke prevention 409–16, 434
atrial septal aneurysm 188–89

## B

"Backpack-sized Ultrasound Device
Detects Neck Artery Blockages"
(American Heart Association) 201n
Baird, Alison E. 237–39
balance information 293–98
balance problems, stroke recovery
356
balloon angioplasty, atherosclerosis
103
Barba, Raquel 181
Barch, Carol A. 73n
Barthel, DW 241n
Barthel index *252*
"Barthel Index" (Mahoney; Barthel)
241n
bathroom activities, stroke recovery
328–30
Baycol (cervistatin) 403, 404
bedroom activities, stroke recovery
326–28
behavioral differences, stroke recovery 356, 358
*Be Independent* (American Parkinson
Disease Association) 325n
beta-2 dependent anticardiolipin antibodies (B2GP1-dependent aCL)
97–99
beta cells, described 133
BIA *see* Brain Injury Association
biomarkers, coronary artery disease
110–11
"Biomarkers and Surrogate Endpoints: Advancing Clinical Research
and Application: Cardiovascular II"
(NIH; FDA) 93n, 101n
bladder control, stroke recovery 356
blood-brain barrier
described 33
stroke 34
blood chemistry tests, described 204–5

blood clots
diagnosis 207
stroke 32
*see also* anticoagulant agents
blood-clotting disorders, mortality
rates *12*
blood lipid tests, described 205
blood oxygen level, test 203
blood pressure (BP)
described 148
test 152–54
*see also* diastolic blood pressure;
systolic blood pressure
"Blood Pressure Drugs Relax Heart,
Reduce Heart Failure Risk" (American Heart Association) 147n
"Blood Tests and Procedures Used for
Stroke Diagnosis" (Internet Stroke
Center) 201n
BMI *see* body mass index
bodily neglect, described 356
body mass index (BMI), heart disease
119
body structure, physical therapy 301–2
Bornstein, Nathan 89
Boston University School of Medicine,
Stroke Research Center, contact information 557
botulinum toxin type A 344
bowel control, stroke recovery 356
Boyd, Douglas P. 111
BP *see* blood pressure
BRAIN *see* Brain Resources and Information Network
brain, described 33
Brain Aneurysm Foundation, Inc.,
contact information 548
brain attack, defined 540
*see also* stroke
The Brain Attack Coalition, stroke
centers publication 257n
brain biopsy, described 202–3
Brain Injury Association (BIA), contact information 551
brain plasticity, described 458
Brain Resources and Information
Network (BRAIN), contact information 287, 547

# Health Reference Series
## COMPLETE CATALOG

## Adolescent Health Sourcebook

*Basic Consumer Health Information about Common Medical, Mental, and Emotional Concerns in Adolescents, Including Facts about Acne, Body Piercing, Mononucleosis, Nutrition, Eating Disorders, Stress, Depression, Behavior Problems, Peer Pressure, Violence, Gangs, Drug Use, Puberty, Sexuality, Pregnancy, Learning Disabilities, and More*

*Along with a Glossary of Terms and Other Resources for Further Help and Information*

Edited by Chad T. Kimball. 658 pages. 2002. 0-7808-0248-9. $78.

"A good starting point for information related to common medical, mental, and emotional concerns of adolescents." — *School Library Journal, Nov '02*

"This book provides accurate information in an easy to access format. It addresses topics that parents and caregivers might not be aware of and provides practical, useable information." — *Doody's Health Sciences Book Review Journal, Sep-Oct '02*

"Recommended reference source." — *Booklist, American Library Association, Sep '02*

■

## AIDS Sourcebook, 1st Edition

*Basic Information about AIDS and HIV Infection, Featuring Historical and Statistical Data, Current Research, Prevention, and Other Special Topics of Interest for Persons Living with AIDS*

*Along with Source Listings for Further Assistance*

Edited by Karen Bellenir and Peter D. Dresser. 831 pages. 1995. 0-7808-0031-1. $78.

"One strength of this book is its practical emphasis. The intended audience is the lay reader . . . useful as an educational tool for health care providers who work with AIDS patients. Recommended for public libraries as well as hospital or academic libraries that collect consumer materials." — *Bulletin of the Medical Library Association, Jan '96*

"This is the most comprehensive volume of its kind on an important medical topic. Highly recommended for all libraries." — *Reference Book Review, '96*

"Very useful reference for all libraries." — *Choice, Association of College and Research Libraries, Oct '95*

"There is a wealth of information here that can provide much educational assistance. It is a must book for all libraries and should be on the desk of each and every congressional leader. Highly recommended." — *AIDS Book Review Journal, Aug '95*

"Recommended for most collections." — *Library Journal, Jul '95*

## AIDS Sourcebook, 2nd Edition

*Basic Consumer Health Information about Acquired Immune Deficiency Syndrome (AIDS) and Human Immunodeficiency Virus (HIV) Infection, Featuring Updated Statistical Data, Reports on Recent Research and Prevention Initiatives, and Other Special Topics of Interest for Persons Living with AIDS, Including New Antiretroviral Treatment Options, Strategies for Combating Opportunistic Infections, Information about Clinical Trials, and More*

*Along with a Glossary of Important Terms and Resource Listings for Further Help and Information*

Edited by Karen Bellenir. 751 pages. 1999. 0-7808-0225-X. $78.

"Highly recommended." — *American Reference Books Annual, 2000*

"Excellent sourcebook. This continues to be a highly recommended book. There is no other book that provides as much information as this book provides." — *AIDS Book Review Journal, Dec-Jan 2000*

"Recommended reference source." — *Booklist, American Library Association, Dec '99*

"A solid text for college-level health libraries." — *The Bookwatch, Aug '99*

Cited in *Reference Sources for Small and Medium-Sized Libraries, American Library Association, 1999*

■

## AIDS Sourcebook, 3rd Edition

*Basic Consumer Health Information about Acquired Immune Deficiency Syndrome (AIDS) and Human Immunodeficiency Virus (HIV) Infection, Including Facts about Transmission, Prevention, Diagnosis, Treatment, Opportunistic Infections, and Other Complications, with a Section for Women and Children, Including Details about Associated Gynecological Concerns, Pregnancy, and Pediatric Care*

*Along with Updated Statistical Information, Reports on Current Research Initiatives, a Glossary, and Directories of Internet, Hotline, and Other Resources*

Edited by Dawn D. Matthews. 664 pages. 2003. 0-7808-0631-X. $78.

■

## Alcoholism Sourcebook

*Basic Consumer Health Information about the Physical and Mental Consequences of Alcohol Abuse, Including Liver Disease, Pancreatitis, Wernicke-Korsakoff Syndrome (Alcoholic Dementia), Fetal Alcohol Syndrome, Heart Disease, Kidney Disorders, Gastrointestinal Problems, and Immune System Compromise and Featuring Facts about Addiction, Detoxification, Alcohol Withdrawal, Recovery, and the Maintenance of Sobriety*

'It is very handy to have information on more than thirty neurological disorders under one cover, and there is no recent source like it." — *Reference Quarterly, American Library Association, Fall '93*

SEE ALSO *Brain Disorders Sourcebook*

■

# Alzheimer's Disease Sourcebook, 2nd Edition

*Basic Consumer Health Information about Alzheimer's Disease, Related Disorders, and Other Dementias, Including Multi-Infarct Dementia, AIDS-Related Dementia, Alcoholic Dementia, Huntington's Disease, Delirium, and Confusional States*

*Along with Reports Detailing Current Research Efforts in Prevention and Treatment, Long-Term Care Issues, and Listings of Sources for Additional Help and Information*

Edited by Karen Bellenir. 524 pages. 1999. 0-7808-0223-3. $78.

"Provides a wealth of useful information not otherwise available in one place. This resource is recommended for all types of libraries."
— *American Reference Books Annual, 2000*

"Recommended reference source."
— *Booklist, American Library Association, Oct '99*

■

# Arthritis Sourcebook

*Basic Consumer Health Information about Specific Forms of Arthritis and Related Disorders, Including Rheumatoid Arthritis, Osteoarthritis, Gout, Polymyalgia Rheumatica, Psoriatic Arthritis, Spondyloarthropathies, Juvenile Rheumatoid Arthritis, and Juvenile Ankylosing Spondylitis*

*Along with Information about Medical, Surgical, and Alternative Treatment Options, and Including Strategies for Coping with Pain, Fatigue, and Stress*

Edited by Allan R. Cook. 550 pages. 1998. 0-7808-0201-2. $78.

". . . accessible to the layperson."
— *Reference and Research Book News, Feb '99*

■

# Asthma Sourcebook

*Basic Consumer Health Information about Asthma, Including Symptoms, Traditional and Nontraditional Remedies, Treatment Advances, Quality-of-Life Aids, Medical Research Updates, and the Role of Allergies, Exercise, Age, the Environment, and Genetics in the Development of Asthma*

*Along with Statistical Data, a Glossary, and Directories of Support Groups, and Other Resources for Further Information*

Edited by Annemarie S. Muth. 628 pages. 2000. 0-7808-0381-7. $78.

"A worthwhile reference acquisition for public libraries and academic medical libraries whose readers desire a quick introduction to the wide range of asthma information." — *Choice, Association of College & Research Libraries, Jun '01*

"Recommended reference source."
— *Booklist, American Library Association, Feb '01*

"Highly recommended." — *The Bookwatch, Jan '01*

"There is much good information for patients and their families who deal with asthma daily."
— *American Medical Writers Association Journal, Winter '01*

"This informative text is recommended for consumer health collections in public, secondary school, and community college libraries and the libraries of universities with a large undergraduate population."
— *American Reference Books Annual, 2001*

■

# Attention Deficit Disorder Sourcebook

*Basic Consumer Health Information about Attention Deficit/Hyperactivity Disorder in Children and Adults, Including Facts about Causes, Symptoms, Diagnostic Criteria, and Treatment Options Such as Medications, Behavior Therapy, Coaching, and Homeopathy*

*Along with Reports on Current Research Initiatives, Legal Issues, and Government Regulations, and Featuring a Glossary of Related Terms, Internet Resources, and a List of Additional Reading Material*

Edited by Dawn D. Matthews. 470 pages. 2002. 0-7808-0624-7. $78.

■

# Back & Neck Disorders Sourcebook

*Basic Information about Disorders and Injuries of the Spinal Cord and Vertebrae, Including Facts on Chiropractic Treatment, Surgical Interventions, Paralysis, and Rehabilitation*

*Along with Advice for Preventing Back Trouble*

Edited by Karen Bellenir. 548 pages. 1997. 0-7808-0202-0. $78.

"The strength of this work is its basic, easy-to-read format. Recommended."
— *Reference and User Services Quarterly, American Library Association, Winter '97*

■

# Blood & Circulatory Disorders Sourcebook

*Basic Information about Blood and Its Components, Anemias, Leukemias, Bleeding Disorders, and Circulatory Disorders, Including Aplastic Anemia, Thalassemia, Sickle-Cell Disease, Hemochromatosis, Hemophilia, Von Willebrand Disease, and Vascular Diseases*

Along with a Special Section on Blood Transfusions and Blood Supply Safety, a Glossary, and Source Listings for Further Help and Information

Edited by Karen Bellenir and Linda M. Shin. 554 pages. 1998. 0-7808-0203-9. $78.

"Recommended reference source."
—Booklist, American Library Association, Feb '99

"An important reference sourcebook written in simple language for everyday, non-technical users. "
—Reviewer's Bookwatch, Jan '99

■

# Brain Disorders Sourcebook

Basic Consumer Health Information about Strokes, Epilepsy, Amyotrophic Lateral Sclerosis (ALS/Lou Gehrig's Disease), Parkinson's Disease, Brain Tumors, Cerebral Palsy, Headache, Tourette Syndrome, and More

Along with Statistical Data, Treatment and Rehabilitation Options, Coping Strategies, Reports on Current Research Initiatives, a Glossary, and Resource Listings for Additional Help and Information

Edited by Karen Bellenir. 481 pages. 1999. 0-7808-0229-2. $78.

"Belongs on the shelves of any library with a consumer health collection."          —E-Streams, Mar '00

"Recommended reference source."
—Booklist, American Library Association, Oct '99

SEE ALSO Alzheimer's Disease Sourcebook, 2nd Edition

■

# Breast Cancer  Sourcebook

Basic Consumer Health Information about Breast Cancer, Including Diagnostic Methods, Treatment Options, Alternative Therapies, Self-Help Information, Related Health Concerns, Statistical and Demographic Data, and Facts for Men with Breast Cancer

Along with Reports on Current Research Initiatives, a Glossary of Related Medical Terms, and a Directory of Sources for Further Help and Information

Edited by Edward J. Prucha and Karen Bellenir. 580 pages. 2001. 0-7808-0244 6. $78.

"Recommended reference source."
—Booklist, American Library Association, Jan '02

"This reference source is highly recommended. It is quite informative, comprehensive and detailed in nature, and yet it offers practical advice in easy-to-read language. It could be thought of as the 'bible' of breast cancer for the consumer."          —E-Streams, Jan '02

"The broad range of topics covered in lay language make the Breast Cancer Sourcebook an excellent addition to public and consumer health library collections."
—American Reference Books Annual 2002

"From the pros and cons of different screening methods and results to treatment options, Breast Cancer Sourcebook provides the latest information on the subject."
—Library Bookwatch, Dec '01

"This thoroughgoing, very readable reference covers all aspects of breast health and cancer. . . . Readers will find much to consider here. Recommended for all public and patient health collections."
—Library Journal, Sep '01

SEE ALSO Cancer Sourcebook for Women, 1st and 2nd Editions, Women's Health Concerns Sourcebook

■

# Breastfeeding Sourcebook

Basic Consumer Health Information about the Benefits of Breastmilk, Preparing to Breastfeed, Breastfeeding as a Baby Grows, Nutrition, and More, Including Information on Special Situations and Concerns Such as Mastitis, Illness, Medications, Allergies, Multiple Births, Prematurity, Special Needs, and Adoption

Along with a Glossary and Resources for Additional Help and Information

Edited by Jenni Lynn Colson. 388 pages. 2002. 0-7808-0332-9. $78.

SEE ALSO Pregnancy & Birth Sourcebook

■

# Burns Sourcebook

Basic Consumer Health Information about Various Types of Burns and Scalds, Including Flame, Heat, Cold, Electrical, Chemical, and Sun Burns

Along with Information on Short-Term and Long-Term Treatments, Tissue Reconstruction, Plastic Surgery, Prevention Suggestions, and First Aid

Edited by Allan R. Cook. 604 pages. 1999. 0-7808-0204-7. $78.

"This is an exceptional addition to the series and is highly recommended for all consumer health collections, hospital libraries, and academic medical centers."
—E-Streams, Mar '00

"This key reference guide is an invaluable addition to all health care and public libraries in confronting this ongoing health issue."
—American Reference Books Annual, 2000

"Recommended reference source."
—Booklist, American Library Association, Dec '99

SEE ALSO Skin Disorders Sourcebook

■

# Cancer Sourcebook, 1st Edition

Basic Information on Cancer Types, Symptoms, Diagnostic Methods, and Treatments, Including Statistics on Cancer Occurrences Worldwide and the Risks Associated with Known Carcinogens and Activities

Edited by Frank E. Bair. 932 pages. 1990. 1-55888-888-8. $78.

Cited in Reference Sources for Small and Medium-Sized Libraries, American Library Association, 1999

"Written in nontechnical language. Useful for patients, their families, medical professionals, and librarians."
—Guide to Reference Books, 1996

"Designed with the non-medical professional in mind. Libraries and medical facilities interested in patient education should certainly consider adding the *Cancer Sourcebook* to their holdings. This compact collection of reliable information . . . is an invaluable tool for helping patients and patients' families and friends to take the first steps in coping with the many difficulties of cancer."
— *Medical Reference Services Quarterly, Winter '91*

"Specifically created for the nontechnical reader . . . an important resource for the general reader trying to understand the complexities of cancer."
— *American Reference Books Annual, 1991*

"This publication's nontechnical nature and very comprehensive format make it useful for both the general public and undergraduate students."
— *Choice, Association of College and Research Libraries, Oct '90*

∎

# New Cancer Sourcebook, 2nd Edition

*Basic Information about Major Forms and Stages of Cancer, Featuring Facts about Primary and Secondary Tumors of the Respiratory, Nervous, Lymphatic, Circulatory, Skeletal, and Gastrointestinal Systems, and Specific Organs; Statistical and Demographic Data; Treatment Options; and Strategies for Coping*

Edited by Allan R. Cook. 1,313 pages. 1996. 0-7808-0041-9. $78.

"An excellent resource for patients with newly diagnosed cancer and their families. The dialogue is simple, direct, and comprehensive. Highly recommended for patients and families to aid in their understanding of cancer and its treatment."
— *Booklist Health Sciences Supplement, American Library Association, Oct '97*

"The amount of factual and useful information is extensive. The writing is very clear, geared to general readers. Recommended for all levels." — *Choice, Association of College & Research Libraries, Jan '97*

∎

# Cancer Sourcebook, 3rd Edition
*Basic Consumer Health Information about Major Forms and Stages of Cancer, Featuring Facts about Primary and Secondary Tumors of the Respiratory, Nervous, Lymphatic, Circulatory, Skeletal, and Gastrointestinal Systems, and Specific Organs*

*Along with Statistical and Demographic Data, Treatment Options, Strategies for Coping, a Glossary, and a Directory of Sources for Additional Help and Information*

Edited by Edward J. Prucha. 1,069 pages. 2000. 0-7808-0227-6. $78.

"This title is recommended for health sciences and public libraries with consumer health collections."
— *E-Streams, Feb '01*

". . . can be effectively used by cancer patients and their families who are looking for answers in a language they can understand. Public and hospital libraries should have it on their shelves."
— *American Reference Books Annual, 2001*

"Recommended reference source."
— *Booklist, American Library Association, Dec '00*

∎

# Cancer Sourcebook for Women, 1st Edition
*Basic Information about Specific Forms of Cancer That Affect Women, Featuring Facts about Breast Cancer, Cervical Cancer, Ovarian Cancer, Cancer of the Uterus and Uterine Sarcoma, Cancer of the Vagina, and Cancer of the Vulva; Statistical and Demographic Data; Treatments, Self-Help Management Suggestions, and Current Research Initiatives*

Edited by Allan R. Cook and Peter D. Dresser. 524 pages. 1996. 0-7808-0076-1. $78.

". . . written in easily understandable, non-technical language. Recommended for public libraries or hospital and academic libraries that collect patient education or consumer health materials."
— *Medical Reference Services Quarterly, Spring '97*

"Would be of value in a consumer health library. . . . written with the health care consumer in mind. Medical jargon is at a minimum, and medical terms are explained in clear, understandable sentences."
— *Bulletin of the Medical Library Association, Oct '96*

"The availability under one cover of all these pertinent publications, grouped under cohesive headings, makes this certainly a most useful sourcebook." — *Choice, Association of College & Research Libraries, Jun '96*

"Presents a comprehensive knowledge base for general readers. Men and women both benefit from the gold mine of information nestled between the two covers of this book. Recommended."
— *Academic Library Book Review, Summer '96*

"This timely book is highly recommended for consumer health and patient education collections in all libraries." — *Library Journal, Apr '96*

∎

# Cancer Sourcebook for Women, 2nd Edition
*Basic Consumer Health Information about Gynecologic Cancers and Related Concerns, Including Cervical Cancer, Endometrial Cancer, Gestational Trophoblastic Tumor, Ovarian Cancer, Uterine Cancer, Vaginal Cancer, Vulvar Cancer, Breast Cancer, and Common Non-Cancerous Uterine Conditions, with Facts about Cancer Risk Factors, Screening and Prevention, Treatment Options, and Reports on Current Research Initiatives*

*Along with a Glossary of Cancer Terms and a Directory of Resources for Additional Help and Information*

Edited by Karen Bellenir. 604 pages. 2002. 0-7808-0226-8. $78.

587

"Highly recommended for academic and medical reference collections." —*Library Bookwatch, Sep '02*

"This is a highly recommended book for any public or consumer library, being reader friendly and containing accurate and helpful information."
—*E-Streams, Aug '02*

"Recommended reference source."
—*Booklist, American Library Association, Jul '02*

*SEE ALSO Breast Cancer Sourcebook, Women's Health Concerns Sourcebook*

■

# Cardiovascular Diseases & Disorders Sourcebook, 1st Edition

*Basic Information about Cardiovascular Diseases and Disorders, Featuring Facts about the Cardiovascular System, Demographic and Statistical Data, Descriptions of Pharmacological and Surgical Interventions, Lifestyle Modifications, and a Special Section Focusing on Heart Disorders in Children*

Edited by Karen Bellenir and Peter D. Dresser. 683 pages. 1995. 0-7808-0032-X. $78.

". . . comprehensive format provides an extensive overview on this subject." —*Choice, Association of College & Research Libraries, Jun '96*

". . . an easily understood, complete, up-to-date resource. This well executed public health tool will make valuable information available to those that need it most, patients and their families. The typeface, sturdy non-reflective paper, and library binding add a feel of quality found wanting in other publications. Highly recommended for academic and general libraries. "
—*Academic Library Book Review, Summer '96*

*SEE ALSO Healthy Heart Sourcebook for Women, Heart Diseases & Disorders Sourcebook, 2nd Edition*

■

# Caregiving Sourcebook

*Basic Consumer Health Information for Caregivers, Including a Profile of Caregivers, Caregiving Responsibilities and Concerns, Tips for Specific Conditions, Care Environments, and the Effects of Caregiving*

*Along with Facts about Legal Issues, Financial Information, and Future Planning, a Glossary, and a Listing of Additional Resources*

Edited by Joyce Brennfleck Shannon. 600 pages. 2001. 0-7808-0331-0. $78.

"Essential for most collections."
—*Library Journal, Apr 1, 2002*

"An ideal addition to the reference collection of any public library. Health sciences information professionals may also want to acquire the *Caregiving Sourcebook* for their hospital or academic library for use as a ready reference tool by health care workers interested in aging and caregiving." —*E-Streams, Jan '02*

"Recommended reference source."
—*Booklist, American Library Association, Oct '01*

# Childhood Diseases & Disorders Sourcebook

*Basic Consumer Health Information about Medical Problems Often Encountered in Pre-Adolescent Children, Including Respiratory Tract Ailments, Ear Infections, Sore Throats, Disorders of the Skin and Scalp, Digestive and Genitourinary Diseases, Infectious Diseases, Inflammatory Disorders, Chronic Physical and Developmental Disorders, Allergies, and More*

*Along with Information about Diagnostic Tests, Common Childhood Surgeries, and Frequently Used Medications, with a Glossary of Important Terms and Resource Directory*

Edited by Chad T. Kimball. 600 pages. 2003. 0-7808-0458-9. $78.

■

# Colds, Flu & Other Common Ailments Sourcebook

*Basic Consumer Health Information about Common Ailments and Injuries, Including Colds, Coughs, the Flu, Sinus Problems, Headaches, Fever, Nausea and Vomiting, Menstrual Cramps, Diarrhea, Constipation, Hemorrhoids, Back Pain, Dandruff, Dry and Itchy Skin, Cuts, Scrapes, Sprains, Bruises, and More*

*Along with Information about Prevention, Self-Care, Choosing a Doctor, Over-the-Counter Medications, Folk Remedies, and Alternative Therapies, and Including a Glossary of Important Terms and a Directory of Resources for Further Help and Information*

Edited by Chad T. Kimball. 638 pages. 2001. 0-7808-0435-X. $78.

"A good starting point for research on common illnesses. It will be a useful addition to public and consumer health library collections."
—*American Reference Books Annual 2002*

"Will prove valuable to any library seeking to maintain a current, comprehensive reference collection of health resources. . . . Excellent reference."
—*The Bookwatch, Aug '01*

"Recommended reference source."
—*Booklist, American Library Association, July '01*

■

# Communication Disorders Sourcebook

*Basic Information about Deafness and Hearing Loss, Speech and Language Disorders, Voice Disorders, Balance and Vestibular Disorders, and Disorders of Smell, Taste, and Touch*

Edited by Linda M. Ross. 533 pages. 1996. 0-7808-0077-X. $78.

"This is skillfully edited and is a welcome resource for the layperson. It should be found in every public and medical library." —*Booklist Health Sciences Supplement, American Library Association, Oct '97*

# Congenital Disorders Sourcebook

Basic Information about Disorders Acquired during Gestation, Including Spina Bifida, Hydrocephalus, Cerebral Palsy, Heart Defects, Craniofacial Abnormalities, Fetal Alcohol Syndrome, and More

Along with Current Treatment Options and Statistical Data

Edited by Karen Bellenir. 607 pages. 1997. 0-7808-0205-5. $78.

"Recommended reference source."
— *Booklist, American Library Association, Oct '97*

*SEE ALSO Pregnancy & Birth Sourcebook*

# Consumer Issues in Health Care Sourcebook

Basic Information about Health Care Fundamentals and Related Consumer Issues, Including Exams and Screening Tests, Physician Specialties, Choosing a Doctor, Using Prescription and Over-the-Counter Medications Safely, Avoiding Health Scams, Managing Common Health Risks in the Home, Care Options for Chronically or Terminally Ill Patients, and a List of Resources for Obtaining Help and Further Information

Edited by Karen Bellenir. 618 pages. 1998. 0-7808-0221-7. $78.

"Both public and academic libraries will want to have a copy in their collection for readers who are interested in self-education on health issues."
— *American Reference Books Annual, 2000*

"The editor has researched the literature from government agencies and others, saving readers the time and effort of having to do the research themselves. Recommended for public libraries."
— *Reference and User Services Quarterly, American Library Association, Spring '99*

"Recommended reference source."
— *Booklist, American Library Association, Dec '98*

# Contagious & Non-Contagious Infectious Diseases Sourcebook

Basic Information about Contagious Diseases like Measles, Polio, Hepatitis B, and Infectious Mononucleosis, and Non-Contagious Infectious Diseases like Tetanus and Toxic Shock Syndrome, and Diseases Occurring as Secondary Infections Such as Shingles and Reye Syndrome

Along with Vaccination, Prevention, and Treatment Information, and a Section Describing Emerging Infectious Disease Threats

Edited by Karen Bellenir and Peter D. Dresser. 566 pages. 1996. 0-7808-0075-3. $78.

# Death & Dying Sourcebook

Basic Consumer Health Information for the Layperson about End-of-Life Care and Related Ethical and Legal Issues, Including Chief Causes of Death, Autopsies, Pain Management for the Terminally Ill, Life Support Systems, Insurance, Euthanasia, Assisted Suicide, Hospice Programs, Living Wills, Funeral Planning, Counseling, Mourning, Organ Donation, and Physician Training

Along with Statistical Data, a Glossary, and Listings of Sources for Further Help and Information

Edited by Annemarie S. Muth. 641 pages. 1999. 0-7808-0230-6. $78.

"Public libraries, medical libraries, and academic libraries will all find this sourcebook a useful addition to their collections."
— *American Reference Books Annual, 2001*

"An extremely useful resource for those concerned with death and dying in the United States."
— *Respiratory Care, Nov '00*

"Recommended reference source."
— *Booklist, American Library Association, Aug '00*

"This book is a definite must for all those involved in end-of-life care." — *Doody's Review Service, 2000*

# Depression Sourcebook

Basic Consumer Health Information about Unipolar Depression, Bipolar Disorder, Postpartum Depression, Seasonal Affective Disorder, and Other Types of Depression in Children, Adolescents, Women, Men, the Elderly, and Other Selected Populations

Along with Facts about Causes, Risk Factors, Diagnostic Criteria, Treatment Options, Coping Strategies, Suicide Prevention, a Glossary, and a Directory of Sources for Additional Help and Information

Edited by Karen Belleni. 602 pages. 2002. 0-7808-0611-5. $78.

# Diabetes Sourcebook, 1st Edition

Basic Information about Insulin-Dependent and Non-insulin-Dependent Diabetes Mellitus, Gestational Diabetes, and Diabetic Complications, Symptoms, Treatment, and Research Results, Including Statistics on Prevalence, Morbidity, and Mortality

Along with Source Listings for Further Help and Information

Edited by Karen Bellenir and Peter D. Dresser. 827 pages. 1994. 1-55888-751-2. $78.

". . . very informative and understandable for the layperson without being simplistic. It provides a comprehensive overview for laypersons who want a general understanding of the disease or who want to focus on various aspects of the disease."
— *Bulletin of the Medical Library Association, Jan '96*

# Diabetes Sourcebook, 2nd Edition

Basic Consumer Health Information about Type 1 Diabetes (Insulin-Dependent or Juvenile-Onset Diabetes), Type 2 (Noninsulin-Dependent or Adult-Onset Diabetes), Gestational Diabetes, and Related Disorders, Including Diabetes Prevalence Data, Management Issues, the Role of Diet and Exercise in Controlling Diabetes, Insulin and Other Diabetes Medicines, and Complications of Diabetes Such as Eye Diseases, Periodontal Disease, Amputation, and End-Stage Renal Disease

Along with Reports on Current Research Initiatives, a Glossary, and Resource Listings for Further Help and Information

Edited by Karen Bellenir. 688 pages. 1998. 0-7808-0224-1. $78.

"An invaluable reference." — *Library Journal, May '00*

Selected as one of the 250 "Best Health Sciences Books of 1999." — *Doody's Rating Service, Mar-Apr 2000*

"This comprehensive book is an excellent addition for high school, academic, medical, and public libraries. This volume is highly recommended."
— *American Reference Books Annual, 2000*

"Provides useful information for the general public."
— *Healthlines, University of Michigan Health Management Research Center, Sep/Oct '99*

". . . provides reliable mainstream medical information . . . belongs on the shelves of any library with a consumer health collection." — *E-Streams, Sep '99*

"Recommended reference source."
— *Booklist, American Library Association, Feb '99*

■

# Diabetes Sourcebook, 3rd Edition

Basic Consumer Health Information about Type 1 Diabetes (Insulin-Dependent or Juvenile-Onset Diabetes), Type 2 Diabetes (Noninsulin-Dependent or Adult-Onset Diabetes), Gestational Diabetes, Impaired Glucose Tolerance (IGT), and Related Complications, Such as Amputation, Eye Disease, Gum Disease, Nerve Damage, and End-Stage Renal Disease, Including Facts about Insulin, Oral Diabetes Medications, Blood Sugar Testing, and the Role of Exercise and Nutrition in the Control of Diabetes

Along with a Glossary and Resources for Further Help and Information

Edited by Dawn D. Matthews. 622 pages. 2003. 0-7808-0629-8. $78.

■

# Diet & Nutrition Sourcebook, 1st Edition

Basic Information about Nutrition, Including the Dietary Guidelines for Americans, the Food Guide Pyramid, and Their Applications in Daily Diet, Nutritional Advice for Specific Age Groups, Current Nutritional Issues and Controversies, the New Food Label and How to Use It to Promote Healthy Eating, and Recent Developments in Nutritional Research

Edited by Dan R. Harris. 662 pages. 1996. 0-7808-0084-2. $78.

"Useful reference as a food and nutrition sourcebook for the general consumer." — *Booklist Health Sciences Supplement, American Library Association, Oct '97*

"Recommended for public libraries and medical libraries that receive general information requests on nutrition. It is readable and will appeal to those interested in learning more about healthy dietary practices."
— *Medical Reference Services Quarterly, Fall '97*

"An abundance of medical and social statistics is translated into readable information geared toward the general reader." — *Bookwatch, Mar '97*

"With dozens of questionable diet books on the market, it is so refreshing to find a reliable and factual reference book. Recommended to aspiring professionals, librarians, and others seeking and giving reliable dietary advice. An excellent compilation." — *Choice, Association of College and Research Libraries, Feb '97*

SEE ALSO *Digestive Diseases & Disorders Sourcebook, Gastrointestinal Diseases & Disorders Sourcebook*

■

# Diet & Nutrition Sourcebook, 2nd Edition

Basic Consumer Health Information about Dietary Guidelines, Recommended Daily Intake Values, Vitamins, Minerals, Fiber, Fat, Weight Control, Dietary Supplements, and Food Additives

Along with Special Sections on Nutrition Needs throughout Life and Nutrition for People with Such Specific Medical Concerns as Allergies, High Blood Cholesterol, Hypertension, Diabetes, Celiac Disease, Seizure Disorders, Phenylketonuria (PKU), Cancer, and Eating Disorders, and Including Reports on Current Nutrition Research and Source Listings for Additional Help and Information

Edited by Karen Bellenir. 650 pages. 1999. 0-7808-0228-4. $78.

"This book is an excellent source of basic diet and nutrition information." — *Booklist Health Sciences Supplement, American Library Association, Dec '00*

"This reference document should be in any public library, but it would be a very good guide for beginning students in the health sciences. If the other books in this publisher's series are as good as this, they should all be in the health sciences collections."
— *American Reference Books Annual, 2000*

"This book is an excellent general nutrition reference for consumers who desire to take an active role in their health care for prevention. Consumers of all ages who select this book can feel confident they are receiving current and accurate information." — *Journal of Nutrition for the Elderly, Vol. 19, No. 4, '00*

"Recommended reference source."
— *Booklist, American Library Association, Dec '99*

SEE ALSO *Digestive Diseases & Disorders Sourcebook, Gastrointestinal Diseases & Disorders Sourcebook*

# Digestive Diseases & Disorders Sourcebook

*Basic Consumer Health Information about Diseases and Disorders that Impact the Upper and Lower Digestive System, Including Celiac Disease, Constipation, Crohn's Disease, Cyclic Vomiting Syndrome, Diarrhea, Diverticulosis and Diverticulitis, Gallstones, Heartburn, Hemorrhoids, Hernias, Indigestion (Dyspepsia), Irritable Bowel Syndrome, Lactose Intolerance, Ulcers, and More*

*Along with Information about Medications and Other Treatments, Tips for Maintaining a Healthy Digestive Tract, a Glossary, and Directory of Digestive Diseases Organizations*

Edited by Karen Bellenir. 335 pages. 2000. 0-7808-0327-2. $78.

"This title would be an excellent addition to all public or patient-research libraries."
—*American Reference Books Annual, 2001*

"This title is recommended for public, hospital, and health sciences libraries with consumer health collections." —*E-Streams, Jul-Aug '00*

"Recommended reference source."
—*Booklist, American Library Association, May '00*

SEE ALSO *Diet & Nutrition Sourcebook, 1st and 2nd Editions, Gastrointestinal Diseases & Disorders Sourcebook*

■

# Disabilities Sourcebook

*Basic Consumer Health Information about Physical and Psychiatric Disabilities, Including Descriptions of Major Causes of Disability, Assistive and Adaptive Aids, Workplace Issues, and Accessibility Concerns*

*Along with Information about the Americans with Disabilities Act, a Glossary, and Resources for Additional Help and Information*

Edited by Dawn D. Matthews. 616 pages. 2000. 0-7808-0389-2. $78.

"It is a must for libraries with a consumer health section." —*American Reference Books Annual 2002*

"A much needed addition to the Omnigraphics *Health Reference Series*. A current reference work to provide people with disabilities, their families, caregivers or those who work with them, a broad range of information in one volume, has not been available until now. . . . It is recommended for all public and academic library reference collections." —*E-Streams, May '01*

"An excellent source book in easy-to-read format covering many current topics; highly recommended for all libraries." —*Choice, Association of College and Research Libraries, Jan '01*

"Recommended reference source."
—*Booklist, American Library Association, Jul '00*

# Domestic Violence & Child Abuse Sourcebook

*Basic Consumer Health Information about Spousal/Partner, Child, Sibling, Parent, and Elder Abuse, Covering Physical, Emotional, and Sexual Abuse, Teen Dating Violence, and Stalking; Includes Information about Hotlines, Safe Houses, Safety Plans, and Other Resources for Support and Assistance, Community Initiatives, and Reports on Current Directions in Research and Treatment*

*Along with a Glossary, Sources for Further Reading, and Governmental and Non-Governmental Organizations Contact Information*

Edited by Helene Henderson. 1,064 pages. 2001. 0-7808-0235-7. $78.

"This is important information. The Web has many resources but this sourcebook fills an important societal need. I am not aware of any other resources of this type." —*Doody's Review Service, Sep '01*

"Recommended for all libraries, scholars, and practitioners." —*Choice, Association of College & Research Libraries, Jul '01*

"Recommended reference source."
—*Booklist, American Library Association, Apr '01*

"Important pick for college-level health reference libraries." —*The Bookwatch, Mar '01*

"Because this problem is so widespread and because this book includes a lot of issues within one volume, this work is recommended for all public libraries."
—*American Reference Books Annual, 2001*

■

# Drug Abuse Sourcebook

*Basic Consumer Health Information about Illicit Substances of Abuse and the Diversion of Prescription Medications, Including Depressants, Hallucinogens, Inhalants, Marijuana, Narcotics, Stimulants, and Anabolic Steroids*

*Along with Facts about Related Health Risks, Treatment Issues, and Substance Abuse Prevention Programs, a Glossary of Terms, Statistical Data, and Directories of Hotline Services, Self-Help Groups, and Organizations Able to Provide Further Information*

Edited by Karen Bellenir. 629 pages. 2000. 0-7808-0242-X. $78.

"Containing a wealth of information . . . . This resource belongs in libraries that serve a lower-division undergraduate or community college clientele as well as the general public." —*Choice, Association of College and Research Libraries, Jun '01*

"Recommended reference source."
—*Booklist, American Library Association, Feb '01*

"Highly recommended." —*The Bookwatch, Jan '01*

"Even though there is a plethora of books on drug abuse, this volume is recommended for school, public, and college libraries."
—*American Reference Books Annual, 2001*

SEE ALSO *Alcoholism Sourcebook, Substance Abuse Sourcebook*

# Ear, Nose & Throat Disorders Sourcebook

*Basic Information about Disorders of the Ears, Nose, Sinus Cavities, Pharynx, and Larynx, Including Ear Infections, Tinnitus, Vestibular Disorders, Allergic and Non-Allergic Rhinitis, Sore Throats, Tonsillitis, and Cancers That Affect the Ears, Nose, Sinuses, and Throat Along with Reports on Current Research Initiatives, a Glossary of Related Medical Terms, and a Directory of Sources for Further Help and Information*

Edited by Karen Bellenir and Linda M. Shin. 576 pages. 1998. 0-7808-0206-3. $78.

**"Overall, this sourcebook is helpful for the consumer seeking information on ENT issues. It is recommended for public libraries."**
—*American Reference Books Annual, 1999*

**"Recommended reference source."**
—*Booklist, American Library Association, Dec '98*

◼

# Eating Disorders Sourcebook

*Basic Consumer Health Information about Eating Disorders, Including Information about Anorexia Nervosa, Bulimia Nervosa, Binge Eating, Body Dysmorphic Disorder, Pica, Laxative Abuse, and Night Eating Syndrome Along with Information about Causes, Adverse Effects, and Treatment and Prevention Issues, and Featuring a Section on Concerns Specific to Children and Adolescents, a Glossary, and Resources for Further Help and Information*

Edited by Dawn D. Matthews. 322 pages. 2001. 0-7808-0335-3. $78.

**"Recommended for health science libraries that are open to the public, as well as hospital libraries. This book is a good resource for the consumer who is concerned about eating disorders."** —*E-Streams, Mar '02*

**"This volume is another convenient collection of excerpted articles. Recommended for school and public library patrons; lower-division undergraduates; and two-year technical program students."** —*Choice, Association of College & Research Libraries, Jan '02*

**"Recommended reference source."** —*Booklist, American Library Association, Oct '01*

◼

# Emergency Medical Services Sourcebook

*Basic Consumer Health Information about Preventing, Preparing for, and Managing Emergency Situations, When and Who to Call for Help, What to Expect in the Emergency Room, the Emergency Medical Team, Patient Issues, and Current Topics in Emergency Medicine Along with Statistical Data, a Glossary, and Sources of Additional Help and Information*

Edited by Jenni Lynn Colson. 494 pages. 2002. 0-7808-0420-1. $78.

# Endocrine & Metabolic Disorders Sourcebook

*Basic Information for the Layperson about Pancreatic and Insulin-Related Disorders Such as Pancreatitis, Diabetes, and Hypoglycemia; Adrenal Gland Disorders Such as Cushing's Syndrome, Addison's Disease, and Congenital Adrenal Hyperplasia; Pituitary Gland Disorders Such as Growth Hormone Deficiency, Acromegaly, and Pituitary Tumors; Thyroid Disorders Such as Hypothyroidism, Graves' Disease, Hashimoto's Disease, and Goiter; Hyperparathyroidism; and Other Diseases and Syndromes of Hormone Imbalance or Metabolic Dysfunction Along with Reports on Current Research Initiatives*

Edited by Linda M. Shin. 574 pages. 1998. 0-7808-0207-1. $78.

**"Omnigraphics has produced another needed resource for health information consumers."**
—*American Reference Books Annual, 2000*

**"Recommended reference source."**
—*Booklist, American Library Association, Dec '98*

◼

# Environmentally Induced Disorders Sourcebook, 1st Edition

*Basic Information about Diseases and Syndromes Linked to Exposure to Pollutants and Other Substances in Outdoor and Indoor Environments Such as Lead, Asbestos, Formaldehyde, Mercury, Emissions, Noise, and More*

Edited by Allan R. Cook. 620 pages. 1997. 0-7808-0083-4. $78.

**"Recommended reference source."**
—*Booklist, American Library Association, Sep '98*

**"This book will be a useful addition to anyone's library."** —*Choice Health Sciences Supplement, Association of College and Research Libraries, May '98*

**". . . a good survey of numerous environmentally induced physical disorders . . . a useful addition to anyone's library."**
—*Doody's Health Sciences Book Reviews, Jan '98*

**". . . provide[s] introductory information from the best authorities around. Since this volume covers topics that potentially affect everyone, it will surely be one of the most frequently consulted volumes in the *Health Reference Series.*"** —*Rettig on Reference, Nov '97*

◼

# Ethnic Diseases Sourcebook

*Basic Consumer Health Information for Ethnic and Racial Minority Groups in the United States, Including General Health Indicators and Behaviors, Ethnic Diseases, Genetic Testing, the Impact of Chronic Diseases, Women's Health, Mental Health Issues, and Preventive Health Care Services Along with a Glossary and a Listing of Additional Resources*

Edited by Joyce Brennfleck Shannon. 664 pages. 2001. 0-7808-0336-1. $78.

"Recommended for health sciences libraries where public health programs are a priority."
—*E-Streams, Jan '02*

"Not many books have been written on this topic to date, and the *Ethnic Diseases Sourcebook* is a strong addition to the list. It will be an important introductory resource for health consumers, students, health care personnel, and social scientists. It is recommended for public, academic, and large hospital libraries."
—*American Reference Books Annual 2002*

"Recommended reference source."
—*Booklist, American Library Association, Oct '01*

"Will prove valuable to any library seeking to maintain a current, comprehensive reference collection of health resources.... An excellent source of health information about genetic disorders which affect particular ethnic and racial minorities in the U.S."
—*The Bookwatch, Aug '01*

■

# Eye Care Sourcebook, 2nd Edition

*Basic Consumer Health Information about Eye Care and Eye Disorders, Including Facts about the Diagnosis, Prevention, and Treatment of Common Refractive Problems Such as Myopia, Hyperopia, Astigmatism, and Presbyopia, and Eye Diseases, Including Glaucoma, Cataract, Age-Related Macular Degeneration, and Diabetic Retinopathy*

*Along with a Section on Vision Correction and Refractive Surgeries, Including LASIK and LASEK, a Glossary, and Directories of Resources for Additional Help and Information*

Edited by Amy L. Sutton. 543 pages. 2003. 0-7808-0635-2. $78.

■

# Family Planning Sourcebook

*Basic Consumer Health Information about Planning for Pregnancy and Contraception, Including Traditional Methods, Barrier Methods, Hormonal Methods, Permanent Methods, Future Methods, Emergency Contraception, and Birth Control Choices for Women at Each Stage of Life*

*Along with Statistics, a Glossary, and Sources of Additional Information*

Edited by Amy Marcaccio Keyzer. 520 pages. 2001. 0-7808-0379-5. $78.

"Recommended for public, health, and undergraduate libraries as part of the circulating collection."
—*E-Streams, Mar '02*

"Information is presented in an unbiased, readable manner, and the sourcebook will certainly be a necessary addition to those public and high school libraries where Internet access is restricted or otherwise problematic." —*American Reference Books Annual 2002*

"Recommended reference source."
—*Booklist, American Library Association, Oct '01*

"Will prove valuable to any library seeking to maintain a current, comprehensive reference collection of health resources.... Excellent reference."
—*The Bookwatch, Aug '01*

SEE ALSO *Pregnancy & Birth Sourcebook*

■

# Fitness & Exercise Sourcebook, 1st Edition

*Basic Information on Fitness and Exercise, Including Fitness Activities for Specific Age Groups, Exercise for People with Specific Medical Conditions, How to Begin a Fitness Program in Running, Walking, Swimming, Cycling, and Other Athletic Activities, and Recent Research in Fitness and Exercise*

Edited by Dan R. Harris. 663 pages. 1996. 0-7808-0186-5. $78.

"A good resource for general readers." —*Choice, Association of College and Research Libraries, Nov '97*

"The perennial popularity of the topic ... make this an appealing selection for public libraries."
—*Rettig on Reference, Jun/Jul '97*

■

# Fitness & Exercise Sourcebook, 2nd Edition

*Basic Consumer Health Information about the Fundamentals of Fitness and Exercise, Including How to Begin and Maintain a Fitness Program, Fitness as a Lifestyle, the Link between Fitness and Diet, Advice for Specific Groups of People, Exercise as It Relates to Specific Medical Conditions, and Recent Research in Fitness and Exercise*

*Along with a Glossary of Important Terms and Resources for Additional Help and Information*

Edited by Kristen M. Gledhill. 646 pages. 2001. 0-7808-0334-5. $78.

"This work is recommended for all general reference collections."
—*American Reference Books Annual 2002*

"Highly recommended for public, consumer, and school grades fourth through college."
—*E-Streams, Nov '01*

"Recommended reference source." —*Booklist, American Library Association, Oct '01*

"The information appears quite comprehensive and is considered reliable.... This second edition is a welcomed addition to the series."
—*Doody's Review Service, Sep '01*

"This reference is a valuable choice for those who desire a broad source of information on exercise, fitness, and chronic-disease prevention through a healthy lifestyle." —*American Medical Writers Association Journal, Fall '01*

"Will prove valuable to any library seeking to maintain a current, comprehensive reference collection of health resources.... Excellent reference."
—*The Bookwatch, Aug '01*

593

# Food & Animal Borne Diseases Sourcebook

Basic Information about Diseases That Can Be Spread to Humans through the Ingestion of Contaminated Food or Water or by Contact with Infected Animals and Insects, Such as Botulism, E. Coli, Hepatitis A, Trichinosis, Lyme Disease, and Rabies

Along with Information Regarding Prevention and Treatment Methods, and Including a Special Section for International Travelers Describing Diseases Such as Cholera, Malaria, Travelers' Diarrhea, and Yellow Fever, and Offering Recommendations for Avoiding Illness

Edited by Karen Bellenir and Peter D. Dresser. 535 pages. 1995. 0-7808-0033-8. $78.

"Targeting general readers and providing them with a single, comprehensive source of information on selected topics, this book continues, with the excellent caliber of its predecessors, to catalog topical information on health matters of general interest. Readable and thorough, this valuable resource is highly recommended for all libraries."
— Academic Library Book Review, Summer '96

"A comprehensive collection of authoritative information." — Emergency Medical Services, Oct '95

■

# Food Safety Sourcebook

Basic Consumer Health Information about the Safe Handling of Meat, Poultry, Seafood, Eggs, Fruit Juices, and Other Food Items, and Facts about Pesticides, Drinking Water, Food Safety Overseas, and the Onset, Duration, and Symptoms of Foodborne Illnesses, Including Types of Pathogenic Bacteria, Parasitic Protozoa, Worms, Viruses, and Natural Toxins

Along with the Role of the Consumer, the Food Handler, and the Government in Food Safety; a Glossary, and Resources for Additional Help and Information

Edited by Dawn D. Matthews. 339 pages. 1999. 0-7808-0326-4. $78.

"This book is recommended for public libraries and universities with home economic and food science programs." — E-Streams, Nov '00

"Recommended reference source." — Booklist, American Library Association, May '00

"This book takes the complex issues of food safety and foodborne pathogens and presents them in an easily understood manner. [It does] an excellent job of covering a large and often confusing topic." — American Reference Books Annual, 2000

■

# Forensic Medicine Sourcebook

Basic Consumer Information for the Layperson about Forensic Medicine, Including Crime Scene Investigation, Evidence Collection and Analysis, Expert Testimony, Computer-Aided Criminal Identification, Digital Imaging in the Courtroom, DNA Profiling, Accident Reconstruction, Autopsies, Ballistics, Drugs and

Explosives Detection, Latent Fingerprints, Product Tampering, and Questioned Document Examination

Along with Statistical Data, a Glossary of Forensics Terminology, and Listings of Sources for Further Help and Information

Edited by Annemarie S. Muth. 574 pages. 1999. 0-7808-0232-2. $78.

"Given the expected widespread interest in its content and its easy to read style, this book is recommended for most public and all college and university libraries."
— E-Streams, Feb '01

"Recommended for public libraries."
— Reference & User Services Quarterly, American Library Association, Spring 2000

"Recommended reference source."
— Booklist, American Library Association, Feb '00

"A wealth of information, useful statistics, references are up-to-date and extremely complete. This wonderful collection of data will help students who are interested in a career in any type of forensic field. It is a great resource for attorneys who need information about types of expert witnesses needed in a particular case. It also offers useful information for fiction and nonfiction writers whose work involves a crime. A fascinating compilation. All levels." — Choice, Association of College and Research Libraries, Jan 2000

"There are several items that make this book attractive to consumers who are seeking certain forensic data. . . . This is a useful current source for those seeking general forensic medical answers."
— American Reference Books Annual, 2000

■

# Gastrointestinal Diseases & Disorders Sourcebook

Basic Information about Gastroesophageal Reflux Disease (Heartburn), Ulcers, Diverticulosis, Irritable Bowel Syndrome, Crohn's Disease, Ulcerative Colitis, Diarrhea, Constipation, Lactose Intolerance, Hemorrhoids, Hepatitis, Cirrhosis, and Other Digestive Problems, Featuring Statistics, Descriptions of Symptoms, and Current Treatment Methods of Interest for Persons Living with Upper and Lower Gastrointestinal Maladies

Edited by Linda M. Ross. 413 pages. 1996. 0-7808-0078-8. $78.

". . . very readable form. The successful editorial work that brought this material together into a useful and understandable reference makes accessible to all readers information that can help them more effectively understand and obtain help for digestive tract problems."
— Choice, Association of College & Research Libraries, Feb '97

SEE ALSO Diet & Nutrition Sourcebook, 1st and 2nd Editions, Digestive Diseases & Disorders

# Genetic Disorders Sourcebook, 1st Edition

Basic Information about Heritable Diseases and Disorders Such as Down Syndrome, PKU, Hemophilia, Von Willebrand Disease, Gaucher Disease, Tay-Sachs Disease, and Sickle-Cell Disease, Along with Information about Genetic Screening, Gene Therapy, Home Care, and Including Source Listings for Further Help and Information on More Than 300 Disorders

Edited by Karen Bellenir. 642 pages. 1996. 0-7808-0034-6. $78.

"Recommended for undergraduate libraries or libraries that serve the public."
— Science & Technology Libraries, Vol. 18, No. 1, '99

"Provides essential medical information to both the general public and those diagnosed with a serious or fatal genetic disease or disorder." —Choice, Association of College and Research Libraries, Jan '97

"Geared toward the lay public. It would be well placed in all public libraries and in those hospital and medical libraries in which access to genetic references is limited." — Doody's Health Sciences Book Review, Oct '96

■

# Genetic Disorders Sourcebook, 2nd Edition

Basic Consumer Health Information about Hereditary Diseases and Disorders, Including Cystic Fibrosis, Down Syndrome, Hemophilia, Huntington's Disease, Sickle Cell Anemia, and More; Facts about Genes, Gene Research and Therapy, Genetic Screening, Ethics of Gene Testing, Genetic Counseling, and Advice on Coping and Caring

Along with a Glossary of Genetic Terminology and a Resource List for Help, Support, and Further Information

Edited by Kathy Massimini. 768 pages. 2001. 0-7808-0241-1. $78.

"Recommended for public libraries and medical and hospital libraries with consumer health collections."
— E-Streams, May '01

"Recommended reference source."
— Booklist, American Library Association, Apr '01

"Important pick for college-level health reference libraries." — The Bookwatch, Mar '01

■

# Head Trauma Sourcebook

Basic Information for the Layperson about Open-Head and Closed-Head Injuries, Treatment Advances, Recovery, and Rehabilitation

Along with Reports on Current Research Initiatives

Edited by Karen Bellenir. 414 pages. 1997. 0-7808-0208-X. $78.

# Headache Sourcebook

Basic Consumer Health Information about Migraine, Tension, Cluster, Rebound and Other Types of Headaches, with Facts about the Cause and Prevention of Headaches, the Effects of Stress and the Environment, Headaches during Pregnancy and Menopause, and Childhood Headaches

Along with a Glossary and Other Resources for Additional Help and Information

Edited by Dawn D. Matthews. 362 pages. 2002. 0-7808-0337-X. $78.

"Highly recommended for academic and medical reference collections." — Library Bookwatch, Sep '02

■

# Health Insurance Sourcebook

Basic Information about Managed Care Organizations, Traditional Fee-for-Service Insurance, Insurance Portability and Pre-Existing Conditions Clauses, Medicare, Medicaid, Social Security, and Military Health Care

Along with Information about Insurance Fraud

Edited by Wendy Wilcox. 530 pages. 1997. 0-7808-0222-5. $78.

"Particularly useful because it brings much of this information together in one volume. This book will be a handy reference source in the health sciences library, hospital library, college and university library, and medium to large public library."
— Medical Reference Services Quarterly, Fall '98

Awarded "Books of the Year Award"
— American Journal of Nursing, 1997

"The layout of the book is particularly helpful as it provides easy access to reference material. A most useful addition to the vast amount of information about health insurance. The use of data from U.S. government agencies is most commendable. Useful in a library or learning center for healthcare professional students."
— Doody's Health Sciences Book Reviews, Nov '97

■

# Health Reference Series Cumulative Index 1999

A Comprehensive Index to the Individual Volumes of the Health Reference Series, Including a Subject Index, Name Index, Organization Index, and Publication Index

Along with a Master List of Acronyms and Abbreviations

Edited by Edward J. Prucha, Anne Holmes, and Robert Rudnick. 990 pages. 2000. 0-7808-0382-5. $78.

"This volume will be most helpful in libraries that have a relatively complete collection of the Health Reference Series." —American Reference Books Annual, 2001

"Essential for collections that hold any of the numerous Health Reference Series titles."
— Choice, Association of College and Research Libraries, Nov '00

# Healthy Aging Sourcebook

Basic Consumer Health Information about Maintaining Health through the Aging Process, Including Advice on Nutrition, Exercise, and Sleep, Help in Making Decisions about Midlife Issues and Retirement, and Guidance Concerning Practical and Informed Choices in Health Consumerism

Along with Data Concerning the Theories of Aging, Different Experiences in Aging by Minority Groups, and Facts about Aging Now and Aging in the Future; and Featuring a Glossary, a Guide to Consumer Help, Additional Suggested Reading, and Practical Resource Directory

Edited by Jenifer Swanson. 536 pages. 1999. 0-7808-0390-6. $78.

"Recommended reference source."
—Booklist, American Library Association, Feb '00

SEE ALSO Physical & Mental Issues in Aging Sourcebook

# Healthy Heart Sourcebook for Women

Basic Consumer Health Information about Cardiac Issues Specific to Women, Including Facts about Major Risk Factors and Prevention, Treatment and Control Strategies, and Important Dietary Issues

Along with a Special Section Regarding the Pros and Cons of Hormone Replacement Therapy and Its Impact on Heart Health, and Additional Help, Including Recipes, a Glossary, and a Directory of Resources

Edited by Dawn D. Matthews. 336 pages. 2000. 0-7808-0329-9. $78.

"A good reference source and recommended for all public, academic, medical, and hospital libraries."
—Medical Reference Services Quarterly, Summer '01

"Because of the lack of information specific to women on this topic, this book is recommended for public libraries and consumer libraries."
—American Reference Books Annual, 2001

"Contains very important information about coronary artery disease that all women should know. The information is current and presented in an easy-to-read format. The book will make a good addition to any library."
—American Medical Writers Association Journal, Summer '00

"Important, basic reference."
—Reviewer's Bookwatch, Jul '00

SEE ALSO Cardiovascular Diseases & Disorders Sourcebook, 1st Edition, Heart Diseases & Disorders Sourcebook, 2nd Edition, Women's Health Concerns Sourcebook

# Heart Diseases & Disorders Sourcebook, 2nd Edition

Basic Consumer Health Information about Heart Attacks, Angina, Rhythm Disorders, Heart Failure, Valve Disease, Congenital Heart Disorders, and More,

Including Descriptions of Surgical Procedures and Other Interventions, Medications, Cardiac Rehabilitation, Risk Identification, and Prevention Tips

Along with Statistical Data, Reports on Current Research Initiatives, a Glossary of Cardiovascular Terms, and Resource Directory

Edited by Karen Bellenir. 612 pages. 2000. 0-7808-0238-1. $78.

"This work stands out as an imminently accessible resource for the general public. It is recommended for the reference and circulating shelves of school, public, and academic libraries."
—American Reference Books Annual, 2001

"Recommended reference source."
—Booklist, American Library Association, Dec '00

"Provides comprehensive coverage of matters related to the heart. This title is recommended for health sciences and public libraries with consumer health collections."
—E-Streams, Oct '00

SEE ALSO Cardiovascular Diseases & Disorders Sourcebook, 1st Edition; Healthy Heart Sourcebook for Women

# Household Safety Sourcebook

Basic Consumer Health Information about Household Safety, Including Information about Poisons, Chemicals, Fire, and Water Hazards in the Home

Along with Advice about the Safe Use of Home Maintenance Equipment, Choosing Toys and Nursery Furniture, Holiday and Recreation Safety, a Glossary, and Resources for Further Help and Information

Edited by Dawn D. Matthews. 606 pages. 2002. 0-7808-0338-8. $78.

"As a sourcebook on household safety this book meets its mark. It is encyclopedic in scope and covers a wide range of safety issues that are commonly seen in the home."
—E-Streams, Jul '02

# Immune System Disorders Sourcebook

Basic Information about Lupus, Multiple Sclerosis, Guillain-Barré Syndrome, Chronic Granulomatous Disease, and More

Along with Statistical and Demographic Data and Reports on Current Research Initiatives

Edited by Allan R. Cook. 608 pages. 1997. 0-7808-0209-8. $78.

# Infant & Toddler Health Sourcebook

Basic Consumer Health Information about the Physical and Mental Development of Newborns, Infants, and Toddlers, Including Neonatal Concerns, Nutrition Recommendations, Immunization Schedules, Common Pediatric Disorders, Assessments and Milestones, Safe-

596

ty Tips, and Advice for Parents and Other Caregivers Along with a Glossary of Terms and Resource Listings for Additional Help

Edited by Jenifer Swanson. 585 pages. 2000. 0-7808-0246-2. $78.

"As a reference for the general public, this would be useful in any library." —E-Streams, May '01

"Recommended reference source." —Booklist, American Library Association, Feb '01

"This is a good source for general use." —American Reference Books Annual, 2001

■

# Injury & Trauma Sourcebook

Basic Consumer Health Information about the Impact of Injury, the Diagnosis and Treatment of Common and Traumatic Injuries, Emergency Care, and Specific Injuries Related to Home, Community, Workplace, Transportation, and Recreation

Along with Guidelines for Injury Prevention, a Glossary, and a Directory of Additional Resources

Edited by Joyce Brennfleck Shannon. 696 pages. 2002. 0-7808-0421-X. $78.

"Practitioners should be aware of guides such as this in order to facilitate their use by patients and their families." —Doody's Health Sciences Book Review Journal, Sep-Oct '02

"Recommended reference source." —Booklist, American Library Association, Sep '02

"Highly recommended for academic and medical reference collections." —Library Bookwatch, Sep '02

■

# Kidney & Urinary Tract Diseases & Disorders Sourcebook

Basic Information about Kidney Stones, Urinary Incontinence, Bladder Disease, End Stage Renal Disease, Dialysis, and More

Along with Statistical and Demographic Data and Reports on Current Research Initiatives

Edited by Linda M. Ross. 602 pages. 1997. 0-7808-0079-6. $78.

■

# Learning Disabilities Sourcebook, 1st Edition

Basic Information about Disorders Such as Dyslexia, Visual and Auditory Processing Deficits, Attention Deficit/Hyperactivity Disorder, and Autism

Along with Statistical and Demographic Data, Reports on Current Research Initiatives, an Explanation of the Assessment Process, and a Special Section for Adults with Learning Disabilities

Edited by Linda M. Shin. 579 pages. 1998. 0-7808-0210-1. $78.

Named "Outstanding Reference Book of 1999." —New York Public Library, Feb 2000

"An excellent candidate for inclusion in a public library reference section. It's a great source of information. Teachers will also find the book useful. Definitely worth reading." —Journal of Adolescent & Adult Literacy, Feb 2000

"Readable . . . provides a solid base of information regarding successful techniques used with individuals who have learning disabilities, as well as practical suggestions for educators and family members. Clear language, concise descriptions, and pertinent information for contacting multiple resources add to the strength of this book as a useful tool." —Choice, Association of College and Research Libraries, Feb '99

"Recommended reference source." —Booklist, American Library Association, Sep '98

"A useful resource for libraries and for those who don't have the time to identify and locate the individual publications." —Disability Resources Monthly, Sep '98

■

# Learning Disabilities Sourcebook, 2nd Edition

Basic Consumer Health Information about Learning Disabilities, Including Dyslexia, Developmental Speech and Language Disabilities, Non-Verbal Learning Disorders, Developmental Arithmetic Disorder, Developmental Writing Disorder, and Other Conditions That Impede Learning Such as Attention Deficit/ Hyperactivity Disorder, Brain Injury, Hearing Impairment, Klinefelter Syndrome, Dyspraxia, and Tourette Syndrome

Along with Facts about Educational Issues and Assistive Technology, Coping Strategies, a Glossary of Related Terms, and Resources for Further Help and Information

Edited by Dawn D. Matthews. 621 pages. 2003. 0-7808-0626-3. $78.

■

# Liver Disorders Sourcebook

Basic Consumer Health Information about the Liver and How It Works; Liver Diseases, Including Cancer, Cirrhosis, Hepatitis, and Toxic and Drug Related Diseases; Tips for Maintaining a Healthy Liver; Laboratory Tests, Radiology Tests, and Facts about Liver Transplantation

Along with a Section on Support Groups, a Glossary, and Resource Listings

Edited by Joyce Brennfleck Shannon. 591 pages. 2000. 0-7808-0383-3. $78.

"A valuable resource." —American Reference Books Annual, 2001

"This title is recommended for health sciences and public libraries with consumer health collections." —E-Streams, Oct '00

"Recommended reference source." —Booklist, American Library Association, Jun '00

# Lung Disorders Sourcebook

Basic Consumer Health Information about Emphysema, Pneumonia, Tuberculosis, Asthma, Cystic Fibrosis, and Other Lung Disorders, Including Facts about Diagnostic Procedures, Treatment Strategies, Disease Prevention Efforts, and Such Risk Factors as Smoking, Air Pollution, and Exposure to Asbestos, Radon, and Other Agents

Along with a Glossary and Resources for Additional Help and Information

Edited by Dawn D. Matthews. 678 pages. 2002. 0-7808-0339-6. $78.

"Highly recommended for academic and medical reference collections." — *Library Bookwatch*, Sep '02 [Pain SB, 2nd ed.]

"A source of valuable information. . . . This book offers help to nonmedical people who need information about pain and pain management. It is also an excellent reference for those who participate in patient education." — *Doody's Review Service*, Sep '02

"Highly recommended for academic and medical reference collections." — *Library Bookwatch*, Sep '02

---

# Medical Tests Sourcebook

Basic Consumer Health Information about Medical Tests, Including Periodic Health Exams, General Screening Tests, Tests You Can Do at Home, Findings of the U.S. Preventive Services Task Force, X-ray and Radiology Tests, Electrical Tests, Tests of Blood and Other Body Fluids and Tissues, Scope Tests, Lung Tests, Genetic Tests, Pregnancy Tests, Newborn Screening Tests, Sexually Transmitted Disease Tests, and Computer Aided Diagnoses

Along with a Section on Paying for Medical Tests, a Glossary, and Resource Listings

Edited by Joyce Brennfleck Shannon. 691 pages. 1999. 0-7808-0243-8. $78.

"Recommended for hospital and health sciences libraries with consumer health collections." — *E-Streams*, Mar '00

"This is an overall excellent reference with a wealth of general knowledge that may aid those who are reluctant to get vital tests performed." — *Today's Librarian*, Jan 2000

"A valuable reference guide." — *American Reference Books Annual, 2000*

---

# Men's Health Concerns Sourcebook

Basic Information about Health Issues That Affect Men, Featuring Facts about the Top Causes of Death in Men, Including Heart Disease, Stroke, Cancers, Prostate Disorders, Chronic Obstructive Pulmonary Disease, Pneumonia and Influenza, Human Immunodeficiency Virus and Acquired Immune Deficiency Syndrome, Diabetes Mellitus, Stress, Suicide, Accidents and Homicides; and Facts about Common

Concerns for Men, Including Impotence, Contraception, Circumcision, Sleep Disorders, Snoring, Hair Loss, Diet, Nutrition, Exercise, Kidney and Urological Disorders, and Backaches

Edited by Allan R. Cook. 738 pages. 1998. 0-7808-0212-8. $78.

"This comprehensive resource and the series are highly recommended."
— *American Reference Books Annual, 2000*

"Recommended reference source."
— *Booklist, American Library Association, Dec '98*

---

# Mental Health Disorders Sourcebook, 1st Edition

Basic Information about Schizophrenia, Depression, Bipolar Disorder, Panic Disorder, Obsessive-Compulsive Disorder, Phobias and Other Anxiety Disorders, Paranoia and Other Personality Disorders, Eating Disorders, and Sleep Disorders

Along with Information about Treatment and Therapies

Edited by Karen Bellenir. 548 pages. 1995. 0-7808-0040-0. $78.

"This is an excellent new book . . . written in easy-to-understand language."
— *Booklist Health Sciences Supplement, American Library Association, Oct '97*

". . . useful for public and academic libraries and consumer health collections."
— *Medical Reference Services Quarterly, Spring '97*

"The great strengths of the book are its readability and its inclusion of places to find more information. Especially recommended." — *Reference Quarterly, American Library Association, Winter '96*

". . . a good resource for a consumer health library."
— *Bulletin of the Medical Library Association, Oct '96*

"The information is data-based and couched in brief, concise language that avoids jargon. . . . a useful reference source." — *Readings, Sep '96*

"The text is well organized and adequately written for its target audience." — *Choice, Association of College and Research Libraries, Jun '96*

". . . provides information on a wide range of mental disorders, presented in nontechnical language."
— *Exceptional Child Education Resources, Spring '96*

"Recommended for public and academic libraries."
— *Reference Book Review, 1996*

---

# Mental Health Disorders Sourcebook, 2nd Edition

Basic Consumer Health Information about Anxiety Disorders, Depression and Other Mood Disorders, Eating Disorders, Personality Disorders, Schizophrenia, and More, Including Disease Descriptions, Treatment Options, and Reports on Current Research Initiatives

Along with Statistical Data, Tips for Maintaining Mental Health, a Glossary, and Directory of Sources for Additional Help and Information

Edited by Karen Bellenir. 605 pages. 2000. 0-7808-0240-3. $78.

"Well organized and well written."
—American Reference Books Annual, 2001

"Recommended reference source."
—Booklist, American Library Association, Jun '00

■

# Mental Retardation Sourcebook

Basic Consumer Health Information about Mental Retardation and Its Causes, Including Down Syndrome, Fetal Alcohol Syndrome, Fragile X Syndrome, Genetic Conditions, Injury, and Environmental Sources

Along with Preventive Strategies, Parenting Issues, Educational Implications, Health Care Needs, Employment and Economic Matters, Legal Issues, a Glossary, and a Resource Listing for Additional Help and Information

Edited by Joyce Brennfleck Shannon. 642 pages. 2000. 0-7808-0377-9. $78.

"Public libraries will find the book useful for reference and as a beginning research point for students, parents, and caregivers."
—American Reference Books Annual, 2001

"The strength of this work is that it compiles many basic fact sheets and addresses for further information in one volume. It is intended and suitable for the general public. This sourcebook is relevant to any collection providing health information to the general public."
—E-Streams, Nov '00

"From preventing retardation to parenting and family challenges, this covers health, social and legal issues and will prove an invaluable overview."
—Reviewer's Bookwatch, Jul '00

■

# Movement Disorders Sourcebook

Basic Consumer Health Information about Neurological Movement Disorders, Including Essential Tremor, Parkinson's Disease, Dystonia, Cerebral Palsy, Huntington's Disease, Myasthenia Gravis, Multiple Sclerosis, and Other Early-Onset and Adult-Onset Movement Disorders, Their Symptoms and Causes, Diagnostic Tests, and Treatments

Along with Mobility and Assistive Technology Information, a Glossary, and a Directory of Additional Resources

Edited by Joyce Brennfleck Shannon. 655 pages. 2003. 0-7808-0628-X. $78.

■

# Obesity Sourcebook

Basic Consumer Health Information about Diseases and Other Problems Associated with Obesity, and Including Facts about Risk Factors, Prevention Issues, and Management Approaches

Along with Statistical and Demographic Data, Information about Special Populations, Research Updates, a Glossary, and Source Listings for Further Help and Information

Edited by Wilma Caldwell and Chad T. Kimball. 376 pages. 2001. 0-7808-0333-7. $78.

"The book synthesizes the reliable medical literature on obesity into one easy-to-read and useful resource for the general public."
— American Reference Books Annual 2002

"This is a very useful resource book for the lay public."
—Doody's Review Service, Nov '01

"Well suited for the health reference collection of a public library or an academic health science library that serves the general population."   —E-Streams, Sep '01

"Recommended reference source."
—Booklist, American Library Association, Apr '01

" Recommended pick both for specialty health library collections and any general consumer health reference collection."   — The Bookwatch, Apr '01

■

# Ophthalmic Disorders Sourcebook, 1st Edition

Basic Information about Glaucoma, Cataracts, Macular Degeneration, Strabismus, Refractive Disorders, and More

Along with Statistical and Demographic Data and Reports on Current Research Initiatives

Edited by Linda M. Ross. 631 pages. 1996. 0-7808-0081-8. $78.

SEE ALSO Eye Care Sourcebook, 2nd Edition

■

# Oral Health Sourcebook, 1st Edition

Basic Information about Diseases and Conditions Affecting Oral Health, Including Cavities, Gum Disease, Dry Mouth, Oral Cancers, Fever Blisters, Canker Sores, Oral Thrush, Bad Breath, Temporomandibular Disorders, and other Craniofacial Syndromes

Along with Statistical Data on the Oral Health of Americans, Oral Hygiene, Emergency First Aid, Information on Treatment Procedures and Methods of Replacing Lost Teeth

Edited by Allan R. Cook. 558 pages. 1997. 0-7808-0082-6. $78.

"Unique source which will fill a gap in dental sources for patients and the lay public. A valuable reference tool even in a library with thousands of books on dentistry. Comprehensive, clear, inexpensive, and easy to read and use. It fills an enormous gap in the health care literature."   — Reference and User Services Quarterly, American Library Association, Summer '98

"Recommended reference source."
— Booklist, American Library Association, Dec '97

599

# Osteoporosis Sourcebook

Basic Consumer Health Information about Primary and Secondary Osteoporosis and Juvenile Osteoporosis and Related Conditions, Including Fibrous Dysplasia, Gaucher Disease, Hyperthyroidism, Hypophosphatasia, Myeloma, Osteopetrosis, Osteogenesis Imperfecta, and Paget's Disease

Along with Information about Risk Factors, Treatments, Traditional and Non-Traditional Pain Management, a Glossary of Related Terms, and a Directory of Resources

Edited by Allan R. Cook. 584 pages. 2001. 0-7808-0239-X. $78.

"This would be a book to be kept in a staff or patient library. The targeted audience is the layperson, but the therapist who needs a quick bit of information on a particular topic will also find the book useful."
— *Physical Therapy, Jan '02*

"This resource is recommended as a great reference source for public, health, and academic libraries, and is another triumph for the editors of Omnigraphics."
— *American Reference Books Annual 2002*

"Recommended for all public libraries and general health collections, especially those supporting patient education or consumer health programs."
— *E-Streams, Nov '01*

"Will prove valuable to any library seeking to maintain a current, comprehensive reference collection of health resources. . . . From prevention to treatment and associated conditions, this provides an excellent survey."
— *The Bookwatch, Aug '01*

"Recommended reference source."
— *Booklist, American Library Association, July '01*

**SEE ALSO** *Women's Health Concerns Sourcebook*

■

# Pain Sourcebook, 1st Edition

Basic Information about Specific Forms of Acute and Chronic Pain, Including Headaches, Back Pain, Muscular Pain, Neuralgia, Surgical Pain, and Cancer Pain

Along with Pain Relief Options Such as Analgesics, Narcotics, Nerve Blocks, Transcutaneous Nerve Stimulation, and Alternative Forms of Pain Control, Including Biofeedback, Imaging, Behavior Modification, and Relaxation Techniques

Edited by Allan R. Cook. 667 pages. 1997. 0-7808-0213-6. $78.

"The text is readable, easily understood, and well indexed. This excellent volume belongs in all patient education libraries, consumer health sections of public libraries, and many personal collections."
— *American Reference Books Annual, 1999*

"A beneficial reference." — *Booklist Health Sciences Supplement, American Library Association, Oct '98*

"The information is basic in terms of scholarship and is appropriate for general readers. Written in journalistic style . . . intended for non-professionals. Quite thorough in its coverage of different pain conditions and summa-

rizes the latest clinical information regarding pain treatment." — *Choice, Association of College and Research Libraries, Jun '98*

"Recommended reference source."
— *Booklist, American Library Association, Mar '98*

■

# Pain Sourcebook, 2nd Edition

Basic Consumer Health Information about Specific Forms of Acute and Chronic Pain, Including Muscle and Skeletal Pain, Nerve Pain, Cancer Pain, and Disorders Characterized by Pain, Such as Fibromyalgia, Shingles, Angina, Arthritis, and Headaches

Along with Information about Pain Medications and Management Techniques, Complementary and Alternative Pain Relief Options, Tips for People Living with Chronic Pain, a Glossary, and a Directory of Sources for Further Information

Edited by Karen Bellenir. 670 pages. 2002. 0-7808-0612-3. $78.

■

# Pediatric Cancer Sourcebook

Basic Consumer Health Information about Leukemias, Brain Tumors, Sarcomas, Lymphomas, and Other Cancers in Infants, Children, and Adolescents, Including Descriptions of Cancers, Treatments, and Coping Strategies

Along with Suggestions for Parents, Caregivers, and Concerned Relatives, a Glossary of Cancer Terms, and Resource Listings

Edited by Edward J. Prucha. 587 pages. 1999. 0-7808-0245-4. $78.

"An excellent source of information. Recommended for public, hospital, and health science libraries with consumer health collections." — *E-Streams, Jun '00*

"Recommended reference source."
— *Booklist, American Library Association, Feb '00*

"A valuable addition to all libraries specializing in health services and many public libraries."
— *American Reference Books Annual, 2000*

■

# Physical & Mental Issues in Aging Sourcebook

Basic Consumer Health Information on Physical and Mental Disorders Associated with the Aging Process, Including Concerns about Cardiovascular Disease, Pulmonary Disease, Oral Health, Digestive Disorders, Musculoskeletal and Skin Disorders, Metabolic Changes, Sexual and Reproductive Issues, and Changes in Vision, Hearing, and Other Senses

Along with Data about Longevity and Causes of Death, Information on Acute and Chronic Pain, Descriptions of Mental Concerns, a Glossary of Terms, and Resource Listings for Additional Help

Edited by Jenifer Swanson. 660 pages. 1999. 0-7808-0233-0. $78.

"This is a treasure of health information for the layperson." — *Choice Health Sciences Supplement, Association of College & Research Libraries, May 2000*

"Recommended for public libraries."
—*American Reference Books Annual, 2000*

"Recommended reference source."
— *Booklist, American Library Association, Oct '99*

*SEE ALSO Healthy Aging Sourcebook*

■

# Podiatry Sourcebook

*Basic Consumer Health Information about Foot Conditions, Diseases, and Injuries, Including Bunions, Corns, Calluses, Athlete's Foot, Plantar Warts, Hammertoes and Clawtoes, Clubfoot, Heel Pain, Gout, and More*

*Along with Facts about Foot Care, Disease Prevention, Foot Safety, Choosing a Foot Care Specialist, a Glossary of Terms, and Resource Listings for Additional Information*

Edited by M. Lisa Weatherford. 380 pages. 2001. 0-7808-0215-2. $78.

"Recommended reference source."
— *Booklist, American Library Association, Feb '02*

"There is a lot of information presented here on a topic that is usually only covered sparingly in most larger comprehensive medical encyclopedias."
— *American Reference Books Annual 2002*

■

# Pregnancy & Birth Sourcebook

*Basic Information about Planning for Pregnancy, Maternal Health, Fetal Growth and Development, Labor and Delivery, Postpartum and Perinatal Care, Pregnancy in Mothers with Special Concerns, and Disorders of Pregnancy, Including Genetic Counseling, Nutrition and Exercise, Obstetrical Tests, Pregnancy Discomfort, Multiple Births, Cesarean Sections, Medical Testing of Newborns, Breastfeeding, Gestational Diabetes, and Ectopic Pregnancy*

Edited by Heather E. Aldred. 737 pages. 1997. 0-7808-0216-0. $78.

"A well-organized handbook. Recommended."
— *Choice, Association of College and Research Libraries, Apr '98*

"Recommended reference source."
— *Booklist, American Library Association, Mar '98*

"Recommended for public libraries."
—*American Reference Books Annual, 1998*

*SEE ALSO Congenital Disorders Sourcebook, Family Planning Sourcebook*

■

# Prostate Cancer Sourcebook

*Basic Consumer Health Information about Prostate Cancer, Including Information about the Associated Risk Factors, Detection, Diagnosis, and Treatment of Prostate Cancer*

*Along with Information on Non-Malignant Prostate*

*Conditions, and Featuring a Section Listing Support and Treatment Centers and a Glossary of Related Terms*

Edited by Dawn D. Matthews. 358 pages. 2001. 0-7808-0324-8. $78.

"Recommended reference source."
— *Booklist, American Library Association, Jan '02*

"A valuable resource for health care consumers seeking information on the subject. . . .All text is written in a clear, easy-to-understand language that avoids technical jargon. Any library that collects consumer health resources would strengthen their collection with the addition of the *Prostate Cancer Sourcebook*."
— *American Reference Books Annual 2002*

■

# Public Health Sourcebook

*Basic Information about Government Health Agencies, Including National Health Statistics and Trends, Healthy People 2000 Program Goals and Objectives, the Centers for Disease Control and Prevention, the Food and Drug Administration, and the National Institutes of Health*

*Along with Full Contact Information for Each Agency*

Edited by Wendy Wilcox. 698 pages. 1998. 0-7808-0220-9. $78.

"Recommended reference source."
— *Booklist, American Library Association, Sep '98*

"This consumer guide provides welcome assistance in navigating the maze of federal health agencies and their data on public health concerns."
— *SciTech Book News, Sep '98*

■

# Reconstructive & Cosmetic Surgery Sourcebook

*Basic Consumer Health Information on Cosmetic and Reconstructive Plastic Surgery, Including Statistical Information about Different Surgical Procedures, Things to Consider Prior to Surgery, Plastic Surgery Techniques and Tools, Emotional and Psychological Considerations, and Procedure-Specific Information*

*Along with a Glossary of Terms and a Listing of Resources for Additional Help and Information*

Edited by M. Lisa Weatherford. 374 pages. 2001. 0-7808-0214-4. $78.

"An excellent reference that addresses cosmetic and medically necessary reconstructive surgeries. . . . The style of the prose is calm and reassuring, discussing the many positive outcomes now available due to advances in surgical techniques."
— *American Reference Books Annual 2002*

"Recommended for health science libraries that are open to the public, as well as hospital libraries that are open to the patients. This book is a good resource for the consumer interested in plastic surgery."
—*E-Streams, Dec '01*

"Recommended reference source."
—*Booklist, American Library Association, July '01*

601

# Rehabilitation Sourcebook

*Basic Consumer Health Information about Rehabilitation for People Recovering from Heart Surgery, Spinal Cord Injury, Stroke, Orthopedic Impairments, Amputation, Pulmonary Impairments, Traumatic Injury, and More, Including Physical Therapy, Occupational Therapy, Speech/ Language Therapy, Massage Therapy, Dance Therapy, Art Therapy, and Recreational Therapy*

*Along with Information on Assistive and Adaptive Devices, a Glossary, and Resources for Additional Help and Information*

Edited by Dawn D. Matthews. 531 pages. 1999. 0-7808-0236-5. $78.

"This is an excellent resource for public library reference and health collections."
— *American Reference Books Annual, 2001*

"Recommended reference source."
— *Booklist, American Library Association, May '00*

∎

# Respiratory Diseases & Disorders Sourcebook

*Basic Information about Respiratory Diseases and Disorders, Including Asthma, Cystic Fibrosis, Pneumonia, the Common Cold, Influenza, and Others, Featuring Facts about the Respiratory System, Statistical and Demographic Data, Treatments, Self-Help Management Suggestions, and Current Research Initiatives*

Edited by Allan R. Cook and Peter D. Dresser. 771 pages. 1995. 0-7808-0037-0. $78.

"Designed for the layperson and for patients and their families coping with respiratory illness. . . . an extensive array of information on diagnosis, treatment, management, and prevention of respiratory illnesses for the general reader." — *Choice, Association of College and Research Libraries, Jun '96*

"A highly recommended text for all collections. It is a comforting reminder of the power of knowledge that good books carry between their covers."
— *Academic Library Book Review, Spring '96*

"A comprehensive collection of authoritative information presented in a nontechnical, humanitarian style for patients, families, and caregivers."
— *Association of Operating Room Nurses, Sep/Oct '95*

∎

# Sexually Transmitted Diseases Sourcebook, 1st Edition

*Basic Information about Herpes, Chlamydia, Gonorrhea, Hepatitis, Nongonoccocal Urethritis, Pelvic Inflammatory Disease, Syphilis, AIDS, and More*

*Along with Current Data on Treatments and Preventions*

Edited by Linda M. Ross. 550 pages. 1997. 0-7808-0217-9. $78.

# Sexually Transmitted Diseases Sourcebook, 2nd Edition

*Basic Consumer Health Information about Sexually Transmitted Diseases, Including Information on the Diagnosis and Treatment of Chlamydia, Gonorrhea, Hepatitis, Herpes, HIV, Mononucleosis, Syphilis, and Others*

*Along with Information on Prevention, Such as Condom Use, Vaccines, and STD Education; And Featuring a Section on Issues Related to Youth and Adolescents, a Glossary, and Resources for Additional Help and Information*

Edited by Dawn D. Matthews. 538 pages. 2001. 0-7808-0249-7. $78.

"Recommended for consumer health collections in public libraries, and secondary school and community college libraries."
— *American Reference Books Annual 2002*

"Every school and public library should have a copy of this comprehensive and user-friendly reference book."
— *Choice, Association of College & Research Libraries, Sep '01*

"This is a highly recommended book. This is an especially important book for all school and public libraries." — *AIDS Book Review Journal, Jul-Aug '01*

"Recommended reference source."
— *Booklist, American Library Association, Apr '01*

"Recommended pick both for specialty health library collections and any general consumer health reference collection." — *The Bookwatch, Apr '01*

∎

# Skin Disorders Sourcebook

*Basic Information about Common Skin and Scalp Conditions Caused by Aging, Allergies, Immune Reactions, Sun Exposure, Infectious Organisms, Parasites, Cosmetics, and Skin Traumas, Including Abrasions, Cuts, and Pressure Sores*

*Along with Information on Prevention and Treatment*

Edited by Allan R. Cook. 647 pages. 1997. 0-7808-0080-X. $78.

"... comprehensive, easily read reference book."
— *Doody's Health Sciences Book Reviews, Oct '97*

SEE ALSO Burns Sourcebook

∎

# Sleep Disorders Sourcebook

*Basic Consumer Health Information about Sleep and Its Disorders, Including Insomnia, Sleepwalking, Sleep Apnea, Restless Leg Syndrome, and Narcolepsy*

*Along with Data about Shiftwork and Its Effects, Information on the Societal Costs of Sleep Deprivation, Descriptions of Treatment Options, a Glossary of Terms, and Resource Listings for Additional Help*

Edited by Jenifer Swanson. 439 pages. 1998. 0-7808-0234-9. $78.

"This text will complement any home or medical library. It is user-friendly and ideal for the adult reader."
— *American Reference Books Annual, 2000*

"A useful resource that provides accurate, relevant, and accessible information on sleep to the general public. Health care providers who deal with sleep disorders patients may also find it helpful in being prepared to answer some of the questions patients ask."
— *Respiratory Care, Jul '99*

"Recommended reference source."
— *Booklist, American Library Association, Feb '99*

■

# Sports Injuries Sourcebook, 1st Edition

*Basic Consumer Health Information about Common Sports Injuries, Prevention of Injury in Specific Sports, Tips for Training, and Rehabilitation from Injury*

*Along with Information about Special Concerns for Children, Young Girls in Athletic Training Programs, Senior Athletes, and Women Athletes, and a Directory of Resources for Further Help and Information*

Edited by Heather E. Aldred. 624 pages. 1999. 0-7808-0218-7. $78.

"While this easy-to-read book is recommended for all libraries, it should prove to be especially useful for public, high school, and academic libraries; certainly it should be on the bookshelf of every school gymnasium."
— *E-Streams, Mar '00*

"Public libraries and undergraduate academic libraries will find this book useful for its nontechnical language."
— *American Reference Books Annual, 2000*

■

# Sports Injuries Sourcebook, 2nd Edition

*Basic Consumer Health Information about the Diagnosis, Treatment, and Rehabilitation of Common Sports-Related Injuries in Children and Adults*

*Along with Suggestions for Conditioning and Training, Information and Prevention Tips for Injuries Frequently Associated with Specific Sports and Special Populations, a Glossary, and a Directory of Additional Resources*

Edited by Joyce Brennfleck Shannon. 614 pages. 2002. 0-7808-0604-2. $78.

■

# Stress-Related Disorders Sourcebook

*Basic Consumer Health Information about Stress and Stress-Related Disorders, Including Stress Origins and Signals, Environmental Stress at Work and Home, Mental and Emotional Stress Associated with Depression, Post-Traumatic Stress Disorder, Panic Disorder, Suicide, and the Physical Effects of Stress on the Cardiovascular, Immune, and Nervous Systems*

*Along with Stress Management Techniques, a Glossary, and a Listing of Additional Resources*

Edited by Joyce Brennfleck Shannon. 610 pages. 2002. 0-7808-0560-7. $78.

"I am impressed by the amount of information. It offers a thorough overview of the causes and consequences of stress for the layperson. . . . A well-done and thorough reference guide for professionals and nonprofessionals alike." — *Doody's Review Service, Dec '02*

■

# Stroke Sourcebook

*Basic Consumer Health Information about Stroke, Including Ischemic, Hemorrhagic, Transient Ischemic Attack (TIA), and Pediatric Stroke, Stroke Triggers and Risks, Diagnostic Tests, Treatments, and Rehabilitation Information*

*Along with Stroke Prevention Guidelines, Legal and Financial Information, a Glossary, and a Directory of Additional Resources*

Edited by Joyce Brennfleck Shannon. 606 pages. 2003. 0-7808-0630-1. $78.

■

# Substance Abuse Sourcebook

*Basic Health-Related Information about the Abuse of Legal and Illegal Substances Such as Alcohol, Tobacco, Prescription Drugs, Marijuana, Cocaine, and Heroin; and Including Facts about Substance Abuse Prevention Strategies, Intervention Methods, Treatment and Recovery Programs, and a Section Addressing the Special Problems Related to Substance Abuse during Pregnancy*

Edited by Karen Bellenir. 573 pages. 1996. 0-7808-0038-9. $78.

"A valuable addition to any health reference section. Highly recommended."
— *The Book Report, Mar/Apr '97*

". . . a comprehensive collection of substance abuse information that's both highly readable and compact. Families and caregivers of substance abusers will find the information enlightening and helpful, while teachers, social workers and journalists should benefit from the concise format. Recommended."
— *Drug Abuse Update, Winter '96/'97*

*SEE ALSO Alcoholism Sourcebook, Drug Abuse Sourcebook*

■

# Surgery Sourcebook

*Basic Consumer Health Information about Inpatient and Outpatient Surgeries, Including Cardiac, Vascular, Orthopedic, Ocular, Reconstructive, Cosmetic, Gynecologic, and Ear, Nose, and Throat Procedures and More*

*Along with Information about Operating Room Policies and Instruments, Laser Surgery Techniques, Hospital Errors, Statistical Data, a Glossary, and Listings of Sources for Further Help and Information*

Edited by Annemarie S. Muth and Karen Bellenir. 596 pages. 2002. 0-7808-0380-9. $78.

# Transplantation Sourcebook

*Basic Consumer Health Information about Organ and Tissue Transplantation, Including Physical and Financial Preparations, Procedures and Issues Relating to Specific Solid Organ and Tissue Transplants, Rehabilitation, Pediatric Transplant Information, the Future of Transplantation, and Organ and Tissue Donation*

*Along with a Glossary and Listings of Additional Resources*

Edited by Joyce Brennfleck Shannon. 628 pages. 2002. 0-7808-0322-1. $78.

**"Recommended for libraries with an interest in offering consumer health information."** — *E-Streams, Jul '02*

**"This is a unique and valuable resource for patients facing transplantation and their families."**
— *Doody's Review Service, Jun '02*

■

# Traveler's Health Sourcebook

*Basic Consumer Health Information for Travelers, Including Physical and Medical Preparations, Transportation Health and Safety, Essential Information about Food and Water, Sun Exposure, Insect and Snake Bites, Camping and Wilderness Medicine, and Travel with Physical or Medical Disabilities*

*Along with International Travel Tips, Vaccination Recommendations, Geographical Health Issues, Disease Risks, a Glossary, and a Listing of Additional Resources*

Edited by Joyce Brennfleck Shannon. 613 pages. 2000. 0-7808-0384-1. $78.

**"Recommended reference source."**
— *Booklist, American Library Association, Feb '01*

**"This book is recommended for any public library, any travel collection, and especially any collection for the physically disabled."**
— *American Reference Books Annual, 2001*

■

# Vegetarian Sourcebook

*Basic Consumer Health Information about Vegetarian Diets, Lifestyle, and Philosophy, Including Definitions of Vegetarianism and Veganism, Tips about Adopting Vegetarianism, Creating a Vegetarian Pantry, and Meeting Nutritional Needs of Vegetarians, with Facts Regarding Vegetarianism's Effect on Pregnant and Lactating Women, Children, Athletes, and Senior Citizens*

*Along with a Glossary of Commonly Used Vegetarian Terms and Resources for Additional Help and Information*

Edited by Chad T. Kimball. 360 pages. 2002. 0-7808-0439-2. $78.

# Women's Health Concerns Sourcebook

*Basic Information about Health Issues That Affect Women, Featuring Facts about Menstruation and Other Gynecological Concerns, Including Endometriosis, Fibroids, Menopause, and Vaginitis; Reproductive Concerns, Including Birth Control, Infertility, and Abortion; and Facts about Additional Physical, Emotional, and Mental Health Concerns Prevalent among Women Such as Osteoporosis, Urinary Tract Disorders, Eating Disorders, and Depression*

*Along with Tips for Maintaining a Healthy Lifestyle*

Edited by Heather E. Aldred. 567 pages. 1997. 0-7808-0219-5. $78.

**"Handy compilation. There is an impressive range of diseases, devices, disorders, procedures, and other physical and emotional issues covered . . . well organized, illustrated, and indexed."** — *Choice, Association of College and Research Libraries, Jan '98*

*SEE ALSO Breast Cancer Sourcebook, Cancer Sourcebook for Women, 1st and 2nd Editions, Healthy Heart Sourcebook for Women, Osteoporosis Sourcebook*

■

# Workplace Health & Safety Sourcebook

*Basic Consumer Health Information about Workplace Health and Safety, Including the Effect of Workplace Hazards on the Lungs, Skin, Heart, Ears, Eyes, Brain, Reproductive Organs, Musculoskeletal System, and Other Organs and Body Parts*

*Along with Information about Occupational Cancer, Personal Protective Equipment, Toxic and Hazardous Chemicals, Child Labor, Stress, and Workplace Violence*

Edited by Chad T. Kimball. 626 pages. 2000. 0-7808-0231-4. $78.

**"As a reference for the general public, this would be useful in any library."** — *E-Streams, Jun '01*

**"Provides helpful information for primary care physicians and other caregivers interested in occupational medicine. . . . General readers; professionals."**
— *Choice, Association of College & Research Libraries, May '01*

**"Recommended reference source."**
— *Booklist, American Library Association, Feb '01*

**"Highly recommended."** — *The Bookwatch, Jan '01*

■

# Worldwide Health Sourcebook

*Basic Information about Global Health Issues, Including Malnutrition, Reproductive Health, Disease Dispersion and Prevention, Emerging Diseases, Risky Health Behaviors, and the Leading Causes of Death*

*Along with Global Health Concerns for Children, Women, and the Elderly, Mental Health Issues, Research and Technology Advancements, and Economic, Environmental, and Political Health Implications, a*

*Glossary, and a Resource Listing for Additional Help and Information*

Edited by Joyce Brennfleck Shannon. 614 pages. 2001. 0-7808-0330-2. $78.

**"Named an Outstanding Academic Title."**
—*Choice, Association of College & Research Libraries, Jan '02*

**"Yet another handy but also unique compilation in the extensive Health Reference Series, this is a useful work because many of the international publications reprinted or excerpted are not readily available. Highly recommended."** —*Choice, Association of College & Research Libraries, Nov '01*

**"Recommended reference source."**
—*Booklist, American Library Association, Oct '01*

# Teen Health Series

## Helping Young Adults Understand, Manage, and Avoid Serious Illness

### Diet Information for Teens
#### Health Tips about Diet and Nutrition

*Including Facts about Nutrients, Dietary Guidelines, Breakfasts, School Lunches, Snacks, Party Food, Weight Control, Eating Disorders, and More*

Edited by Karen Bellenir. 399 pages. 2001. 0-7808-0441-4. $58.

"Full of helpful insights and facts throughout the book. ... An excellent resource to be placed in public libraries or even in personal collections."
*—American Reference Books Annual 2002*

"Recommended for middle and high school libraries and media centers as well as academic libraries that educate future teachers of teenagers. It is also a suitable addition to health science libraries that serve patrons who are interested in teen health promotion and education."
*— E-Streams, Oct '01*

"This comprehensive book would be beneficial to collections that need information about nutrition, dietary guidelines, meal planning, and weight control. ... This reference is so easy to use that its purchase is recommended."
*— The Book Report, Sep-Oct '01*

"This book is written in an easy to understand format describing issues that many teens face every day, and then provides thoughtful explanations so that teens can make informed decisions. This is an interesting book that provides important facts and information for today's teens."
*—Doody's Health Sciences Book Review Journal, Jul-Aug '01*

"A comprehensive compendium of diet and nutrition. The information is presented in a straightforward, plain-spoken manner. This title will be useful to those working on reports on a variety of topics, as well as to general readers concerned about their dietary health."
*— School Library Journal, Jun '01*

### Drug Information for Teens
#### Health Tips about the Physical and Mental Effects of Substance Abuse

*Including Facts about Alcohol, Anabolic Steroids, Club Drugs, Cocaine, Depressants, Hallucinogens, Herbal Products, Inhalants, Marijuana, Narcotics, Stimulants, Tobacco, and More*

Edited by Karen Bellenir. 452 pages. 2002. 0-7808-0444-9. $58.

"This is an excellent resource for teens and their parents. Education about drugs and substances is key to discouraging teen drug abuse and this book provides this much needed information in a way that is interesting and factual." *—Doody's Review Service, Dec '02*

### Mental Health Information for Teens
#### Health Tips about Mental Health and Mental Illness

*Including Facts about Anxiety, Depression, Suicide, Eating Disorders, Obsessive-Compulsive Disorders, Panic Attacks, Phobias, Schizophrenia, and More*

Edited by Karen Bellenir. 406 pages. 2001. 0-7808-0442-2. $58.

"In both language and approach, this user-friendly entry in the *Teen Health Series* is on target for teens needing information on mental health concerns." *— Booklist, American Library Association, Jan '02*

"Readers will find the material accessible and informative, with the shaded notes, facts, and embedded glossary insets adding appropriately to the already interesting and succinct presentation."
*—School Library Journal, Jan '02*

"This title is highly recommended for any library that serves adolescents and parents/caregivers of adolescents." *— E-Streams, Jan '02*

"Recommended for high school libraries and young adult collections in public libraries. Both health professionals and teenagers will find this book useful."
*— American Reference Books Annual 2002*

"This is a nice book written to enlighten the society, primarily teenagers, about common teen mental health issues. It is highly recommended to teachers and parents as well as adolescents."
*— Doody's Review Service, Dec '01*

### Sexual Health Information for Teens
#### Health Tips about Sexual Development, Human Reproduction, and Sexually Transmitted Diseases

*Including Facts about Puberty, Reproductive Health, Chlamydia, Human Papillomavirus, Pelvic Inflammatory Disease, Herpes, AIDS, Contraception, Pregnancy, and More*

Edited by Deborah A. Stanley. 400 pages. 2003. 0-7808-0445-7. $58.

# Health Reference Series